Endoscopy in Obesity Management

Bipan Chand
Editor

Endoscopy in Obesity Management

A Comprehensive Guide

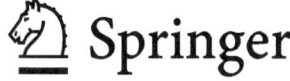 Springer

Editor
Bipan Chand
Gastrointestinal/Minimally Invasive Surgery
Stritch School of Medicine
Loyola University Medical Center
Maywood, IL, USA

ISBN 978-3-319-63527-9   ISBN 978-3-319-63528-6   (eBook)
DOI 10.1007/978-3-319-63528-6

Library of Congress Control Number: 2017952611

Printed on acid-free paper

This Springer imprint is published by Springer Nature
The registered company is Springer International Publishing AG
The registered company address is: Gewerbestrasse 11, 6330 Cham, Switzerland

Preface

Obesity rates continue to increase throughout the world and are more often found in industrialized societies and countries influenced by Western culture. Interventions to counteract this chronic disease epidemic have focused on population-based education, early identification of at-risk groups, prevention through better education, and both medical and surgical treatments. Treatments vary but are more often patient directed and less medically supervised. Obesity is now recognized as a disease and has various degrees and forms, ultimately leading to impaired quality of life and increased morbidity, mortality, and healthcare costs. Studies have shown that with an increasing body mass index, successful amelioration of obesity and comorbid conditions is often better achieved through multidisciplinary obesity-focused programs. To date, programs focusing on diet alone have had limited success. Medically supervised programs emphasize behavior modification, dietary counseling, and the use of various pharmacological agents. Medically supervised program success is often best achieved in overweight and lower classes of obese individuals.

Bariatric and metabolic surgery has provided decades of effective and sustained weight loss for many individuals with morbid obesity. Most weight loss procedures are performed laparoscopically in accredited centers with increasing standardization in technique and pathways. Each individual seeking obesity treatment should have a goal, in terms of both the amount of weight loss and improvement in obesity-related comorbidities. Expectations from patients, the medical community, and the obesity program must be in alignment with the planned therapy or procedure. Success must also be weighed against the risk for each individual, as well as the risks associated with each procedure. Currently, most surgical procedures have inherent risks and are associated with unique challenges and complications. It is imperative that clinicians caring for obese patients are knowledgeable about the history of therapy, treatment options, and endoscopic management.

Endoscopy is currently used in the diagnosis and treatment of preoperative conditions in patients seeking surgery and postoperative complications from surgery. This textbook covers the full spectrum of endoluminal obesity care. Chapters will cover the background of bariatric surgery, indications for endoscopy, and anesthesia considerations in the obese patient. The anatomy of common and uncommon bariatric procedures will be discussed, as well as the management of acute and chronic complications. Endoscopic therapy may also become the mainstay for surgical revisions to optimize postsurgical anatomy and provide the means of reestablishing the anatomy of the primary obesity surgery.

Finally, this textbook will allow the endoscopist to establish the foundation for future endoluminal therapy, including primary endoscopic obesity procedures.

Maywood, IL, USA   Bipan Chand

Contents

Contributors

Jawad Tahir Ali, MD Department of Surgery, University of California at Davis, Sacramento, CA, USA

Department of Surgery, University of California, Davis Medical Center, Sacramento, CA, USA

Matthew T. Allemang, MD Section of Surgical Endoscopy, Department of General Surgery, Digestive Disease and Surgery Institute, Cleveland Clinic Foundation, Cleveland, OH, USA

Julius Balogh, MD MHA Department of Anesthesiology, Memorial Hermann Hospital, University of Texas at Houston Health Science Center, Houston, TX, USA

Diego R. Camacho, MD, FACS Department of Surgery, Minimally Invasive and Laparoscopic General Surgery, Montefiore Medical Center, Montefiore Greene Medical Arts Pavilion, Bronx, NY, USA

Aaron D. Carr, MD Department of Surgery, University of California Davis Medical Center, Sacramento, CA, USA

Bipan Chand, MD Gastrointestinal/Minimally Invasive Surgery, Stritch School of Medicine, Loyola University Medical Center, Maywood, IL, USA

Salvatore Docimo, Jr, DO MSc Division of Bariatric, Foregut, and Advanced Gastrointestinal Surgery, Department of Surgery, Stony Brook School of Medicine, Stony Brook, NY, USA

Sofiane El Djouzi, MD, MSc Division of GI/Minimally Invasive Surgery, Strich School of Medicine, Loyola University Medical Center, Chicago, IL, USA

Kevin M. El-Hayek, MD Section of Surgical Endoscopy, Department of General Surgery, Digestive Disease and Surgery Institute, Cleveland Clinic Foundation, Cleveland, OH, USA

Cleveland Clinic Lerner College of Medicine, Case Western Reserve University, Cleveland, OH, USA

Melissa Felinski, DO Department of Surgery, McGovern Medical School, University of Texas Health, Houston, TX, USA

Manoel Galvao Neto, MD Department of General Surgery, Herbert Wertheim College of Medicine, Florida International University, Miami, FL, USA

Maamoun A. Harmouch, MD Department of Surgery, McGovern Medical School, University of Texas Health, Houston, TX, USA

Pichamol Jirapinyo, MD Division of Gastroenterology, Hepatology and Endoscopy, Brigham and Women's Hospital/Harvard Medical School, Boston, MA, USA

Amanda M. Johner, BSc, MD, MHSc, FRCSC General Surgery, Lions Gate Hospital, North Vancouver, BC, Canada

Mojdeh S. Kappus, MD Department of Surgery, Montefiore Medical Center, Bronx, NY, USA

Leena Khaitan, MD, MPH Department of Surgery, University Hospitals Cleveland Medical Center, Cleveland, OH, USA

Adil Haleem Khan, MD Department of Surgery, University Hospitals Cleveland Medical Center, Cleveland, OH, USA

Matthew D. Kroh, MD Section of Surgical Endoscopy, Department of General Surgery, Digestive Disease and Surgery Institute, Cleveland Clinic, Cleveland Clinic Lerner College of Medicine, Cleveland, OH, USA

Digestive Disease Institute, Cleveland Clinic Abu Dhabi, Abu Dhabi, United Arab Emirates

Jihad Kudsi, MD Department of Surgery, Houston Methodist Hospital, Houston, TX, USA

Eric Marcotte, MD, MSc Department of Surgery, Stritch School of Medicine, Loyola University Medical Center, Maywood, IL, USA

Dean J. Mikami, MD Department of Surgery, The Queen's Medical Center, University of Hawaii John A. Burns School of Medicine, Honolulu, HI, USA

Kenric M. Murayama, MD Department of Surgery, John A. Burns School of Medicine, University of Hawaii at Manoa, Honolulu, HI, USA

Aurora D. Pryor, MD Division of Bariatric, Foregut, and Advanced Gastrointestinal Surgery, Department of Surgery, Stony Brook School of Medicine, Stony Brook, NY, USA

Kevin M. Reavis, MD Foregut and Bariatric Surgery, Department of Gastrointestinal and Minimally Invasive Surgery, The Oregon Clinic, Portland, OR, USA

Shinil K. Shah, DO Department of Surgery, McGovern Medical School, University of Texas Health, Houston, TX, USA

Michael E. DeBakey Institute for Comparative Cardiovascular Science and Biomedical Devices, Texas A&M University, College Station, TX, USA

Andrew T. Strong, MD Section of Surgical Endoscopy, Department of General Surgery, Digestive Disease and Surgery Institute, Cleveland Clinic, Cleveland Clinic Lerner College of Medicine, Cleveland, OH, USA

Nabil Tariq, MD Department of Surgery, Houston Methodist Hospital, Houston, TX, USA

Christopher C. Thompson, MD, MSc, FACG, FASGE, AGAF Division of Gastroenterology, Hepatology and Endoscopy, Brigham and Women's Hospital/Harvard Medical School, Boston, MA, USA

Hung P. Truong, MD Department of Surgery, The Queen's Medical Center, University of Hawaii John A. Burns School of Medicine, Honolulu, HI, USA

Leonard K. Welsh, Jr., MD Department of Surgery, John A. Burns School of Medicine, University of Hawaii at Manoa, Honolulu, HI, USA

Erik B. Wilson, MD Department of Surgery, McGovern Medical School, University of Texas Health, Houston, TX, USA

Natan Zundel, MD Department of General Surgery, Herbert Wertheim College of Medicine, Florida International University, Miami, FL, USA

Leonard K. Welsh, Jr. and Kenric M. Murayama

Introduction

The journey of the surgical treatment of morbid obesity largely stemmed from observations of secondary effects of other operations for unrelated pathology. The problem of incapacitating obesity found its primary treatment from the effects observed in individuals that underwent resection of a portion of their small intestine or stomach and the resulting weight loss, even if the individual was of normal weight at the outset.

Recognition of an obesity health crisis and its many comorbidities is only a few decades old. For many centuries, as a consequence of chronic scarcity of food, obesity was associated with affluence, power, health, and prosperity. It was only after the technologic advances of the eighteenth century that food became more affordable and readily available. As the world exited the Second World War, farming in many areas became increasingly mechanized and industrialized. Manpower was more available resulting in decreased costs and food commodities became more affordable. The birth of the fast-food industry emerged and thrived, as did the urbanization

of not only the United States, but also the world. This environment established conditions in which the prevalence of obesity skyrocketed. Late in the nineteenth century, obesity was recognized only as an aesthetic issue, and it was not until the twentieth century that it was later accepted as a significant health problem [1].

Early attempts to curtail obesity were trivial. Surgical limitation of oral intake with jaw wiring was one of the earliest attempts to alleviate obesity [2]. Historical reports claim that the earliest bariatric surgery was performed in Spain in the tenth century. Accounts report that Sancho I, King of León, was so obese that he could not walk, ride a horse, or pick up a sword. He eventually lost his throne and was escorted by his grandmother to Cordoba to see the famous Jewish doctor Hasdai Ibn Shaprut where he sutured the king's lips, limiting him to a liquid diet. King Sancho lost half his body weight, returned to León on his horse, and triumphantly retook his throne [3, 4].

Other jaw wiring techniques proved to be unsuccessful, as patients would continue to consume high calorie liquids only to lead to weight regain. In addition, patients had difficulty maintaining oral hygiene and suffered from dental complications. Emesis and aspiration with resulting respiratory tract infections were also significant concerns [5]. Jaw wiring was abandoned, but an important concept in bariatric management was recognized: caloric restriction coupled with the need to provide permanent results.

L.K. Welsh, Jr., M.D. • K.M. Murayama, M.D. (✉)
Department of Surgery, John A. Burns School of
Medicine, University of Hawaii at Manoa,
1356 Lusitana Street, 6th floor, Honolulu, HI 96817,
USA
e-mail: lkwelsh@hawaii.edu; kenricm@hawaii.edu

© Springer International Publishing AG 2018
B. Chand (ed.), *Endoscopy in Obesity Management*, DOI 10.1007/978-3-319-63528-6_1

Weight loss operations and interventions were sparsely reported in the literature during the early twentieth century and largely remained in obscurity until the 1980s. It was not until the obesity epidemic was finally recognized that the medical community started considering surgical approaches, bringing surgery to the forefront as a durable and respected treatment [6, 7].

Obesity Epidemic

At present, obesity is recognized as a major public health crisis and many improvements in public health have come to a halt due to its effects. For the first time in decades, the life span of the next generation is predicted to be shorter than their parents [8]. Morbidly obese patients (body mass index, BMI > 40 kg/m²) are clearly disadvantaged in our society. Not only are they afflicted by health conditions associated with morbid obesity, e.g., diabetes, sleep apnea, and cardiovascular diseases, but also struggle with many of life's simple activities, such as sitting in a chair or walking normal distances. A great deal of social marginalization is placed on the obese creating complex social and psychological burdens.

Obesity is an increasing public health challenge in both economically developed and developing regions of the world. 33.0% of the world's adult population is overweight or obese [9]. In 2008, more than 1.4 billion adults and more than 40 million children under the age of 5 were overweight. If current trends continue, by 2030 over half of the world's adult population (nearly 3.3 billion people) will be either overweight or obese [10]. While the prevalence of obesity is higher in economically developed countries compared with economically developing countries [10], the absolute number of obese children is greater in the developing world [9]. This represents a significant current and future burden on the developing world and the prevalence of obesity only continues to rise in developing countries, particularly in urban settings where unhealthy "fast food" has become common. Additionally, urbanization and mechanization, coupled with an increased sedentary lifestyle, results in sharp increases in obesity and metabolic syndrome.

Obesity in the United States

Some of the most compelling data on obesity prevalence rates over time in the United States come from figures released by the National Health and Nutrition Examination Surveys (NHANES) program of the National Center for Health Statistics of the Centers for Disease Control and Prevention. These surveys contain data from a national cross-section beginning in 1960 [11–15] in which representative samples of the US population were selected. Adult data suggested a steady prevalence of obesity from the 1960s through the 1980s, with a noticeable increase in beginning in the late 1980s from 23.0% in 1988 to 36.0% in 2010 [14, 15]. Interestingly, the rate of those classified as overweight has been relatively stable, but there has a significant increase in the rate of obesity. Projections based on NHANES data predict that more than half of US adults are likely to be obese and 86.3% are likely to be overweight or obese by 2030 [16]. Similar dramatic projections have been made for children, creating a critical outlook for this progressive epidemic. The global dilemma of obesity requires multiple actions, but for the already affected, bariatric surgery has become a valid option.

Early Pioneers

Soon after World War II, many young physicians returned from the call of duty to complete their training. Several institutions channeled a large part of this workforce into research, including investigating the mysteries of the gastrointestinal tract. It was in this setting that A.J. Kremen and John Linner at the University of Minnesota examined transposing segments of the small intestine to understand the physiology of the jejunum as compared to the ileum. They performed the first metabolic surgery by creating a jejunoileal bypass of various lengths in dogs [17]. They discovered that the animals were not only able to survive with a significant portion of the intestine bypassed, but also that lipid absorption was greatly impacted leading to weight loss. Their canine studies were of such high quality that they were presented at the American Surgical Association Spring Meeting in 1954 [17]. During their presentation, a member of the audience commented that a woman had undergone a similar operation to bypass the majority of her small intestine. She had lost a significant amount of weight and interestingly her cardiac disease had improved [18]. Around the same time, the Swedish surgeon Viktor Henriksson had been performing an intestinal bypass procedure in a small group of patients resulting in notable weight loss; however, each had experienced "difficult situations of nutritional balance" [18]. In the groups operated upon by Linner and Henriksson, it was noticed that patients had experienced long-term control of obesity and associated conditions. Several surgeons would later adapt these intestinal bypass procedures in the 1960s and initiated the birth of the surgical treatment of obesity.

Boom in Surgical Techniques

In 1963, Payne, DeWind, and Commons formed a multidisciplinary group that conducted a large study on morbidly obese patients. Payne even coined the term "morbid obesity" to help persuade insurance providers to pay for the operation. They performed an end-to-side jejunocolic shunt in ten patients [19]. This purely malabsorptive procedure involved dividing the jejunum 35–50 cm distal to the ligament of Treitz and creating an end-to-side anastomosis to the proximal transverse colon. The distal end was simply closed leaving a long blind loop. The procedure was later modified by moving the anastomosis to the proximal ascending colon to help decrease the degree of diarrhea. Weight loss occurred in each of the patients after surgery, with the majority of weight loss observed in the first postoperative year. Decreased absorption of fats and resultant decreased serum cholesterol

and lipoprotein levels were also noted in each patient [20].

Their protocol called for the reestablishment of continuity of the gastrointestinal tract when optimal weight had been achieved. In the six patients in whom continuity of the gastrointestinal tract was restored, all regained their previous obese state. Three patients had their jejunocolic shunt revised to an end-to-side jejunoileal shunt and one patient died from complications related to a pulmonary embolism [19].

The patients were plagued with many postoperative complications including poor absorption of essential vitamins and minerals, which required arduous continuous replacement [19, 20]. All experienced fatty stools, significant diarrhea, and anal excoriations [20]. Other complications included dehydration, electrolyte imbalance, postural hypotension, tetany, anemia, cholelithiasis, nephrolithiasis, fatty infiltration of the liver, hepatic cirrhosis, and hepatic failure [21]. The authors concluded that if a reasonable amount of jejunum, around 14 in., and a smaller portion of about 4 in. of terminal ileum were left in continuity with ingested food, weight loss could be better maintained. Other surgeons found similar results with intestinal bypass operations. In 1964, Henry Buchwald demonstrated that a similar ileal bypass with a jejunocolic anastomosis would lower the lipid levels in those with familial hypercholesterolemia and that the effect was sustainable for many years [22, 23]. These benefits were overshadowed by the severe complications, and the jejunocolic bypass was ultimately abandoned, and many patients were later converted to alternative operations [21].

In 1969, Payne and DeWind [24] reported the effects of another intestinal bypass operation—a jejunoileostomy bypass. This procedure again involved dividing the small intestine 35 cm distal to the ligament of Treitz, but was altered with an anastomosis at the terminal ileum, 10 cm proximal to the ileocecal valve rather than to the colon. These operations provided acceptable weight loss results in a large number of patients in addition to other favorable physiologic effects, while limiting some of the side effects seen in jejunocolic bypasses [24].

By the late 1960s and early 1970s, additional reports of successful weight loss from jejunoileal or jejunocolic shunt were being published. These studies were quick to identify complications directly associated with the intestinal bypass procedure and allowed researchers fertile ground to investigate the mechanisms of action that produced the aberrations. In Payne's original protocol, all of the patients had liver biopsies and the vast majority demonstrated steatosis of the liver with pathology that looked identical to alcohol-induced cirrhosis. Interestingly, if the excluded limb of intestine was resected, liver failure did not occur. Certain investigators demonstrated bacterial overgrowth of gram-negatives and anaerobic bacteria in the excluded limb of intestine along with morphological changes in the intestinal wall [25]. These investigators coined the term "enterohepatic syndrome" to describe this phenomenon.

Although the benefits of these intestinal bypass operations were profound, they continued to be limited by severe complications. The second National Institutes of Health (NIH) Consensus Development Conference was held in 1978 [26] with a primary focus on the treatment of morbid obesity, including investigations into surgical interventions. Although the recommendations were favorable for certain operative procedures, it was felt that the risk–benefit ratio for intestinal shunting was too high to recommend its routine use. This conclusion was combined with a sentiment that surgeons investigating weight loss operations were outsiders merely involved in the treatment of a condition not recognized as a disease, but simply the result of poor self-control. This prejudice intensified discrimination against the patients, their disease, and the surgeons dedicated to treating them. Continued pursuits in surgical obesity treatments were often viewed as a waste of resources that could be better used in the treatment of "real" surgical problems like cancer and ulcer disease [18].

In the following years, many surgeons became sensitive to the complications of malabsorptive procedures and started to look for alternatives. In 1967, Edward Mason, a surgeon from the University of Iowa with strong connections to Linner at the University of Minnesota, published a paper in which he observed that patients with subtotal gastrectomy for cancer and peptic ulcer disease lost a considerable amount of weight after resection. From this observation he proposed the first true "bariatric surgery," the gastric bypass [27]. Working with Chikashi "Chick" Ito, Mason was routinely performing a side-to-side anastomosis between the upper third of the divided stomach and a loop of jejunum to treat duodenal ulcer disease. A number of their patients were obese and it was noticed that although the procedure did not effectively control the ulcers, it was associated with significant weight loss [27]. His findings came at the peak of popularity for the jejunoileal bypass [27]and represented a fresh approach. The procedure was later optimized with a smaller gastric pouch and stoma size [28] and due to severe bile reflux, the reconstruction was adapted by Alden with a "Roux-en-Y" gastrojejunostomy [29]. Compared to the earlier jejunoileal bypass operation, gastric bypass resulted in less diarrhea, kidney stones and gallstones, and improvements in liver fat content [30].

The procedure was not without its own challenges. It required operating high in the abdomen and therefore was technically demanding and often the enlarged left lobe of the liver proved problematic. Staplers were not available and two hand-sewn anastomoses were technically challenging and time consuming. Postoperative complications often included dumping syndrome, anastomotic failure, marginal ulcers, bile reflux, and various nutritional deficiencies.

Several modifications to this technique were implemented to improve weight loss, such as the Fobi-Capella banded gastric bypass, which consisted of the application of a ring to the gastric pouch in order to limit its enlargement and possible weight regain [31, 32]. Mason himself continued to modify his procedure and explore alternatives and by the mid-1970s he performed a gastric partitioning procedure in which he stapled the stomach transversely toward the greater curvature, leaving a small orifice of communication between the two gastric channels [33]. This procedure was later modified by several surgeons to various configurations. Over then following year, vertical gastric partitioning along the lesser curvature in conjunction with controlling the outlet using a variety of devices grew in popularity [34]. Mason further modified this approach by placing an end-to-end anastomosis stapler through the stomach at the distal end of the lesser curvature and placing a piece of mesh through the hole and back up through an aperture at the stomach [35]. This variation of vertical banded gastroplasty rapidly gained popularity and was arguably the most commonly performed bariatric operation in the United States in the 1980s.

Ironically, the same NIH Consensus Conference that led to the fall of the jejunoileal bypass also provided a new life for gastric restrictive procedures [18]. Various pioneers began to tirelessly work on adapting the operative techniques surrounding the gastric bypass procedures. Investigators published many comparison studies between the intestinal bypass procedure and gastric bypass [30, 36], demonstrating that complications were clearly less in the gastric procedures and weight loss was equivalent. During the 1980s, Mason continued to champion gastric restriction with variations of the banded gastroplasty.

In an ingenious modification of gastroplasty, in the 1980s Kuzmak invented a silastic ring with a small balloon embedded on the inner aspect of the ring that could be accessed from a subcutaneously placed reservoir [37]. This allowed calibration and adjustment of the outflow obstruction, and thus adjustable gastric banding was born. At this time gastric restrictive procedures, including gastric bypass, which was classified as a primarily restrictive procedure, and banding were commonly associated with less postoperative complications compared to previous shunts while providing satisfactory weight loss. These restrictive procedures benefited enormously from advances in technology, especially with improved stapling devices.

Investigations into obesity and bariatric surgery were not unique to North America as the field was becoming more recognized in Europe, Latin America, and to a lesser degree in Asia. In 1979, Italian surgeon Nicola Scopinaro devised

an operation he termed the biliopancreatic diversion [38]. This operation consisted of a generous distal gastrectomy combined with dividing the small intestine near the midpoint. The distal end of the divided ileum is anastomosed to the proximal stomach remnant and the proximal biliopancreatic limb channeling the digestive excretions was anastomosed to the side of the ileum 50–120 cm proximal from the ileocecal valve [39]. This produced a shortened common channel for ingested food contact with digestive juices resulting in further decreased absorption. Scopinaro reported excellent weight loss results and his patients underwent a battery of metabolic studies that demonstrated resolution of many comorbidities associated with morbid obesity [40, 41]. As with previous operations, biliopancreatic diversion was not without many of the side effects observed in other malabsorptive procedures, especially related to iron and fat-soluble vitamin absorption. Many patients experienced frequent voluminous and malodorous stools and flatus in addition to postgastrectomy syndrome symptoms such as dumping. Regardless of these effects, Scopinaro reported excellent long-term results and the procedure remains popular outside the United States today, commonly resulting in 70% long-term weight loss in more than 90% of patients.

The high incidence of postgastrectomy syndrome after biliopancreatic diversion lead to several modifications and alterations of the operation. In 1986, Hess and Hess devised an alteration by changing to a pylorus-sparing gastrectomy to the original biliopancreatic bypass procedure and modified the anastomosis to a duodenojejunal configuration [42]. A similar operation was later described by Marceau in 1993 combining a pylorus-sparing gastrectomy along the greater curvature of the stomach, leaving a tube-like gastric remnant in order to preserve pyloric function and its innervation [43]. Similar to Scopinaro's reconstruction, the jejunum was divided approximately 250 cm distal to the ligament of Treitz; however, the Roux limb was anastomosed to the postpyloric duodenum. The long biliopancreatic limb was attached to the distal bowel 50 cm proximal to the ileocecal valve [39]. This operation, aptly named a "duodenal switch," was and still is an effective surgery for weight loss, often reserved for super-obese patients [44]. It also allows patients to lose weight without significantly altering their eating habits, resulting in durable long-term weight loss [45]. Although the incidence of postgastrectomy syndrome decreased with the duodenal switch modification, other complications and postoperative effects are similar to those seen in patients with a biliopancreatic diversion [39].

Interest and investment in developing safer and more effective procedures continued and in 1987 Johnston performed an operation described as the Magenstrasse and Mill procedure in search for a safe and simple alternative to gastric bypass and vertical banded gastroplasty [46]. Similar to Marceau, the "Magenstrasse" referred to a thin tube created from the lesser curvature of the stomach while the "Mill" referred to the antrum; however, the operation performed using a circular stapler to create a defect in the antrum and then creating a narrow tube along the lesser curvature initially over a bougie. The technique was later modified by resecting the greater curvature of the stomach in same fashion as Hess in the duodenal switch and also Marceau in his series [42, 43]. This created a shift in thought as the sleeve gastrectomy was initially used as part of a two-step procedure in high-risk (BMI > 60) patients. Follow-up of these patients demonstrated substantial weight loss and resolution of comorbidities with the sleeve gastrectomy alone [47] eventually leading to popularity of sleeve gastrectomy as a stand-alone procedure, further aided with the progression of laparoscopy [48].

Minimally Invasive Revolution

On a second front, many pivotal technological advancements in general surgery found fertile ground in bariatric surgery. From the time Bozzini developed the Lichtleiter in the late eighteenth century, light conductors offered improved illumination allowing improved exploration and illumination of internal cavities. Initially these devices were limited to urologic and gynecologic procedures, the Lichtleiter and other viewing devices had limited application for the next 100 years until Edison's invention of the incandescent light, igniting a new chapter of minimally invasive surgery.

In 1901, Kelling used light and rudimentary optical technology to examine the abdominal cavity of dogs [49]. This was quickly followed by a report by Jacobeus, a surgeon from Stockholm, who coined the phrases *laparoscopie* and *thoracoscopie*, and who was the first to publish a series of abdominal and thoracic examination in humans using minimally invasive techniques [50]. Berheim at Johns Hopkins was the first in 1911 to perform laparoscopy in the United States [49]. These events were followed by numerous advancements in fiberoptics and insufflation over the next 70 years until this surgical approach would become a standard treatment and chisel the role of minimally invasive techniques into the surgical world. Surgeons committed to the treatment of obesity had also begun to explore the application of laparoscopic approaches to procedures.

The first laparoscopic gastric bypass operation in the United States was performed by Wittgrove and Clark in October 1993 after developing their technique in the laboratory. With a six-trocar technique, they created a retrocolic Roux limb using a circular stapler anastomosis for the gastrojejunostomy [51]. The anvil of the circular stapler was passed transorally, using a proprietary technique. The procedure was principally the same as its open counterpart with three common key components: creation of a small gastric pouch, a restrictive gastrojejunal anastomosis, and the creation of a long Roux limb for malabsorption. Their initial results were excellent, and the authors reported on 500 patients who maintained 73% excess body weight loss at 54 months [52]. The leak rate was low (2.2%) and comparable to open procedures at that time. The overall complication rate was less than 10%, which indicated that the laparoscopic approach was indeed feasible and safe.

Swedish surgeon Lönroth pioneered a manual suturing technique to connect an antecolic jejunal loop to the proximal stomach pouch [53] and in

2003, the Gothenburg group reported comparable long-term weight loss in laparoscopic gastric bypass patients compared to open [54]. In a large series of 400 patients, Higa et al. reported favorable complication rates with no leakages at the gastrojejunal anastomosis in addition to impressive long-term weight loss [55, 56].

The technical constraints of laparoscopy proved these operations very difficult, but as experience and more advanced devices became available, the learning curve proved manageable. The popularity of laparoscopic gastric bypass increased rapidly and by the late 1990s almost every major center had devoted a division for minimally invasive bariatric procedures. This era of minimally invasive surgery truly revolutionized the surgical treatment of obesity. Laparoscopy allowed surgeons to perform complex gastrointestinal operations with an improved level of safety. Operative mortality for many open bariatric operations had been around 1%, only to fall to less than 0.2% with a laparoscopic approach and complication rates fell by two-thirds [57]. Other benefits including decreased hospital length of stay, improved pulmonary function, less blood loss, decreased wound infections, and fewer incisional hernias were reported [58, 59].

Gastric bypass was not the only operation to benefit from laparoscopy. Although various reports date back to 1992 by Forsell and Cadière [60, 61], the first successful laparoscopic banding procedure is commonly credited to Broadbent in 1993 with the placement of a nonadjustable gastric band in a 16-year-old female [62]. Catona also published a series of patients who underwent nonadjustable gastric banding using a laparoscopic approach at around the same time [63]. During the same time, Belachew designed an adjustable gastric band that could be placed using laparoscopic techniques in a porcine model using a device similar to the band patented by Kuzmak a decade earlier [64]. Banding operations presented a favorable option for many patients and surgeons as an alternative to more dramatic bypass operations. In the 1990s and 2000s, a large number of bands were placed worldwide prior to FDA approval in the United States. In clinical practice, laparoscopic adjustable gastric banding boomed during the decade, yet eventually fell out of favor due to technical problems with slippage and pouch dilatation as well as reflux problems and disappointing long-term results [65].

Other operations found life in minimally invasive approaches. The first laparoscopic duodenal switch was performed by Ren and Gagner in 1999, as a modification of the original Scopinaro procedure [66]. A laparoscopic biliopancreatic diversion-duodenal switch is a technically demanding operation even for laparoscopic experts, but has been associated with larger weight loss when compared to other bariatric procedures and often remains reserved for patients with a BMI of 60 or greater. The operative mortality for open biliopancreatic diversion with duodenal switch was approximately 1% and the rate is slightly higher (2.5%) with a laparoscopic approach. This mortality rate may decrease as the surgeon gains expertise with the technical aspects of this procedure and overcomes the associated learning curve [44]. Due to technical difficulty as well as concerns for nutritional deficiency, the procedure has not been widely adopted in the United States. In 2003, the possibility of a two-stage procedure in super-super obese patients was suggested to overcome technical difficulties [67]. The idea was to first perform a sleeve gastrectomy, leading to sufficient weight loss to later facilitate to second stage division of the duodenum. Many patients elected not to proceed to the planned second stage, satisfied by their initial weight loss after the gastrectomy alone. From this a new stand-alone procedure was born, the laparoscopic sleeve gastrectomy. The number of laparoscopic sleeve gastrectomies continues to increase dramatically in the United States; however, long-term studies on effectiveness and difficult to treat complications, such as leak, require further evaluation.

In the end of the 1990s and into the 2000s, several high-profile celebrities underwent laparoscopic bariatric surgery. In 1999, singer Carnie Wilson famously under laparoscopic gastric bypass broadcasted live on the Internet, exposing the public to the operation [68]. This acceptance and publicity was in great contrast to what the pioneers had endured in prior years and consequently the number of bariatric procedures dramatically increased. In consecutive reviews, Buchwald et al. presented fascinating worldwide data on all bariatric surgery performed in nations belonging to the International Federation for the Surgery of Obesity, IFSO. The proportion of laparoscopic bariatric surgery increased from 63% in 2003 to over 90% in 2008 [69, 70]. During the same time frame, the annual number of bariatric procedures worldwide increased from 146,000 to 340,000 with nearly 200,000 operations annually in the United States alone [70].

Laparoscopy adds many advantages to bariatric surgery including but not limited to reduced wound-related complications and improved patient recovery [71] with adverse event rates comparable to common procedures such as laparoscopic cholecystectomy and appendectomy [72]. In a systematic review of fast-track laparoscopic bariatric surgery, next-day discharge was possible in 81–100% of patients after laparoscopic gastric bypass [73], an impossible idea only a decade earlier in the area of open bariatric surgery when postoperative complications and prolonged hospital stays were the norm.

Metabolic Discoveries

Throughout the late twentieth century as the field of bariatric surgery reached new heights and knowledge about the disease had advanced substantially, the understanding of hormonal mechanisms and physiology grew. The majority of procedures focused on some variation of a gastric restrictive operation and the benefits of weight loss were clearly apparent and well documented on a macroscopic level. Microscopically, the effects remained largely unknown. In a report MacDonald and Pories published in 1995, the beneficial effects on type II diabetes in patients who had undergone a Roux-en-Y gastric bypass were examined [74]. The positive effects of weight loss on diabetes was already well known, but the metabolic effects of surgery had only occurred as an anecdotal observation until sev-

eral authors reported decreases in insulin resistance and improved glucose metabolism after intestinal shunting procedures, often well before any weight loss had occurred [75]. Unfortunately these reports did not gain much notoriety partly because intestinal shunting procedures were falling out of favor. Decades later, Schauer reported similar results in a large cohort of gastric bypass patients who had either impaired testing glucose levels or type 2 diabetes [76]. Subsequent studies confirmed the positive effects of Roux-en-Y gastric bypass on treating type 2 diabetes, establishing the role of surgery in the treatment of diabetes and metabolic syndrome [77, 78].

A summit was convened in 2010 in Rome by a multidisciplinary group with an interest in type 2 diabetes where a consensus was reached and published outlining the creation of a research agenda in order to focus attention and efforts into understanding the mechanisms by which diabetes can be controlled with surgical intervention [79]. It was observed that something intrinsic was occurring physiologically that surpasses simply diverting and bypassing the flow of food in the intestines. Greater emphasis was placed on the distinction of "metabolic" surgery [80]. A third NIH consensus conference on obesity was held in 1991 that concluded that surgical intervention of morbid obesity significantly treated or resolved many of the comorbidities associated with obesity [81]. As further evidence of this shift in understanding, the American Society of Bariatric Surgery elected at the 2008 annual business meeting to change the name of the society by adding "Metabolic" to the organization's title. This change stressed the efforts on understanding how these procedures worked on a metabolic level and in many ways validated the work of earlier surgeons who had recommended that patients be followed long term to track metabolic parameters of success.

Conclusion

As demonstrated, bariatric surgery has come a long way from a king unfit to mount a horse to complex operations with significant metabolic impact. Several operations born out of observation have paved the way to a more thorough knowledge and understanding of digestive physiology. The growth of laparoscopic surgery with reduced morbidity and mortality has ushered bariatric surgery to the forefront of innovation and treatment to combat the growing obesity epidemic. Today's surgeons are indebted to the pioneers that have sought for an ideal procedure in order to relieve morbidly obese patients from comorbid conditions, and to increase life expectancy and quality of life. In only a matter of a couple decades, laparoscopic techniques have revolutionized bariatric surgery and further technological advancements by the way of robotics await. The number of bariatric procedures performed worldwide continues to rise and will continue to increase as the indications and benefits for metabolic operations are further understood.

References

1. Eknoyan G. A history of obesity, or how what was good became ugly and then bad. Adv Chronic Kidney Dis. 2006;13(4):421–7.
2. Rodgers S, Burnet R, Goss A, Phillips P, Goldney R, Kimber C, et al. Jaw wiring in treatment of obesity. Lancet. 1977;1(8024):1221–2.
3. Tavares A, Viveiros F, Cidade C, Maciel J. Bariatric surgery: epidemic of the XXI century. Acta Medica Port. 2011;24(1):111–6.
4. Hopkins KD, Lehmann ED. Successful medical treatment of obesity in 10th century Spain. Lancet. 1995;346(8972):452.
5. Garrow JS, Gardiner GT. Maintenance of weight loss in obese patients after jaw wiring. Br Med J (Clin Res Ed). 1981;282(6267):858–60.
6. Baker MT. The history and evolution of bariatric surgical procedures. Surg Clin North Am. 2011;91(6):1181–201, viii.
7. Dietz WH. The response of the US Centers for Disease Control and Prevention to the obesity epidemic. Annu Rev Public Health. 2015;36:575–96.
8. Xu JQ, Murphy SL, Kochanek KD, Arias E. Mortality in the United States, 2015. NCHS data brief, no 267. Hyattsville: National Center for Health Statistics. 2016. https://www.cdc.gov/nchs/data/databriefs/db267.pdf. Accessed 25 Apr 2017.
9. World Health Organization. Obesity and overweight fact sheet. Updated Jun 2016. http://www.who.int/mediacentre/factsheets/fs311/en/. Accessed 5 Apr 2017.
10. Kelly T, Yang W, Chen CS, Reynolds K, He J. Global burden of obesity in 2005 and projections to 2030. Int J Obes. 2008;32(9):1431–7.
11. Ogden CL, Carroll MD. Prevalence of overweight, obesity, and extreme obesity among adults: United States, trends 1960–1962 through 2007–2008. Hyattsville: National Center for Health Statistics. 2011. http://www.cdc.gov/nchs/data/hestat/obesity_adult_07_08/obesity_. Accessed 26 Apr 2017.
12. Ogden CL, Lamb MM, Carroll MD, Flegal KM. Obesity and socioeconomic status in adults: United States, 2005–2008. NCHS Data Brief. 2010;(50):1–8.
13. Ogden CL, Lamb MM, Carroll MD, Flegal KM. Obesity and socioeconomic status in children and adolescents: United States, 2005–2008. NCHS Data Brief. 2010;(51):1–8.
14. Fryar C, Carroll MD, Ogden CL. Prevalence of obesity among children and adolescents: United States, trends 1963–1965 through 2009–2010. Hyattsville: National Center for Health Statistics. 2012. http://www.cdc.gov/nchs/data/hestat/obesity_child_09_10/obesity_child_09_10.htm. Accessed 26 Apr 2017.
15. Fryar C, Carrol MD, Ogden CL. Prevalence of overweight, obesity, and extreme obesity among adults: United States, trends 1960–1962 through 2009–2010. Hyattsville: National Center for Health Statistics. 2012. http://www.cdc.gov/nchs/data/hestat/obesity_adult_09_10/obesity_adult_09_10.htm. Accessed 26 Apr 2017.
16. Wang Y, Beydoun MA, Liang L, Caballero B, Kumanyika SK. Will all Americans become overweight or obese? Estimating the progression and cost of the US obesity epidemic. Obesity (Silver Spring). 2008;16(10):2323–30.
17. Kremen AJ, Linner JH, Nelson CH. An experimental evaluation of the nutritional importance of proximal and distal small intestine. Ann Surg. 1954;140(3):439–48.
18. Nguyen NT, Blackstone RP, Morton JM, Ponce J, Rosenthal RJ, editors. The ASMBS textbook of bariatric surgery. 1st ed. New York: Springer; 2014.
19. Payne JH, DeWind LT, Commons RR. Metabolic observations in patients with jejunocolic shunts. Am J Surg. 1963;106:273–89.
20. Lewis LA, Turnbull RB Jr, Page IH. Effects of jejunocolic shunt on obesity, serum lipoproteins, lipids, and electrolytes. Arch Intern Med. 1966;117(1):4–16.
21. Mir-Madjlessi SH, Mackenzie AH, Winkelman EI. Articular complications in obese patients after jejunocolic bypass. Cleve Clin Q. 1974;41(3):119–33.
22. Buchwald H, Varco RL. Ileal bypass in lowering high cholesterol levels. Surg Forum. 1964;15:289–91.
23. Buchwald H, Varco RL. Ileal bypass in patients with hypercholesterolemia and atherosclerosis. Preliminary report on therapeutic potential. JAMA. 1966;196(7):627–30.
24. Payne JH, DeWind LT. Surgical treatment of obesity. Am J Surg. 1969;118(2):141–7.

25. O'Leary JP. Historical perspective on intestinal bypass procedures. In: Griffen WO, Printen KJ, editors. Surgical management of morbid obesity. New York: Marcel Dekker; 1987. p. 1–27.

26. Symposium on surgical treatment of morbid obesity. Proceedings of a consensus conference sponsored by the National Institute of Arthritis, Metabolism, and Digestive Diseases of the National Institutes of Health; held in December 1978 at Bethesda, Maryland. Am J Clin Nutr. 1980;33(2 Suppl):353–530.

27. Mason EE, Ito C. Gastric bypass in obesity. Surg Clin North Am. 1967;47(6):1345–51.

28. Mason EE, Printen KJ, Hartford CE, Boyd WC. Optimizing results of gastric bypass. Ann Surg. 1975;182(4):405–14.

29. Alden JF. Gastric and jejunoileal bypass. A comparison in the treatment of morbid obesity. Arch Surg. 1977;112(7):799–806.

30. Griffen WO Jr, Young VL, Stevenson CC. A prospective comparison of gastric and jejunoileal bypass procedures for morbid obesity. Ann Surg. 1977;186(4):500–9.

31. Fobi MA, Fleming AW. Vertical banded gastroplasty vs gastric bypass in the treatment of obesity. J Natl Med Assoc. 1986;78(11):1091–8.

32. Capella RF, Capella JF, Mandec H, Nath P. Vertical banded gastroplasty-gastric bypass: preliminary report. Obes Surg. 1991;1(4):389–95.

33. Mason EE, Doherty C, Cullen JJ, Scott D, Rodriguez EM, Maher JW. Vertical gastroplasty: evolution of vertical banded gastroplasty. World J Surg. 1998;22(9):919–24.

34. O'Leary JP. Partition of the lesser curvature of the stomach in morbid obesity. Surg Gynecol Obstet. 1982;154(1):85–6.

35. Mason EE, Printen KJ, Blommers TJ, Scott DH. Gastric bypass for obesity after ten years experience. Int J Obes. 1978;2(2):197–206.

36. Buckwalter JA. A prospective comparison of the jejunoileal and gastric bypass operations for morbid obesity. World J Surg. 1977;1(6):757–66.

37. Kuzmak L. Silicone gastric banding: a simple and effective operation for morbid obesity. Contemp Surg. 1986;28(1):13–8.

38. Scopinaro N, Gianetta E, Civalleri D, Bonalumi U, Bachi V. Bilio-pancreatic bypass for obesity: II. Initial experience in man. Br J Surg. 1979;66(9):618–20.

39. Fobi MA. Surgical treatment of obesity: a review. J Natl Med Assoc. 2004;96(1):61–75.

40. Scopinaro N, Adami GF, Marinari GM, Gianetta E, Traverso E, Friedman D, et al. Biliopancreatic diversion. World J Surg. 1998;22(9):936–46.

41. Scopinaro N. Thirty-five years of biliopancreatic diversion: notes on gastrointestinal physiology to complete the published information useful for a better understanding and clinical use of the operation. Obes Surg. 2012;22(3):427–32.

42. Hess DS, Hess DW. Biliopancreatic diversion with a duodenal switch. Obes Surg. 1998;8(3):267–82.

43. Marceau P, Biron S, Bourque RA, Potvin M, Hould FS, Simard S. Biliopancreatic diversion with a new type of gastrectomy. Obes Surg. 1993;3(1):29–35.

44. Sudan R, Jacobs DO. Biliopancreatic diversion with duodenal switch. Surg Clin North Am. 2011;91(6):1281–93, ix.

45. Carucci LR, Turner MA. Imaging following bariatric procedures: roux-en-Y gastric bypass, gastric sleeve, and biliopancreatic diversion. Abdom Imaging. 2012;37(5):697–711.

46. Johnston D, Dachtler J, Sue-Ling HM, King RF, Martin I. The Magenstrasse and mill operation for morbid obesity. Obes Surg. 2003;13(1):10–6.

47. Rosenthal RJ, International Sleeve Gastrectomy Expert Panel, Diaz AA, Arvidsson D, Baker RS, Basso N, et al. International sleeve gastrectomy expert panel consensus statement: best practice guidelines based on experience of >12,000 cases. Surg Obes Relat Dis. 2012;8(1):8–19.

48. Talebpour M, Amoli BS. Laparoscopic total gastric vertical plication in morbid obesity. J Laparoendosc Adv Surg Tech A. 2007;17(6):793–8.

49. St. Peter SD, Holcomb GWI. History of minimally invasive surgery. In: Holcomb GW, Georgeson KE, Rothenberg SS, editors. Endoscopic surgery in infants and children. Philadelphia: Saunders Elsevier; 2009. p. 1–5.

50. Hatzinger M, Kwon ST, Langbein S, Kamp S, Hacker A, Alken P. Hans Christian Jacobaeus: inventor of human laparoscopy and thoracoscopy. J Endourol. 2006;20(11):848–50.

51. Wittgrove AC, Clark GW, Tremblay LJ. Laparoscopic gastric bypass, roux-en-Y: preliminary report of five cases. Obes Surg. 1994;4(4):353–7.

52. Wittgrove AC, Clark GW. Laparoscopic gastric bypass, roux-en-Y-500 patients: technique and results, with 3-60 month follow-up. Obes Surg. 2000;10(3):233–9.

53. Lonroth H, Dalenback J, Haglind E, Lundell L. Laparoscopic gastric bypass. Another option in bariatric surgery. Surg Endosc. 1996;10(6):636–8.

54. Olbers T, Lonroth H, Fagevik-Olsen M, Lundell L. Laparoscopic gastric bypass: development of technique, respiratory function, and long-term outcome. Obes Surg. 2003;13(3):364–70.

55. Higa KD, Boone KB, Ho T, Davies OG. Laparoscopic Roux-en-Y gastric bypass for morbid obesity: technique and preliminary results of our first 400 patients. Arch Surg. 2000;135(9):1029–33; discussion 1033–4.

56. Higa KD, Boone KB, Ho T. Complications of the laparoscopic roux-en-Y gastric bypass: 1,040 patients—what have we learned? Obes Surg. 2000;10(6):509–13.

57. Miller MR, Choban PS. Surgical management of obesity: current state of procedure evolution and strategies to optimize outcomes. Nutr Clin Pract. 2011;26(5):526–33.

58. Nguyen NT, Lee SL, Goldman C, Fleming N, Arango A, McFall R, et al. Comparison of pulmonary function and postoperative pain after laparoscopic versus

open gastric bypass: a randomized trial. J Am Coll Surg. 2001;192(4):469–76; discussion 476–7.

59. Nguyen NT, Hinojosa M, Fayad C, Varela E, Wilson SE. Use and outcomes of laparoscopic versus open gastric bypass at academic medical centers. J Am Coll Surg. 2007;205(2):248–55.

60. Forsell P, Hellers G. The Swedish adjustable gastric banding (SAGB) for morbid obesity: 9 year experience and a 4-year follow-up of patients operated with a new adjustable band. Obes Surg. 1997;7(4):345–51.

61. Cadiere GB, Bruyns J, Himpens J, Favretti F. Laparoscopic gastroplasty for morbid obesity. Br J Surg. 1994;81(10):1524.

62. Broadbent R, Tracey M, Harrington P. Laparoscopic gastric banding: a preliminary report. Obes Surg. 1993;3(1):63–7.

63. Catona A, Gossenberg M, La Manna A, Mussini G. Laparoscopic gastric banding: preliminary series. Obes Surg. 1993;3(2):207–9.

64. Belachew M, Legrand MJ, Defechereux TH, Burtheret MP, Jacquet N. Laparoscopic adjustable silicone gastric banding in the treatment of morbid obesity. A preliminary report. Surg Endosc. 1994;8(11):1354–6.

65. Morino M, Toppino M, Garrone C, Morino F. Laparoscopic adjustable silicone gastric banding for the treatment of morbid obesity. Br J Surg. 1994;81(8):1169–70.

66. Ren CJ, Patterson E, Gagner M. Early results of laparoscopic biliopancreatic diversion with duodenal switch: a case series of 40 consecutive patients. Obes Surg. 2000;10(6):514–23; discussion 524.

67. Silecchia G, Rizzello M, Casella G, Fioriti M, Soricelli E, Basso N. Two-stage laparoscopic biliopancreatic diversion with duodenal switch as treatment of high-risk super-obese patients: analysis of complications. Surg Endosc. 2009;23(5):1032–7.

68. The Weight Loss Surgery Foundation of America (WLSFA.ORG). WLSFA National Ambassador of Hope Carnie Wilson. 2016. http://www.wlsfa.org/about/ambassadors-of-hope/carnie-wilson/. Accessed 25 Apr 2017.

69. Buchwald H, Williams SE. Bariatric surgery worldwide 2003. Obes Surg. 2004;14(9):1157–64.

70. Buchwald H, Oien DM. Metabolic/bariatric surgery worldwide 2008. Obes Surg. 2009;19(12):1605–11.

71. Kendrick ML, Dakin GF. Surgical approaches to obesity. Mayo Clin Proc. 2006;81(10):S18–24.

72. Woodham BL, Cox MR, Eslick GD. Evidence to support the use of laparoscopic over open appendicectomy for obese individuals: a meta-analysis. Surg Endosc. 2012;26(9):2566–70.

73. Elliott JA, Patel VM, Kirresh A, Ashrafian H, Le Roux CW, Olbers T, et al. Fast-track laparoscopic bariatric surgery: a systematic review. Updat Surg. 2013;65(2):85–94.

74. Pories WJ, Swanson MS, MacDonald KG, Long SB, Morris PG, Brown BM, et al. Who would have thought it? An operation proves to be the most effective therapy for adult-onset diabetes mellitus. Ann Surg 1995;222(3):339–50; discussion 350–2.

75. O'Leary JP, Duerson MC. Changes in glucose metabolism after jejunoileal bypass. Surg Forum. 1980;31:87.

76. Schauer PR, Burguera B, Ikramuddin S, Cottam D, Gourash W, Hamad G, et al. Effect of laparoscopic Roux-en Y gastric bypass on type 2 diabetes mellitus. Ann Surg. 2003;238(4):467–84; discussion 484–5.

77. Schauer PR, Kashyap SR, Wolski K, Brethauer SA, Kirwan JP, Pothier CE, et al. Bariatric surgery versus intensive medical therapy in obese patients with diabetes. N Engl J Med. 2012;366(17):1567–76.

78. Schauer PR, Bhatt DL, Kirwan JP, Wolski K, Aminian A, Brethauer SA, et al. Bariatric surgery versus intensive medical therapy for diabetes—5-year outcomes. N Engl J Med. 2017;376(7):641–51.

79. Rubino F, Kaplan LM, Schauer PR, Cummings DE, Diabetes Surgery Summit Delegates. The diabetes surgery summit consensus conference: recommendations for the evaluation and use of gastrointestinal surgery to treat type 2 diabetes mellitus. Ann Surg. 2010;251(3):399–405.

80. Starkloff GB, Donovan JF, Ramach KR, Wolfe BM. Metabolic intestinal surgery. Its complications and management. Arch Surg. 1975;110(5):652–7.

81. NIH conference. Gastrointestinal surgery for severe obesity. Consensus Development Conference Panel. Ann Intern Med. 1991;115(12):956–61.

Jawad Tahir Ali and Aaron D. Carr

General Endoscopic Indications

Screening colonoscopy, for average-risk individuals, is recommended at age 50 and every 10 years thereafter unless pathology is discovered that increases the need for more frequent screening (i.e., adenomatous polyps). If an individual has a first-degree relative that was diagnosed with colon cancer when younger than 60 years old, then that person should be screened at age 40 or 10 years younger than the age of diagnosis of that first-degree relative. Patients with familial adenomatous polyposis (FAP), hereditary nonpolyposis colorectal cancer, and inflammatory bowel disease should also be screened much earlier and more frequent than the average-risk individual [1].

Upper endoscopy in the general population is indicated for patients with dyspepsia and gastro-esophageal reflux disease (GERD) with high-risk features or in patients with increased risk factors for Barrett's esophagus (BE). Generally recommended surveillance for BE includes repeat upper endoscopy in 6 months for low grade dysplasia (LGD), then annual surveillance thereafter using a standard screening protocol. Some experts advocate ablative therapy for LGD, which is more typically used for flat high grade dysplasia [2].

Dyspepsia defined by the Rome IV criteria consists of one or more of the following features: epigastric pain or burning, postprandial fullness, and early satiety. These symptoms must occur 3 or more days per week for the past 3 months with onset at least 6 months prior to diagnosis [3]. Dyspepsia high-risk features include the following (Table 2.1): age > 50 years, family history of gastrointestinal (GI) malignancy in first-degree relative, unintended weight loss, GI bleeding or anemia, dysphagia, odynophagia, and persistent vomiting [4].

The Montreal definition of GERD defines it as a chronic condition caused by the reflux of stomach contents that adversely affects an individual's well-being. This must occur more than twice a week with symptoms of heartburn or regurgitation [5]. GERD high-risk features include the following (see Table 2.1): symptoms that are persistent or progressive despite medical therapy, multiple risk factors for BE, dysphagia, odynophagia, unintended weight loss, GI bleeding or anemia, and persistent vomiting [6].

J.T. Ali, M.D.
Department of Surgery, University of California at Davis, 4223 J St, Unit #3, Sacramento, CA 95819, USA

Department of Surgery, University of California, Davis Medical Center, 2221 Stockton Boulevard, Sacramento, CA 95817, USA
e-mail: jawada@gmail.com

A.D. Carr, M.D. (✉)
Department of Surgery, University of California, Davis Medical Center, 2221 Stockton Boulevard, Sacramento, CA 95817, USA
e-mail: acarr067@gmail.com

© Springer International Publishing AG 2018
B. Chand (ed.), *Endoscopy in Obesity Management*, DOI 10.1007/978-3-319-63528-6_2

Table 2.1 High-risk features of dyspepsia and GERD that should prompt upper endoscopic screening

Dyspepsia	GERD
Age > 50	Persistent symptoms on medications
Family history of malignancy (first-degree relative)	Multiple risk factors for Barrett's esophagus
Weight loss	Weight loss
GI bleeding or anemia	GI bleeding or anemia
Dysphagia or odynophagia	Dysphagia or odynophagia
Persistent vomiting	Persistent vomiting

GERD gastroesophageal reflux disease, *GI* gastrointestinal

Table 2.2 Barrett's esophagus risk factors

Caucasian race
Men
Age > 50
BMI > 25 kg/m^2
GERD > 5 years
Nocturnal reflux
Hiatal hernia
Tobacco use
Family history of BE or adenocarcinoma

BMI body mass index, *GERD* gastroesophageal reflux disease, *BE* Barrett's esophagus

Table 2.3 Obesity risk for gastrointestinal pathology

Conditions	Odds ratio
GERD	2.0
Hiatal hernia	4.2
Esophagitis	1.8
Gastric ulcer	4.1
Esophageal cancer	2.8
Gastric cancer	1.7
Colorectal cancer	1.5 in women
	2.0 in men

GERD gastroesophageal reflux disease

Barrett's esophagus is defined as intestinal metaplastic change in the tubular esophagus, which is known to increase the risk for esophageal adenocarcinoma. BE confers a relative risk of 11.3 over the general population in the development of esophageal adenocarcinoma [7]. Risk factors for BE include the following (Table 2.2): Caucasian race, men, age > 50 years old, body mass index (BMI) >25 kg/m^2, GERD symptoms present for more than 5 years, nocturnal reflux, hiatal hernia, tobacco use, and family history of BE or adenocarcinoma of the esophagus [6]. Non-steroidal anti-inflammatory drug (NSAID) use and old age are also considered independent risk factors for foregut pathology as well [8–10].

Obesity: A Risk Factor for Pathology

There is good observational data that obesity increases the risk of gastroesophageal pathology and colorectal cancer (Table 2.3). We will define obesity based on body mass index (BMI) criteria used by the Centers for Disease Control and World Health Organization. Obesity is defined as BMI >30 kg/m^2, with class I ranging from 30.0 to 34.9 kg/m^2; class II from 35.0 to 39.9 kg/m^2; and class III greater than 40 kg/m^2. One meta-analysis of studies done between 1966 and 2004 found that obesity was associated with an odds ratio (OR) of 2 for GERD symptoms and 1.8 for erosive esophagitis when compared to normal weight people. Furthermore, the odds ratio for esophageal adenocarcinoma was increased to 2.1 for BMI > 25 kg/m^2 and 2.78 for BMI > 30 kg/m^2. Adenocarcinoma of the gastric cardia was also increased in obese patients with OR of 1.68 [10]. Obesity has also been linked to hiatal hernia with an OR of 4.2 [11]. Some studies have noted an increased rate of gastritis and ulcers in obese patients, leading some to propose a new subtype of gastritis, "obesity-related gastritis" [12, 13]. The Kalixanda study randomly surveyed and performed endoscopy on 1001 people in Northern Sweden, and they found that obesity was an independent risk factor for gastric ulcer with an OR of 4.15. The study also found smoking and aspirin use to be independent risk factors as well, OR 3.12 and 7.44, respectively [14].

In addition to foregut pathology, overweight and obese individuals are known to have an increased risk of colorectal cancer. In overweight individuals (BMI 25–29.9 kg/m^2), the relative risk is 1.5 for men and 1.2 for women. Obesity increases the relative risk to 2.0 for men and 1.5 for women [15]. Obesity has also been linked to increased mortality in all types of cancer. The relative risk (RR) of death from colorectal cancer with BMI 30–34.9 kg/m^2 is 1.47 and for BMI

$35–39.9$ kg/m^2 it is 1.85. Death from esophageal cancer follows a similar pattern with RR 1.28 and 1.63, for BMI 30–34.9 and 35–39.9 kg/m^2, respectively. Gastric cancer death carries a RR of 1.2 and 1.94 for the same BMI distributions [16].

The increased risk of reflux and hiatal hernia in obese patients is one likely mechanism for their increased risk of esophageal cancer. Wu et al. found that the risk of esophageal adenocarcinoma was three times higher in those with reflux symptoms, six times higher in those with hiatal hernia, and eight times higher in those that had both when compared to control subjects [17]. There is also a correlation with between obesity and gastritis. As previously described, a Japanese study looking at routine health records found that serum adiponectin, an anti-inflammatory cytokine protective against erosive gastritis, was found in reduced concentrations in the obese population, leading to increased rate of ulcers [13]. A related factor may also be higher rates of *Helicobacter pylori (H. pylori)* found in obese patients. A study of 103 obese people that compared them to 111 healthy controls found the rate of *H. pylori* seropositivity to be 57.2% in the obese population and 27.0% in the control group [18]. A US study also found increased positive serologies for *H. pylori* in obese patients, 61.3%, as compared to 48.2% in their control group [19].

Endoscopy in Bariatric Surgery

Preoperative Indications

Even with the increased risk for upper gastrointestinal disease, there is debate on routine versus selective preoperative endoscopy prior to bariatric surgery with data for each position. Proponents for routine endoscopy cite high rates of pathologic findings that require additional preoperative treatment and sometimes, although rarely, change the surgery to be performed or even contraindicate a bariatric operation. Proponents for selective endoscopy cite the low rates of significant pathology that would change a bariatric operation. In this vein, *H. pylori* prevalence has been shown to be more variable in this population (Class II and III obesity). One study found a

22.4% rate of seropositivity in 259 obese patients scheduled to undergo gastric bypass [20]. They also performed an analysis of selected studies between 1996 and 2006 measuring prevalence of *H. pylori* in patients undergoing weight loss surgery and found a combined prevalence of 30.3% in 2,717 patients, which is comparable to the general population in industrialized countries [20]. Another study found a 30.1% rate of *H. pylori* in their bariatric patients, and were able to decrease the rate of marginal ulcer to 2.4% in the 206 patients that were tested and treated for *H. pylori*, versus 6.8% in the 354 patients that were not treated [21]. One study of 159 patients undergoing laparoscopic Roux-en-Y gastric bypass (LRYGB) found that routine upper endoscopy either delayed surgery, mostly to treat *H. pylori*, or altered the management in 9.4% of those patients [22]. DeMoura et al. concurred with this conclusion after analysis of their 162 patient series showing a 77% rate of positive findings, primarily gastritis and esophagitis [23]. Another review article concurred with the importance of preoperative endoscopy, due to the fact that it is difficult to examine the bypassed portion of the stomach, duodenum, and small bowel after procedures such as the LRYGB or duodenal switch [24]. Lee et al., in their series of 268 Chinese patients, found a 51.1% rate of pathology with significant risk factors identified as NSAID use, old age, and reflux symptoms. They concluded that routine preoperative endoscopy was warranted in the Asian population [8]. Proponents for selective endoscopy cite data that show, although it is likely to have a positive finding, the incidence of clinically significant findings is low. One clinical review of 448 preoperative endoscopies found that while 18% resulted in additional medical management, less than 1% actually changed the technique or timing of surgery [25]. A review of 523 patients that underwent routine endoscopy before RYGB or sleeve gastrectomy in the Netherlands in which they classified pathology based on the need for intervention or change in treatment. In this study they found 17.2% had abnormalities without treatment consequence, 26.8% were positive for *H. pylori*, 14.3% needed preoperative treatment with proton pump inhibitors, and 1.1% needed an additional endoscopy before surgery. Only one patient, 0.2%, actually required cancelling the operation due to BE with carcinoma [26]. Another study examined 272 preoperative endoscopy records for the purpose of assessing the utility of the procedure; they found only a 12% rate of pathology. Their conclusion was that although incidence of significant findings was low, 12% in their series, the findings are still useful and the practice improves the skillset of the operator, which sets the stage for more advanced endoscopic procedures [27]. A study looking specifically at the population receiving laparoscopic adjustable gastric banding (LAGB) that underwent routine endoscopy on 145 patients found that only 10% had abnormal findings, with the majority being hiatal hernia. Patients reporting symptoms had a higher likelihood of having an abnormality. The 18 patients who reported gastroesophageal symptoms were more likely to have abnormal findings with a sensitivity of 80% and a specificity of 98% in the preoperative history and physical [28].

Intraoperative Indications

Intraoperative endoscopy has been used to recognize and address sources of postoperative morbidity. The most common application is to use the endoscope across the gastrojejunostomy to evaluate, and possibly prevent narrowing, and to test whether the anastomosis is airtight. Other applications have been to check hemostasis and alignment in sleeve gastrectomy. No data has conclusively shown better outcomes with the use of intraoperative endoscopy, but its application is self-evident in specific clinical scenarios. What follows in this chapter is a review of the available literature regarding the utility and effectiveness of intraoperative endoscopy (IOE). Laparoscopic Roux-en-Y gastric bypass is the most common anastomotic bariatric operation performed today. There are several opportunities for problems including stricture, leak, marginal ulcer, twisting of the Roux limb, internal hernia, and bleeding from any of the transection sites. Though the incidence of complications is low, some advocate

IOE as a means to prevent or lower the incidence of these complications. The Scandinavian Obesity Surgery Registry database was analyzed for early (<30 days) complications after LRYGB between 2007 and 2012. Out of 26,173 patients, the overall risk of serious complication was 3.4% and the leak rate was 1.8% [29]. In the United States, large series have reported leak rates between 0.1 and 8.3% [30]. The position statement from the American Society for Metabolic and Bariatric Surgery in 2015 states that intraoperative leak tests, including via endoscopy, have not been found to reduce the incidence of leak after gastric bypass or sleeve gastrectomy [30]. Though the position statement is clear and well reasoned, many surgeons continue to perform intraoperative leak tests, claiming that their low leak rates are due to addressing positive leak tests intraoperatively. One series of 825 procedures reported identification of 29 positive intraoperative leak tests, all of which were repaired, and resulted in only three postoperative leaks (0.36%) [31]. Haddad et al. proposed the same hypothesis, when they reported their series of 2,311 patients with a leak rate of 0.2% and a stricture rate of 1.1% [32]. Similarly, a series of 340 patients without a single incidence of postoperative leak, but with 56 patients (16.4%) having a positive leak test during IOE [33]. One paper included bleeding from the gastric pouch as another modifiable risk that is able to be detected with IOE and addressed intraoperative. In their series of 290 patients, 11 (3.7%) had positive leak tests that were repaired intraoperatively and 10 patients (3.4%) developed intraoperative pouch bleeding that was controlled laparoscopically. No documented postoperative leak or bleeding was noted in this series of patients [34]. Overall, routine endoscopy for LRYGB has been proposed by many as a means to decrease leaks, detect bleeding, and examine the construction of the gastric pouch and gastrojejunostomy. Whether it definitively improves outcomes is difficult to state conclusively. The literature regarding intraoperative endoscopy during sleeve gastrectomy (SG) is not as large as for LRYGB. Frezza et al. reported on SG with endoscopic guidance in 2008 using a 29French endoscope instead of a bougie to size the stapling of the stomach. The endoscope was used during stapling and then to perform a leak test with air insufflation as well as to visualize the "sleeved" stomach. In their series of 20 patients, they had no significant nausea, stenosis, or leaks [35]. A larger, more recent series in 2015 with 100 patients undergoing SG under endoscopic guidance found only 2 patients (2%) had stenosis that was successfully treated with dilation [36]. The use of smaller bougies has been theorized to create higher-pressure sleeves that may predispose to increased leak [37, 38]. Again, they did not have any leaks in their series. They concluded that endoscopic guidance is at least as safe and effective as using bougies of larger diameter. A recent, multicenter series from Israel reported on 3,284 patients. They had 44 patients (1.5%) with gastric leaks, of these 33 had positive intraoperative leak tests. Therefore, they recommended that intraoperative leak testing is not sensitive for leak after SG and should perhaps be reserved for cases in which a technical issue is suspected that is amenable to intraoperative repair [39]. Another paper reported on 1550 sleeve gastrectomy patients [40]. Of these, 1,329 had an intraoperative leak test, of which none were positive. There was no difference in leak rate (1% in each group) or complication rate [40]. They noted an increased operative time of 7.6 min for the leak test group and concluded that intraoperative leak test does not have a correlation with ensuing leak and concurred with Sakran et al. that it should be reserved for cases with technical concerns. There may be a role for endoscopic guidance for stapler placement during sleeve gastrectomy as well as to identify stenosis intraoperatively as this can be difficult to address postoperatively. Others have had success without endoscopic guidance and using larger bougie sizes (>32F) and not stapling close to the incisura [37].

Postoperative Indications

The indication for postoperative endoscopy often varies by the type of operation. For example, after Roux-en-Y gastric bypass (RYGB), patients can have leaks, marginal ulcers, gastro-gastric fistula, and gastrojejunal stenosis among other pathologies. Sleeve gastrectomy (SG) has rapidly gained popularity and prevalence in bariatric surgical practice patterns. While SG was 17.8% of a total 158,000 bariatric operations in 2011, it had grown to 53.8% of a total 196,000 operations by 2015 [41]. Reasons for postoperative endoscopy after SG include stenosis or luminal twisting, leak, ulcers, and staple line bleeding. After sleeve gastrectomy, the type of pathology may not be as numerous, but are notoriously more difficult to treat. Although adjustable gastric band (AGB) placement is not as frequently performed, only 5.7% of bariatric cases in 2015, there are still many existing patients that have had them placed. A recent meta-analysis showed mean rates of erosion and slippage at 1.03% and 4.93%, respectively [42]. Some series report complication rates as high as 32.1% [43]. Endoscopy is an excellent tool to evaluate for both of these possible complications. Band erosion can present with abdominal pain, nausea/vomiting, port site infection, weight gain, and even bleeding [44]. Endoscopy is sensitive in detecting erosion and, in cases of at least 50% erosion of the circumference into the gastric lumen, can be used to remove the band [45].

The most common use for stents after gastric bypass has been to treat anastomotic leaks [46–49]. In the past, treatment options consisted of drain placement and surgical revision. Endoscopic stenting using covered self-expanding metal stents (SEMS) is a promising alternative that has shown efficacy in several series with closure rates as high as 80%, though some of those patients also required additional procedures like percutaneous drain placement or additional stents. The major concern with stents is migration, which can occur from 8 to 66% of the time, depending on the type of stent [49–51].

Sleeve gastrectomy leaks can be more challenging to treat with stents due to the anatomy [52, 53]. Of those that are amenable to stents, closure rates of 55–76% have been reported using stent placement with external drainage [39, 53, 54]. Endoscopic internal drainage has also been proposed as a method to drain the fluid collection that forms as a result of the leak and to close the enterotomy. Early results in 67 patients show a 98.5%

success in placing a double pigtail stent across the orifice leak and a 78.2% cure rate at a mean time of 57.5 days [55].

Stricture or stenosis at the gastrojejunostomy is another known complication after RYGB. Smaller circular staplers (21 mm or less) have stricture rates as high as 27% compared to 4–6% with the linear staple technique [56–58]. Endoscopy is the recommended diagnostic and therapeutic approach. Balloon dilation has a near 100% success rate for relief of symptoms in many series, though multiple dilations are often required [59–61]. One study found that a balloon of at least 11 mm in diameter might decrease the need for repeat dilation without an increase in perforation rate [62]. This is contrasted to the esophagus where most patients with an esophageal lumen less than 13 mm will have dysphagia [63]. Perforation is the most serious complication after dilation, although the risk is relatively low, around 2.2% [61]. Savary-Gilliard dilators were used with success in a series of 71 procedures, up to a size of #11. They were advanced over an endoscopically placed guidewire with 75.5% of patients experiencing relief of symptoms with one dilation and no clinically significant perforations [64]. Refractory strictures have usually been treated with surgical revision of the gastrojejunostomy [65]. Recently, expandable stents have been proposed as adjunct in treating refractory strictures [66–68]. Post-SG stenosis is a relatively rare complication with an incidence of 0.5–4% [69, 70]. It is notoriously difficult to treat and the classic dictum was to revise the operation to a gastric bypass. A recent study presented 18 patients with mid-sleeve stricture and had a 94.4% success rate in endoscopic management with a combination of dilation and stenting [69]. In their algorithm, "functional" stenosis that allowed the passage of the endoscope was treated with an achalasia balloon inflated to a pressure of 25 psi while "mechanical" stenosis that restricted the scope passage was treated with 18 mm stent placement. Both groups were re-scoped at 3 weeks for possible repeat dilation. If there was no improvement, the patient was treated with surgical revision

[38]. Other studies have shown reasonable success (60%) with dilation alone [70].

Marginal ulcer is a known long-term complication of LRYGB. It is defined as ulceration on the jejunal aspect of the gastrojejunal anastomosis [71]. While the true incidence is difficult to know, reported rates vary from <1 to 16% [71]. Symptoms most commonly consist of epigastric pain followed by dysphagia and nausea [71]. Endoscopy is considered a very reliable means of diagnosis [72]. Fortunately, most respond to medical therapy and the surgical intervention rate has been reported between 0 and 44% [71–74]. Bleeding from ulcers can be treated endoscopically with injection of epinephrine, clipping, or thermocoagulation [75]. Initial hemostasis is obtained in almost all cases although the rebleeding rate can be as high as 33%, with one study showing a 5% rate of recurrent bleeding with clips and 33% with epinephrine injection and thermocoagulation [75]. Dual therapy is still recommended when bleeding from ulcers is encountered.

A less common complication after LRYGB is gastro-gastric fistula (GGF). These can be found in the setting of marginal ulcer and they can be difficult to detect endoscopically as the opening may be very small. If bile is encountered in the gastric pouch, a high suspicion for a fistula should be entertained. Oral contrast enhanced imaging is also often used as a diagnostic test. As with fistulae in other GI locations, various methods to attempt closure have been proposed. Various endoscopic techniques have been utilized, including hemostatic clips, suture closure, and over the scope clips. The available series are small observational studies with a successful closure rate between 32 and 44% [76–78].

Weight recidivism occurs in up to 20% of patients in the first 10 years after bariatric surgery and long-term rates reported as high as 34.9% [79, 80]. Initial therapy should focus on ruling out pathology, like gastro-gastric fistulae, along with diet and lifestyle management. For those that do not have pathology and do not respond to non-interventional attempts, various endoscopic techniques to decrease pouch volume or diameter of gastrojejunostomy have been proposed in order to avoid the morbidity of revisional surgery. One randomized, blinded, sham controlled trial compared transoral outlet reduction (TORe), in 50 patients, with a sham procedure, in 27 patients. The TORe was performed with superficial sutures placed with the aid of suction to achieve partial closure of the gastrojejunostomy. In the TORe group, there was greater mean percentage weight loss (3.9%) as compared to the sham group (0.2%) [81]. Another method of using argon plasma coagulation (APC) to cause reduction in the gastrojejunostomy was reported by Baretta et al. and showed an average weight loss of 15.48 kg in 30 patients with an average BMI of 45.63 [82]. One study demonstrated the effectiveness of combining sclerotherapy with suture tightening of the gastrojejunostomy [83]. When compared suturing had improved results as compared to sclerotherapy alone with those patients losing 10.4% of total body weight (TBW) as compared to 2.7%, respectively [84].

Due to the anatomical changes after RYGB, it is difficult to access the remnant stomach or the duodenum. Solutions have included transgastrostomy tube access and double balloon enteroscopy [85, 86]. A more direct approach is transgastric endoscopy. One group described the technique of establishing pneumoperitoneum, placing ports, performing a purse-string suture with a gastrotomy laparoscopically and then placing a 15 mm trocar into the bypassed stomach through which the endoscope can pass. This access allows for evaluating the remnant, duodenum and biliopancreatic limb. It also allows for performing ERCP (endoscopic retrograde cholangiopancreatogram) or EUS (endoscopic ultrasound) to evaluate the pancreas and ductal system of the pancreas and bile duct. The gastrotomy is stapled closed at the end of the procedure [87].

Conclusion

Endoscopy is critical in the evaluation of the obese patient. Obesity should be considered a high-risk feature for patients with GERD, dyspepsia, and BE. Most studies show increased prevalence of gastritis, reflux, hiatal hernia, esophageal, gastric and colorectal cancer, and possibly *H. pylori*. In bariatric patients with Class II and III obesity, the incidence of significant pathology is variable, but patients undergoing bariatric surgery should have endoscopic evaluation if they have symptoms of dyspepsia, GERD, consume NSAIDs or have other risk factors for BE. These same patients should also undergo screening colonoscopy. Obesity should cause medical and surgical professionals to have a lower threshold to screen for GI pathology. Endoscopy continues to play a vital role in the postsurgical patient, both intraoperatively and more importantly after surgery. In the operating room, endoscopy can allow for the detection of bleeding, leaks from staple and suture lines, and poor anatomic configuration. Postoperatively, endoscopy plays a crucial role in functional gastrointestinal symptoms, detecting anatomic abnormalities that may be leading to poor oral intake, dysphagia, abdominal pain, anemia, and weight recidivism.

References

1. Levin B, Lieberman DA, McFarland B, Smith RA, Brooks D, Andrews KS, et al. Screening and surveillance for the early detection of colorectal cancer and adenomatous polyps, 2008: a joint guideline from the American Cancer Society, the US multi-society task force on colorectal cancer, and the American College of Radiology. CA Cancer J Clin. 2008;58(3):130–60.
2. Evans JA, Early DS, Fukami N, Ben-Menachem T, Chandrasekhara V, Chathadi KV, et al. The role of endoscopy in Barrett's esophagus and other premalignant conditions of the esophagus. Gastrointest Endosc. 2012;76(6):1087–94.
3. Talley NJ, Walker MM, Holtmann G. Functional dyspepsia. Curr Opin Gastroenterol. 2016;32(6):467–73.
4. Shaukat A, Wang A, Acosta RD, Bruining DH, Chandrasekhara V, Chathadi KV, et al. The role of endoscopy in dyspepsia. Gastrointest Endosc. 2015;82(2):227–32.
5. Vakil N, van Zanten SV, Kahrilas P, Dent J, Jones R, Global Consensus G. The Montreal definition and classification of gastroesophageal reflux disease: a global evidence-based consensus. Am J Gastroenterol. 2006;101(8):1900–20.
6. Muthusamy VR, Lightdale JR, Acosta RD, Chandrasekhara V, Chathadi KV, Eloubeidi MA, et al. The role of endoscopy in the management of GERD. Gastrointest Endosc. 2015;81(6):1305–10.

7. Hvid-Jensen F, Pedersen L, Drewes AM, Sorensen HT, Funch-Jensen P. Incidence of adenocarcinoma among patients with Barrett's esophagus. N Engl J Med. 2011;365(15):1375–83.
8. Lee J, Wong SK, Liu SY, Ng EK. Is preoperative upper gastrointestinal endoscopy in obese patients undergoing bariatric surgery mandatory? An Asian perspective. Obes Surg. 2017;27(1):44–50.
9. Bhatt DL, Scheiman J, Abraham NS, Antman EM, Chan FKL, Furberg CD, et al. ACCF/ACG/AHA 2008 expert consensus document on reducing the gastrointestinal risks of antiplatelet therapy and NSAID use: a report of the American College of Cardiology Foundation task force on clinical expert consensus documents. J Am Coll Cardiol. 2008;52(18):1502.
10. Hampel H, Abraham NS, El-Serag HB. Meta-analysis: obesity and the risk for gastroesophageal reflux disease and its complications. Ann Intern Med. 2005;143(3):199–211.
11. Wilson LJ, Ma M, Hirschowitz BI. Association of obesity with hiatal hernia and esophagitis. Am J Gastroenterol. 1999;94(10):2840–4.
12. Yamamoto S, Watabe K, Takehara T. Is obesity a new risk factor for gastritis? Digestion. 2012;85(2):108–10.
13. Yamamoto S, Watabe K, Tsutsui S, Kiso S, Hamasaki T, Kato M, et al. Lower serum level of adiponectin is associated with increased risk of endoscopic erosive gastritis. Dig Dis Sci. 2011;56(8):2354–60.
14. Aro P, Storskrubb T, Ronkainen J, Bolling-Sternevald E, Engstrand L, Vieth M, et al. Peptic ulcer disease in a general adult population: the Kalixanda study: a random population-based study. Am J Epidemiol. 2006;163(11):1025–34.
15. Calle EE, Kaaks R. Overweight, obesity and cancer: epidemiological evidence and proposed mechanisms. Nat Rev Cancer. 2004;4(8):579–91.
16. Calle EE, Rodriguez C, Walker-Thurmond K, Thun MJ. Overweight, obesity, and mortality from cancer in a prospectively studied cohort of U.S. adults. N Engl J Med. 2003;348(17):1625–38.
17. Wu AH, Tseng CC, Bernstein L. Hiatal hernia, reflux symptoms, body size, and risk of esophageal and gastric adenocarcinoma. Cancer. 2003;98(5):940–8.
18. Arslan E, Atılgan H, Yavaşoğlu İ. The prevalence of Helicobacter pylori in obese subjects. Eur J Intern Med. 2009;20(7):695–7.
19. Erim T, Cruz-Correa MR, Szomstein S, Velis E, Rosenthal R. Prevalence of Helicobacter pylori seropositivity among patients undergoing bariatric surgery: a preliminary study. World J Surg. 2008;32(9):2021–5.
20. Papasavas PK, Gagné DJ, Donnelly PE, Salgado J, Urbandt JE, Burton KK, et al. Prevalence of Helicobacter pylori infection and value of preoperative testing and treatment in patients undergoing laparoscopic roux-en-Y gastric bypass. Surg Obes Relat Dis. 2008;4(3):383–8.
21. Schirmer B, Erenoglu C, Miller A. Flexible endoscopy in the management of patients undergoing roux-en-Y gastric bypass. Obes Surg. 2002;12(5):634–8.
22. Zeni TM, Frantzides CT, Mahr C, Denham EW, Meiselman M, Goldberg MJ, et al. Value of preoperative upper endoscopy in patients undergoing laparoscopic gastric bypass. Obes Surg. 2006;16(2):142–6.
23. de Moura AA, Cotrim HP, Santos AS, Bitencourt AGV, Barbosa DBV, Lobo AP, et al. Preoperative upper gastrointestinal endoscopy in obese patients undergoing bariatric surgery: is it necessary? Surg Obes Relat Dis. 2008;4(2):144–9.
24. Greenwald D. Preoperative gastrointestinal assessment before bariatric surgery. Gastroenterol Clin N Am. 2010;39(1):81–6.
25. Loewen M, Giovanni J, Barba C. Screening endoscopy before bariatric surgery: a series of 448 patients. Surg Obes Relat Dis. 2008;4(6):709–12.
26. Schigt A, Coblijn U, Lagarde S, Kuiken S, Scholten P, van Wagensveld B. Is esophagogastroduodenoscopy before Roux-en-Y gastric bypass or sleeve gastrectomy mandatory? Surg Obes Relat Dis. 2014;10(3):411–7; quiz 565–6.
27. Mong C, Van Dam J, Morton J, Gerson L, Curet M, Banerjee S. Preoperative endoscopic screening for laparoscopic roux-en-Y gastric bypass has a low yield for anatomic findings. Obes Surg. 2008;18(9):1067–73.
28. Korenkov M, Sauerland S, Shah S, Junginger T. Is routine preoperative upper endoscopy in gastric banding patients really necessary? Obes Surg. 2006;16(1):45–7.
29. Stenberg E, Szabo E, Agren G, Naslund E, Boman L, Bylund A, et al. Early complications after laparoscopic gastric bypass surgery: results from the Scandinavian obesity surgery registry. Ann Surg. 2014;260(6):1040–7.
30. Kim J, Azagury D, Eisenberg D, DeMaria E, Campos GM. ASMBS position statement on prevention, detection, and treatment of gastrointestinal leak after gastric bypass and sleeve gastrectomy, including the roles of imaging, surgical exploration, and nonoperative management. Surg Obes Relat Dis. 2015;11(4):739–48.
31. Champion JK, Hunt T, DeLisle N. Role of routine intraoperative endoscopy in laparoscopic bariatric surgery. Surg Endosc. 2002;16(12):1663–5.
32. Haddad A, Tapazoglou N, Singh K, Averbach A. Role of intraoperative esophagogastroenteroscopy in minimizing gastrojejunostomy-related morbidity: experience with 2,311 laparoscopic gastric bypasses with linear stapler anastomosis. Obes Surg. 2012;22(12):1928–33.
33. Sekhar N, Torquati A, Lutfi R, Richards WO. Endoscopic evaluation of the gastrojejunostomy in laparoscopic gastric bypass: a series of 340 patients without postoperative leak. Surg Endosc. 2006;20(2):199–201.
34. Alasfar F, Chand B. Intraoperative endoscopy for laparoscopic roux-en-Y gastric bypass: leak test and beyond. Surg Laparosc Endosc Percutan Tech. 2010;20(6):424–7.
35. Frezza EE, Barton A, Herbert H, Wachtel MS. Laparoscopic sleeve gastrectomy with endoscopic guidance in morbid obesity. Surg Obes Relat Dis. 2008;4(5):575–9.
36. Andreas A, Adamantios M, Antonios A, Theofilos R, Christos T, Theodoros D. Laparoscopic sleeve gastrectomy for morbid obesity with intra-operative endoscopy: lessons we learned after 100 consecutive patients. Obes Surg. 2015;25(7):1223–8.

37. Bellanger DE, Greenway FL. Laparoscopic sleeve gastrectomy, 529 cases without a leak: short-term results and technical considerations. Obes Surg. 2011;21(2):146–50.
38. Yehoshua RT, Eidelman LA, Stein M, Fichman S, Mazor A, Chen J, et al. Laparoscopic sleeve gastrectomy—volume and pressure assessment. Obes Surg. 2008;18(9):1083–8.
39. Sakran N, Goitein D, Raziel A, Keidar A, Beglaibter N, Grinbaum R, et al. Gastric leaks after sleeve gastrectomy: a multicenter experience with 2,834 patients. Surg Endosc. 2013;27(1):240–5.
40. Sethi M, Zagzag J, Patel K, Magrath M, Somoza E, Parikh MS, et al. Intraoperative leak testing has no correlation with leak after laparoscopic sleeve gastrectomy. Surg Endosc. 2016;30(3):883–91.
41. Ponce J, Nguyen NT, Hutter M, Sudan R, Morton JM. American Society for Metabolic and Bariatric Surgery estimation of bariatric surgery procedures in the United States, 2011-2014. Surg Obes Relat Dis. 2015;11(6):1199–200.
42. Singhal R, Bryant C, Kitchen M, Khan KS, Deeks J, Guo B, et al. Band slippage and erosion after laparoscopic gastric banding: a meta-analysis. Surg Endosc. 2010;24(12):2980–6.
43. Owers C, Ackroyd R. A study examining the complications associated with gastric banding. Obes Surg. 2013;23(1):56–9.
44. Evans JA, Muthusamy VR, Acosta RD, Bruining DH, Chandrasekhara V, Chathadi KV, et al. The role of endoscopy in the bariatric surgery patient. Gastrointest Endosc. 2015;81(5):1063–72.
45. Lattuada E, Zappa MA, Mozzi E, Fichera G, Granelli P, Ruberto FD, et al. Band erosion following gastric banding: how to treat it. Obes Surg. 2007;17(3):329–33.
46. Varban OA, Cassidy RB, Sheetz KH, Cain-Nielsen A, Carlin AM, Schram JL, et al. Technique or technology? Evaluating leaks after gastric bypass. Surg Obes Relat Dis. 2016;12(2):264–72.
47. Fullum TM, Aluka KJ, Turner PL. Decreasing anastomotic and staple line leaks after laparoscopic roux-en-Y gastric bypass. Surg Endosc. 2009;23(6):1403–8.
48. Schiesser M, Kressig P, Bueter M, Nocito A, Bauerfeind P, Gubler C. Successful endoscopic management of gastrointestinal leakages after laparoscopic roux-en-Y gastric bypass surgery. Dig Surg. 2014;31(1):67–70.
49. van Wezenbeek MR, de Milliano MM, Nienhuijs SW, Friederich P, Gilissen LP. A specifically designed stent for anastomotic leaks after bariatric surgery: experiences in a tertiary referral hospital. Obes Surg. 2016;26(8):1875–80.
50. Puli SR, Spofford IS, Thompson CC. Use of self-expandable stents in the treatment of bariatric surgery leaks: a systematic review and meta-analysis. Gastrointest Endosc. 2012;75(2):287–93.
51. Murino A, Arvanitakis M, Le Moine O, Blero D, Devière J, Eisendrath P. Effectiveness of endoscopic management using self-expandable metal stents in a large cohort of patients with post-bariatric leaks. Obes Surg. 2015;25(9):1569–76.
52. Parikh M, Issa R, McCrillis A, Saunders JK, Ude-Welcome A, Gagner M. Surgical strategies that may decrease leak after laparoscopic sleeve gastrectomy a systematic review and meta-analysis of 9,991 cases. Ann Surg. 2013;257(2):231–7.
53. Simon F, Siciliano I, Gillet A, Castel B, Coffin B, Msika S. Gastric leak after laparoscopic sleeve gastrectomy: early covered self-expandable stent reduces healing time. Obes Surg. 2013;23(5):687–92.
54. Alazmi W, Al-Sabah S, Ali DA, Almazeedi S. Treating sleeve gastrectomy leak with endoscopic stenting: the kuwaiti experience and review of recent literature. Surg Endosc. 2014;28(12):3425–8.
55. Donatelli G, Ferretti S, Vergeau BM, Dhumane P, Dumont J-L, Derhy S, et al. Endoscopic internal drainage with enteral nutrition (EDEN) for treatment of leaks following sleeve gastrectomy. Obes Surg. 2014;24(8):1400–7.
56. Higa KD, Boone KB, Ho T. Complications of the laparoscopic roux-en-y gastric bypass: 1,040 patients—what have we learned? Obes Surg. 2000;10(6):509–13.
57. Schauer PR, Ikramuddin S, Gourash W, Ramanathan R, Luketich J. Outcomes after laparoscopic roux-en-Y gastric bypass for morbid obesity. Ann Surg. 2000;232(4):515–29.
58. Nguyen NT, Stevens CM, Wolfe BM. Incidence and outcome of anastomotic stricture after laparoscopic gastric bypass. J Gastrointest Surg. 2003;7(8):997–1003; discussion.
59. Barba CA, Butensky MS, Lorenzo M, Newman R. Endoscopic dilation of gastroesophageal anastomosis stricture after gastric bypass. Surg Endosc. 2003;17(3):416–20.
60. Takata MC, Ciovica R, Cello JP, Posselt AM, Rogers SJ, Campos GM. Predictors, treatment, and outcomes of gastrojejunostomy stricture after gastric bypass for morbid obesity. Obes Surg. 2007;17(7):878–84.
61. Ukleja A, Afonso BB, Pimentel R, Szomstein S, Rosenthal R. Outcome of endoscopic balloon dilation of strictures after laparoscopic gastric bypass. Surg Endosc. 2008;22(8):1746–50.
62. Ryskina KL, Miller KM, Aisenberg J, Herron DM, Kini SU. Routine management of stricture after gastric bypass and predictors of subsequent weight loss. Surg Endosc. 2010;24(3):554–60.
63. Tobin RW. Esophageal rings, webs, and diverticula. J Clin Gastroenterol. 1998;27(4):285–95.
64. Escalona A, Devaud N, Boza C, Pérez G, Fernández J, Ibáñez L, et al. Gastrojejunal anastomotic stricture after roux-en-Y gastric bypass: ambulatory management with the Savary–Gilliard dilator. Surg Endosc. 2007;21(5):765–8.
65. Cusati D, Sarr M, Kendrick M, Que F, Swain JM. Refractory strictures after roux-en-Y gastric bypass: operative management. Surg Obes Relat Dis. 2011;7(2):165–9.
66. Uchima H, Abu-Suboh M, Mata A, Cruz M, Espinos J. Lumen-apposing metal stent for the treat-

ment of refractory gastrojejunal anastomotic stricture after laparoscopic gastric bypass. Gastrointest
Endosc. 2016;83(1):251.
67. Marcotte E, Comeau E, Meziat-Burdin A,
    Ménard C, Rateb G. Early migration of fully cov-
    ered double-layered metallic stents for post-gastric
    bypass anastomotic strictures. Int J Surg Case Rep.
    2012;3(7):283–6.
68. Yimcharoen P, Heneghan HM, Tariq N,
    Brethauer SA, Kroh M, Chand B. Endoscopic
    stent management of leaks and anastomotic stric-
    tures after foregut surgery. Surg Obes Relat Dis.
    2011;7(5):628–36.
69. Manos T, Nedelcu M, Cotirlet A, Eddbali I,
    Gagner M, Noel P. How to treat stenosis after sleeve
    gastrectomy? Surg Obes Relat Dis. 2017;13(2):150–4.
70. Donatelli G, Dumont J-L, Pourcher G, Tranchart H,
    Tuszynski T, Dagher I, et al. Pneumatic dilation for
    functional helix stenosis after sleeve gastrectomy:
    long-term follow-up (with videos). Surg Obes Relat
    Dis. 2016;13(6):943–50. http://dx.doi.org/10.1016/j.
    soard.2016.09.023
71. El-Hayek K, Timratana P, Shimizu H,
    Chand B. Marginal ulcer after roux-en-Y gastric
    bypass: what have we really learned? Surg Endosc.
    2012;26(10):2789–96.
72. Gumbs AA, Duffy AJ, Bell RL. Incidence and man-
    agement of marginal ulceration after laparoscopic
    roux-en-Y gastric bypass. Surg Obes Relat Dis.
    2006;2(4):460–3.
73. Moon RC, Teixeira AF, Goldbach M,
    Jawad MA. Management and treatment outcomes of
    marginal ulcers after roux-en-Y gastric bypass at a
    single high volume bariatric center. Surg Obes Relat
    Dis. 2014;10(2):229–34.
74. Azagury DE, Abu Dayyeh BK, Greenwalt IT, Thompson
    CC. Marginal ulceration after roux-en-Y gastric bypass
    surgery: characteristics, risk factors, treatment, and
    outcomes. Endoscopy. 2011;43(11):950–4.
75. Lee YC, Wang HP, Yang CS, Yang TH, Chen JH,
    Lin CC, et al. Endoscopic hemostasis of a bleeding
    marginal ulcer: hemoclipping or dual therapy with
    epinephrine injection and heater probe thermocoagu-
    lation. J Gastroenterol Hepatol. 2002;17(11):1220–5.
76. Niland B, Brock A. Over-the-scope clip for endo-
    scopic closure of gastrogastric fistulae. Surg Obes
    Relat Dis. 2017;13(1):15–20.
77. Mukewar S, Kumar N, Catalano M, Thompson C,
    Abidi W, Harmsen W, et al. Safety and efficacy of
fistula closure by endoscopic suturing: a multi-center
study. Endoscopy. 2016;48(11):1023–8.
78. Fernandez-Esparrach G, Lautz DB, Thompson
    CC. Endoscopic repair of gastrogastric fistula after
    roux-en-Y gastric bypass: a less-invasive approach.
    Surg Obes Relat Dis. 2010;6(3):282–8.
79. Mikami D, Needleman B, Narula V, Durant J,
    Melvin WS. Natural orifice surgery: initial U.S. expe-
    rience utilizing the StomaphyXTM device to reduce
    gastric pouches after roux-en-Y gastric bypass. Surg
    Endosc. 2010;24(1):223–8.
80. Goyal V, Holover S, Garber S. Gastric pouch reduc-
    tion using StomaphyX™ in post roux-en-Y gas-
    tric bypass patients does not result in sustained
    weight loss: a retrospective analysis. Surg Endosc.
    2013;27(9):3417–20.
81. Thompson CC, Chand B, Chen YK, Demarco DC,
    Miller L, Schweitzer M, et al. Endoscopic suturing for
    transoral outlet reduction increases weight loss after
    roux-en-Y gastric bypass surgery. Gastroenterology.
    2013;145(1):129–137.e3.
82. Baretta GAP, Alhinho HCAW, Matias JEF,
    Marchesini JB, de Lima JHF, Empinotti C, et al.
    Argon plasma coagulation of gastrojejunal anastomo-
    sis for weight regain after gastric bypass. Obes Surg.
    2015;25(1):72–9.
83. Riva P, Perretta S, Swanstrom L. Weight regain fol-
    lowing RYGB can be effectively treated using a com-
    bination of endoscopic suturing and sclerotherapy.
    Surg Endosc. 2017;31(4):1891–5.
84. Jirapinyo P, Dayyeh BKA, Thompson
    CC. Gastrojejunal anastomotic reduction for weight
    regain in roux-en-Y gastric bypass patients: physi-
    ological, behavioral, and anatomical effects of endo-
    scopic suturing and sclerotherapy. Surg Obes Relat
    Dis. 2016;12(10):1810–6.
85. Fobi MAL, Chicola K, Lee H. Access to the
    bypassed stomach after gastric bypass. Obes Surg.
    1998;8(3):289–95.
86. Sakai P, Kuga R, Safatle-Ribeiro AV, Faintuch J,
    Gama-Rodrigues JJ, Ishida RK, et al. Is it fea-
    sible to reach the bypassed stomach after roux-
    en-Y gastric bypass for morbid obesity? The use
    of the double-balloon enteroscope. Endoscopy.
    2005;37(6):566.
87. Ceppa FA, Gagné DJ, Papasavas PK,
    Caushaj PF. Laparoscopic transgastric endoscopy
    after roux-en-Y gastric bypass. Surg Obes Relat Dis.
    2007;3(1):21–4.

Jihad Kudsi, Julius Balogh, and Nabil Tariq

Initial Assessment and Pre-procedure Preparation

Obesity is increasingly prevalent in the world and especially in the United States where 34.9% of adults are obese [1]. In 2014, the World Health Organization reported that 13% of adults worldwide were obese [2]. There is also an increased prevalence of gastrointestinal disorders in obesity such as gallbladder disease and esophageal and colon cancer [3]. This means that endoscopists are going to increasingly encounter obese patients, thus a thorough understanding of the implications of sedation in obesity is warranted.

Patient safety should always be the priority and pre-procedure risk assessment and planning are key components for success. It also involves appropriate informed consent and education regarding expectations.

Consent

Appropriate informed consent is an extremely important part of any procedural planning. It addresses the ethical principle of patient autonomy. It allows patients to be involved in the decision-making process and allows then to ask appropriate questions. This discussion should involve sedation-related risks as well and not be limited to the endoscopic procedure. Sedation can help increase patient comfort and allow better performance of the procedure. The risks of cardiopulmonary complications and reactions to medications should also be discussed. Even if the endoscopist is not the one administering the sedation, a discussion should be held. Ideally, it should be done in a quiet environment where the patient has an opportunity to ask questions and the discussion should not be rushed [4].

History and Physical Exam

A detailed history and physical exam are crucial for initial risk assessment. The history should be focused especially on eliciting any history of

J. Kudsi, M.D. • N. Tariq, M.D. (✉)
Department of Surgery, Houston Methodist Hospital, 6550 Fannin Street, SM 1661, Houston, TX 77030, USA
e-mail: j.kudsi@gmail.com; ntariq@houstonmethodist.org

J. Balogh, M.D., M.H.A
Department of Anesthesiology, Memorial Hermann Hospital, University of Texas at Houston Health Science Center, 6431 Fannin St, MSB 5.020, Houston, TX 77030, USA
e-mail: Julius.g.balogh@uth.tmc.edu

© Springer International Publishing AG 2018
B. Chand (ed.), *Endoscopy in Obesity Management*, DOI 10.1007/978-3-319-63528-6_3

current GI disorder that may affect sedation/procedure such as gastrointestinal obstruction or gastroparesis. These clinical scenarios can lead to a risk of aspiration if the stomach is full of content and the patient cannot protect their airway. It also needs to elucidate if there is any major organ dysfunction, and a screening for obstructive sleep apnea should be performed. Information should be gathered regarding current medications, any allergies, or prior reactions to anesthesia or sedation. Social history regarding substance abuse, alcohol, or narcotic dependence can affect the amount of sedation as well. Time and type of oral intake should also be asked. Women of childbearing age should be asked about pregnancy and a pregnancy test obtained.

A complete physical examination should be done with emphasis on the cardiopulmonary system, the neck, and the airway. A common component of this exam is determining the Mallampati score [3, 5, 6]. This score was developed in 1985 to predict the difficulty of endotracheal intubation. It is a visual assessment of the distance from the base of the tongue to the roof of the mouth. It is defined as follows: Class I - Soft palate, uvula, fauces, pillars visible, Class II - Soft palate, uvula, fauces visible, Class III - Soft palate, base of uvula visible, Class IV - Only hard palate visible (From UpToDate [5]). A higher body mass index (BMI) has been associated with a higher Mallampati score; however, no studies to date demonstrate an increased risk of sedation with an increased score. However, the Mallampati score is used as a predictor of a difficult airway in cases of rescue.

Risk Assessment

With a good history and physical exam, the patient should be able to be risk stratified for better sedation planning. A commonly used method is the American Society of Anesthesiologists (ASA) score. The ASA score is a subjective assessment of a patient's overall health and is based on six classes [7, 8]:

I. A normal healthy patient
II. A patient with mild systemic disease
III. A patient with severe systemic disease
IV. A patient with severe systemic disease that is a constant threat to life
V. A moribund patient who is not expected to survive without the operation
VI. A declared brain-dead patient whose organs are being removed for donor purposes

Specific cardiopulmonary risk stratification with respect to obstructive sleep apnea (OSA), pulmonary hypertension, and other cardiac conditions can determine the sedation plan and even the location of where to perform the procedure. Procedures can be performed in a hospital setting as opposed to an ambulatory surgery center. Levels of sedation planned include moderate sedation or deep sedation and are described below.

Timeout

The *timeout* is not just an institutional or Joint Commission requirement, but also a very important aspect of patient safety. It is done before sedation is started with patient participation. Sedation plan, any relevant comorbidities, patient allergies, anticipated length of procedure, equipment needed, or any other concerns are just some of the vital issues to be touched upon during this portion of the procedure. This is especially important when several back-to-back endoscopies are planned, on multiple patients with similar conditions.

Intra-procedure Monitoring

Intra-procedure monitoring can detect changes in blood pressure, pulse, oxygenation, cardiac electrical activity, and neurological status before clinically significant events occur. A trained healthcare professional other than the endoscopist should be monitoring the patient throughout the entire procedure. This person should be trained to monitor and interpret physiological changes and be able to initiate appropriate countermeasures. They should be certified in advanced cardiac life support (ACLS). In the USA, when an anesthesia provider is not being used, the majority of sites use a registered nurse for this purpose. During moderate sedation, this person can perform brief interruptible tasks. If deep sedation is administered, another person in the room, such as the endoscopist, should also be ACLS certified and be able to bag-mask ventilate and secure an airway [9].

Electrocardiogram Monitoring

In the USA, electrocardiogram (ECG) monitoring is routinely used during an endoscopic procedure. The American Society of Anesthesiology (ASA) guidelines recommend ECG monitoring of all patients undergoing deep sedation. In moderate sedation, it is recommended for those with significant cardiopulmonary disease, elderly individuals, and when a prolonged procedure is anticipated [8]. Though there may not be significant data supporting routine ECG monitoring in young, healthy patients undergoing moderate sedation, it seems prudent to use it routinely, especially in obese patients where there may be underlying cardiopulmonary disease.

Blood Pressure Monitoring

Blood pressure and heart rate monitoring is an essential component of ensuring hemodynamic stability throughout the procedure. This is recommended for all patients. Blood pressure should be measured every 3–5 min if not more frequently. Appropriate bariatric sized cuffs or thigh cuffs may have to be used in obese patients for accurate measurements and should be available.

Pulse Oximetry

Pulse oximetry is a good indicator of arterial oxygen saturation but an insensitive marker for ventilation. Arterial oxygen saturation may not drop for several minutes after inadequate ventilation sets in, especially if a high amount of supplemental oxygen is being administered. Hypercapnia can set in before significant desaturation. Risk factors for significant desaturations include emergency procedures, procedures of prolonged duration, presence of preexisting cardiopulmonary disease, difficulty with esophageal intubation, and baseline saturations of less than 95% [8]. Although it seems intuitive that pulse oximetry monitoring should decrease adverse events, this has been hard to demonstrate. A Cochrane review and a large randomized trial with over 20,000 patients failed to demonstrate improved outcomes with continuous pulse oximetry [10, 11].

However, it seems that knowing any desaturation events as soon as possible may certainly initiate corrective maneuvers early. This is especially important in morbidly obese patients in whom rescue maneuvers can be difficult and can take longer. That is why the ASA and the American Society of Gastrointestinal Endoscopy (ASGE) recommend using it for all endoscopy procedures [12].

The ASA recommends supplemental oxygen for all deep sedation cases and that it be considered for moderate sedation cases.

Capnography

Capnography is a noninvasive way of detecting the adequacy of ventilation by measuring exhaled carbon dioxide. It may detect ventilation problems sooner, resulting in less hypoxemic episodes. This is especially true with procedures requiring deep sedation like endoscopic retrograde cholangiopancreatography (ERCP) [13]. It can also be very useful in obese patients with OSA in whom pulmonary ventilator reserve may be low and significant respiratory acidosis can occur. The ASA recommends capnography for all patients receiving deep sedation, for patients undergoing moderate sedation whose ventilation can be difficult to assess, and for those with OSA [14].

BIS Monitoring

In bispectral index monitoring (BIS), electroencephalographic (EEG) waveforms from a forehead adhesive probe are captured and analyzed using a complex algorithm. This results in display of an index that ranges from 0 to 100. A fully awake person correlates with a score of 100. Moderate sedation can result in a BIS of 70–90, deep sedation with 60–69, and general anesthesia 40–59 [15]. Though the concept seems appropriate, the results of using BIS monitoring to titrate sedation, when compared to clinical assessment, have been equivocal [15–18]. It may end up becoming more useful if there is an increase in the use of propofol by non-anesthesia providers. It may also have value in some of the closed loop automated sedation systems that are being developed [15].

Sedation

Sedation is a drug-induced state of depressed consciousness that provides relief of discomfort and anxiety for the patient and allows the endoscopist to focus on the procedure. Four levels have been described:

Minimal

A drug-induced state in which the patient responds to verbal commands. Coordination and cognitive function can be impaired; however, cardiovascular and respiratory functions are unaffected.

Moderate

A drug-induced depression of consciousness during which the patient can respond purposefully to verbal commands, either alone or accompanied by light stimulation. Cardiovascular and spontaneous ventilation is usually maintained.

Deep

A drug-induced depression of consciousness during which a patient cannot be easily aroused but may respond purposefully to painful stimulation. Patients may require assistance to maintain a patent airway. Spontaneous ventilation is depressed; however, cardiovascular function is not affected.

General Anesthesia

Patients are not arousable, even with painful stimulation, and require assistance in maintaining patent airway. Positive pressure ventilation may be required secondary to neuromuscular blockade and respiratory depression. Cardiovascular function may be impaired.

Sedation can be evaluated using several tools (Tables 3.1, 3.2, and 3.3) [19, 20].

In a study by Consales et al. [21], the Ramsey level of 6 corresponded to a BIS value ranging from 32 to 68. Previous studies demonstrated that BIS scores of 90–100 correspond to the awake state, 80–70 to light sedation, 60 to moderate sedation, while BIS values of less than 40 indicate progressively deeper levels of sedation [22].

Table 3.1 Definition of general anesthesia and levels of sedation/analgesia (From the American Society of Anesthesiologists [19])

	Minimal sedation/ anxiolysis	Moderate sedation/ analgesia ("conscious sedation")	Deep sedation/analgesia	General anesthesia
Responsiveness	Normal response to verbal stimulation	Purposeful response to verbal or tactile stimulation	Purposeful response following repeated or painful stimulation	Unarousable even with painful stimulus
Airway	Unaffected	No intervention required	Intervention may be required	Intervention often required
Spontaneous ventilation	Unaffected	Adequate	May be inadequate	Frequently inadequate
Cardiovascular function	Unaffected	Usually maintained	May be inadequate	May be impaired

Table 3.2 Inova sedation scale (From Nisbet and Mooney-Cotter [20], with permission)

1	Alert
2	Occasionally drowsy, easy to rouse
3	Dozing intermittently
4	Asleep, easy to waken
5	Difficult to awaken
6	Unresponsive

Table 3.3 Ramsey sedation scale

Sedation level	Description
1	Anxious patient, agitated or restless or both
2	Cooperative patient, oriented, and tranquil
3	Responds to commands only
4	Patient responds to light glabellar tap or loud auditory stimulus
5	Patient exhibits sluggish response to light glabellar tap or loud auditory stimulus
6	No response

Table 3.4 Aldrete recovery scale score (From Hasanein and El-Sayed [23], with permission)

Activity: able to move voluntarily or on command	
4 extremities	2
2 extremities	1
0 extremities	0
Respiration	
Able to deep breathe and cough freely	2
Dyspnea, shallow or limited breathing	1
Apnea	0
Circulation	
BP ± 20 mmHg of preanesthetic level	2
BP ± 20–50 mmHg of preanesthetic level	1
BP > 50 mmHg of preanesthetic level	0
Consciousness	
Fully awake	2
Arousable on calling	1
Not responding	0
Oxygen saturation	
Able to maintain O_2 saturation > 92% on room air	2
Needs O_2 inhalation to maintain O_2 saturation > 90%	1
O_2 saturation < 90% even with O_2 supplementation	0

BP blood pressure

Recovery from Sedation

Once the procedure is completed, the patient is taken to the recovery area. Specialized nurses monitor the patient during recovery from sedation. Prior to discharge, the patient should attain an Aldrete Recovery Scale Score of 9–10 (Table 3.4) [23].

Drugs Used for Sedation (Table 3.5) [24]

Propofol. Propofol is an anesthetic agent that is FDA approved for the induction and maintenance of general anesthesia and for sedation [25]. It is classified as an ultrashort-acting hypnotic agent. Propofol possesses sedative, amnestic, and hypnotic properties with minimal analgesia [26].

Table 3.5 The pharmacologic profile of common sedation drugs (From Da and Buxbaum [24], with permission)

Drug	Onset of action (min)	Peak effect (min)	Duration of effect (min)	Side effects	Antagonism
Midazolam	1–2	3–4	15–80	Respiratory depression	Flumazenil
				Disinhibition reactions	
				Cardiac dysrhythmia	
Diazepam	2–3	3–5	360	Respiratory depression	Flumazenil
				Disinhibition reactions	
Propofol	<1	1–2	4–8	Hypoxemia	None
				Apnea	
				Hypotension	
				Bradycardia	
				Upper airway obstruction	
				Injection site pain	
				Propofol infusion syndrome	
Meperidine	3–6	5–7	60–180	Synergistic respiratory depression	Naloxone
				Cardiovascular instability	
				Nausea and vomiting	
				Neurotoxicity with renal failure	
Fentanyl	1–2	3–5	30–60	Synergistic respiratory depression	Naloxone
				Chest wall rigidity	
				Skeletal muscle hypertonicity	

Propofol is 98% plasma-protein bound, and is metabolized primarily by the liver. The drug is lipophilic and is prepared as an oil/water emulsion consisting of 1% propofol, 10% soybean oil, 2.25% glycerol, and 1.2% egg lecithin. Propofol is contra-indicated in patients with hypersensitivity to eggs or soybean. A generic formulation can contain sodium metabisulfite and is therefore also contra-indicated in patients with sulfite allergies [27, 28].

Propofol increases the likelihood of satisfactory deep sedation. In addition, the risk of rapid and profound decrease in the level of consciousness and cardiorespiratory function can occur, which may culminate in general anesthesia. Propofol crosses the blood–brain barrier and causes a depression in consciousness that is thought to be related to potentiation of the gamma-aminobutyric acid (GABA) activity in the brain. Typically, the time from injection to the onset of sedation is 30–60 s. The plasma half-life ranges from 1.3 to 4.13 min.

Propofol potentiates the effects of benzodiazepines, barbiturates, and opioids [26, 29]. The pharmacokinetic properties do not significantly change in patients with chronic liver disease or renal failure [26, 30]. Dose reduction is required in patients with cardiac dysfunction and in the elderly due to decreased clearance of the drug [31]. The narrow therapeutic window of propofol separates it from "conventional" sedation used in endoscopy and increases the risk for complications if it is not administered appropriately. Hence, additional training and monitoring may be needed to allow the safe administration of propofol (Table 3.6) [32–35].

Midazolam. Midazolam is a water-soluble, short-acting benzodiazepine central nervous system (CNS) depressant for intravenous or intramuscular injection. The effects of midazolam on the CNS are dependent on the dose administered, the route of administration, and the presence or absence of additional medications. Onset time of

Table 3.6 Dosing recommendations for propofol

Author	Loading dose (mg)	Subsequent dosing (mg)	Minimum dosing frequency (min)
Walker et al. [33]	30–50	10–20	0.5–1.0
Vargo et al. [34]	40 (<60 kg)	10–20	Not mentioned
	50 (>60 kg)		
Rex et al. [35]	20–40	10–20	Not mentioned
Heuss et al. [36]	20	10–20 (Asa I–ii)	0.33 min
		10 (if ASA III–IV)	

sedation effects after intramuscular administration in adults is 15 min, with peak sedation occurring 30–60 min following injection. As an anesthetic induction agent, induction of anesthesia occurs in approximately 1.5 min when narcotic premedication has been administered and in 2–2.5 min without narcotic premedication or another sedative premedication.

Midazolam's activity is primarily due to the parent drug. Elimination of the parent drug takes place via hepatic metabolism of midazolam to hydroxylated metabolites that are conjugated and excreted in the urine. Elimination half-life is 1.8–6.4 h (mean approximately 3 h); total clearance (Cl), 0.25 to 0.54 L/h/kg.

Sedation with IV midazolam does not adversely affect the mechanics of respiration; total lung capacity and peak expiratory flow decrease significantly, but static compliance and maximum expiratory flow at 50% of awake total lung capacity (V_{max}) increase. Impairment of ventilatory response to carbon dioxide is more marked in adult patients with chronic obstructive pulmonary disease (COPD).

Intravenous induction of general anesthesia with midazolam hydrochloride was associated with a slight to moderate decrease in mean arterial pressure, cardiac output, stroke volume, and systemic vascular resistance. Slow heart rates (less than 65/min), particularly in patients taking propranolol for angina, tended to rise slightly; faster heart rates (e.g., 85/min) tended to slow slightly.

Benzodiazepines are contraindicated in patients with acute narrow-angle glaucoma. Benzodiazepines may be used in patients with open-angle glaucoma only if they are receiving appropriate therapy. Intravenous doses of midazolam hydrochloride should be decreased for both elderly and debilitated patients. These patients will also take longer recovery times after midazolam administration for the induction of anesthesia.

Fentanyl. Fentanyl is a synthetic opioid with rapid onset and short duration of action. It is a potent μ-opioid agonist. Fentanyl is 50–100 times more potent than morphine; however, response to parenteral fentanyl is variable. Fentanyl's lipophilic structure allows it to cross the blood–brain barrier and results in delta wave appearance on EEG. Fentanyl is used during general anesthesia to dampen cardiovascular response to noxious stimulation from laryngoscopy, intubation, skin incision, and surgical stress. When combining fentanyl with propofol, the required amount of both drugs is reduced to prevent movement and hemodynamic changes to surgical stress and laryngoscopy. Dosing should be repeated at regular intervals to maintain a comfortable analgesic state; however, continuous infusion can result in accumulation of the drug, as its 50% context sensitive half-time increases rapidly with the duration of infusion. Frequent dosing also causes accumulation. Rapid administration can rarely be associated with chest wall rigidity and compromised ventilation. The exact mechanism is not known but is thought to be centrally mediated. Bag-mask ventilation, even with an oral or nasal airway, can be difficult. It needs to be rapidly treated with administration of naloxone or even neuromuscular blockers if needed.

Emerging Sedation Technologies

Patient-controlled sedation and analgesia (PCSA) allows for a tailored approach to procedural sedation. A pump delivers a preset bolus dose and a lockout interval is used to prevent oversedation. Prerequisites include both a cooperative patient and a planned moderate level of sedation. Deep sedation or general anesthesia disqualifies patients from this approach.

PCSA usually involves the administration of a rapidly acting narcotic coupled with propofol. Initial results have focused on patients undergoing colonoscopy. Currently, there are no studies of the obese patient for either upper or lower endoscopy. Recovery time is usually improved when compared with standard sedation, with equivalent to improved satisfaction and no appreciable difference in cardiopulmonary parameters [36, 37].

Target-controlled infusion (TCI) typically involves a computer-aided infusion of sedation agents that is designed to achieve a steady-state effect of drug concentration and is based on pharmacologic modeling. Since this is population-based, variances in the response can be expected, and adjustments in infusion rates are accomplished by some type of physiologic feedback. Feedback can be from bispectral index monitoring (closed loop) or via physician (open loop). As opposed to patient-controlled sedation, TCI can be cut targeted to deeper levels of sedation for extended intervals. A case series by Gillham and colleagues exhibited a 15% rate of undersedation and a 20% rate of oversedation using TCI [37]. A much larger study by Fanti and colleagues used target-controlled propofol infusion during monitored anesthesia in patients undergoing ERCP [38]. Excellent sedation was seen in 201 of the 205 patients. Stonell et al. compared anesthesiologist-administered propofol sedation with patient-controlled sedation using propofol [39]. Endoscopist and patient satisfaction were similar between the two sedation arms.

Computer-assisted personalized sedation (CAPS) is a form of target-controlled infusion that enables the non-anesthesiologist administration of propofol with a target of moderate sedation. This platform utilizes both an infusion and bolus administration of propofol. Physiologic feedback includes capnography, pulse oximetry, electrocardiography, and blood pressure monitoring. In addition, automated responsiveness monitoring is employed, which measures the patient's ability to respond to tactile and/or auditory stimulation. A multicenter study involving 1000 patients undergoing elective upper endoscopy and colonoscopy has recently been published [40]. Subjects were randomized to receive either standard sedation with the combination of an opioid and benzodiazepine or sedation with the CAPS device. Patients with a BMI between 30 and 35 kg/m^2 were enrolled but not targeted for a specific analysis. Subjects in the CAPS arm exhibited significantly less hypoxemia and improved recovery times when compared with standard sedation.

Challenges and Risks of Sedation in Obesity

Data are sparse on the actual risk of sedation on obese patients. In recent studies, BMI was found to be an independent risk factor for sedation-related adverse events and was significantly correlated with the number of hypoxemic episodes during a variety of procedures with endoscopist-directed sedation [41–44].

The risk of sedation in obese patients can be attributed to one of the following factors:

Sleep Apnea

Definition. Sleep apnea is defined by pauses in breathing during sleep lasting for a few seconds to several minutes many times a night [45].

There are three forms of sleep apnea: obstructive (OSA), central (CSA), and a combination of the two, or *mixed.* OSA is the most common type and is caused by complete or partial obstructions of the upper airway and is usually associated with a reduction in blood oxygen saturation [46].

Prevalence of OSA in obese patients. Studies estimate 1–5% of the Western adult population experiences OSA [47]. It is estimated that 80–90% of patients with moderate to severe sleep apnea are undiagnosed [48]. The prevalence of OSA is 39–71% in bariatric patients [49, 50]. Initial screening for OSA in bariatric patients is done with a history and physical examination and a daytime sleepiness evaluation, such as the Epworth sleepiness scale or the STOP-BANG (SB) questionnaire; many patients end up being referred for polysomnography or a formal sleep study. Almost 80% of those who are referred for a sleep study are diagnosed with sleep apnea [49].

How to screen for OSA. Many screening tools are available to screen for OSA. One screening tool that is simple and has a high sensitivity is the SB questionnaire. The SB (see Table 3.4) utilizes four questions and four clinical characteristics to stratify patients into high- and low-risk groups for OSA. A positive SB (score R3) has a sensitivity of almost 80% in predicting mild sleep apnea and 90% in predicting moderate to severe apnea on full polysomnography [51].

In patients undergoing advanced endoscopic procedures, who are high risk on the SB score, the frequency of hypoxemia and the rate of advanced airway maneuvers (chin lift, modified mask ventilation, nasal airway, bag-mask ventilation, and endotracheal intubation) are significantly higher than among patients with low-risk SB score [52]. Validity of the SB questionnaire has not been duplicated in routine esophagogastroduodenoscopy (EGD) and colonoscopy (Table 3.7) [3, 41, 53].

OSA, sedation and post-op complications. Several studies were evaluated in a recent published guidelines from the Society of Anesthesia and Sleep Medicine on preoperative screening and assessment of adult patients with obstructive sleep apnea [54]. Some studies showed worse outcomes with OSA and others showed no difference (Table 3.8).

Pulmonary Hypertension

Pulmonary hypertension (PH) is formally defined by a mean pulmonary artery pressure of 25 mmHg on right heart catheterization. However echocardiography, given its noninvasive nature, is usually used to screen for PH. Echocardiography provides estimates of peak pulmonary artery systolic pressure (PASP). PASP greater than 40 mmHg is considered abnormal [55].

Obesity/pulmonary hypertension association. The prevalence of PH is about 15 individuals per million [56]. There are limited data on the prevalence of PH in the obese population, but there is a significant overall association between BMI and mean PASP. A PASP >40 mmHg is found in 5% of those with a BMI >30 kg/m^2 [57].

Pulmonary hypertension/perioperative morbidity correlation. Data are sparse on the actual risk of sedation in patients with pulmonary hypertension. Still the presence of underlying PH can have a significant negative impact on perioperative outcomes [58, 59]. Given the correlation between obesity and PH, special consideration should be paid to the clinical symptoms and signs of PH, including fatigue,

Table 3.7 STOP-BANG questions and scoring[a] (From Jirapinyo and Thompson [3], with permission)

S	Snoring: Do you snore loudly (louder than talking or loud enough to be heard through closed doors)?	Yes/no
T	Tired: Do you often feel tired, fatigued, or sleepy during the daytime	Yes/no
O	Observed: Has anyone observed you stop breathing during your sleep?	Yes/no
P	Blood pressure: Have you been or are you being treated for high blood pressure?	Yes/no
B	BMI: >35 kg/m^2	Yes/no
A	Age: Older than 50 years	Yes/no
N	Neck circumference: >40 cm	Yes/no
G	Gender: Male	Yes/no

[a]High risk of OSA: yes to three or more questions; low risk of OSA: yes to less than three questions

Table 3.8 Studies evaluating the association of obstructive sleep apnea and postoperative complications, resource utilization and mortality in cases utilizing sedation only (From Chung et al. [54], with permission)

Impact of OSA on outcomes	Studies (no.)	OSA (n)	Non-OSA (n)	Detrimental impact of OSA (no. studies)	Beneficial impact of OSA (no. studies)	No significant impact of OSA (no. studies)	GRADE quality of evidence
Oxygen desaturation	7	610	713	3	0	4	Moderate
Airway maneuvers	7	263	297	1	0	2	Very low
Combined complications	3	978	808	0	0	3	Low

GRADE grading of recommendation, assessment, development, and evaluation, *OSA* obstructive sleep apnea

dyspnea on exertion, chest pain, palpitations, syn-
cope, and lower extremity edema. Common physical exam findings include a pulsatile liver, sternal
lift, right-sided S4, loud P2, and a murmur of tricus-
pid regurgitation with giant v-waves [60].

Restrictive Lung Disease

The excess fat externally and internally in obese
patients compresses the thoracic cavity, and the
fatty infiltration of the accessory muscles can
decrease compliance of the chest wall. Central
adiposity causes increased intra-abdominal
pressure leading to cephalad displacement of
the diaphragm causing a chronic abdominal
compartment syndrome and resulting in dimin-
ished lung volumes. The increased pulmonary
blood volume in obese patients competes for
space in the chest cavity, further decreasing
lung volumes [61].

There is an established link between the dose-
dependent depression of muscle activity and
increased collapsibility of the upper airway with
increasing dosages of propofol [62]. Using opioids in combination with propofol causes further
respiratory depression, and opioids may impair
respiratory function in the postoperative period,
leading to obstructive apnea and oxygen desaturation [63].

Difficult Bag-Mask Ventilation

Mask ventilation is an essential component of
airway management and is commonly used as a
rescue technique during unsuccessful attempts
at laryngoscopy and unanticipated difficult airway situations. The data are limited on mask
ventilation in obese patients, but some studies
have shown that obese patients are more difficult to mask ventilate [64–66]. Ventilation is
often difficult due to increased mass of tissue
around the face and jaw, poor mask fit,
increased pharyngeal and palatal tissue, and
decreased chest wall compliance due to
increased chest wall mass.

Difficult Airway

Obese patients have many anatomic limitations
that make intubation potentially difficult. Many
obese patients have a small mouth opening,
increased submental fat, increased pharyngeal tissue, and a large tongue. All of these cause a narrowing of the airway. The increased cervical and
thoracic fat pads cause limitations in neck extension. Also obese patients have increased prevalence of OSA and decreased functional residual
capacity. This decreases the time that an obese
patient can be apneic or hypoventilating prior to
becoming hypoxic [67]. The incidence of difficult
intubation in normal patients is around 6% [64,
68], whereas in obese patients, it varies between 10
to 15% [64, 69–71] with a higher risk of desaturation with difficult intubation [69]. Difficult tracheal
intubation contributes to significant morbidity and
mortality. Nearly 30% of anesthesia deaths can be
attributed to a compromised airway [72].

Difficult intra-procedure monitoring. Body
habitus in obese patients can make intraoperative
monitoring very challenging. Most commonly,
providers have problems with blood pressure
cuffs frequently not fitting well, which might lead
to inaccurate readings. If the arm circumference is
very large, an alternative approach is to place the
cuff on the forearm. Providers should pay attention that forearm measurement might overesti-
mate both systolic and diastolic pressure [73].

Nonresponse to usual rescue. Obese patients
are at increased risk of adverse airway events.
Reasons include mechanical difficulty in securing the airway, as discussed earlier in this chapter
(mask ventilation, tracheal intubation, and emergency surgical airway), increased risk of aspiration, and accelerated speed and extent of oxygen
desaturation [69].

There is limited information on the effect of
obesity on the pharmacology of commonly used
anesthetic drugs. Much of the excess weight is
fat, which has relatively low blood flow. While
lipophilic drugs will have a larger volume of distribution than hydrophilic ones, the current evi-

dence indicates that changes in volume of distribution in the obese are drug-specific, so generalizations are difficult. Besides the more complicated airway management, obese patients might have drug-specific changes in volume of distribution. Also elimination half-life for some of the medications can be longer in obese patients [74]. In addition to having adequate experience in airway support techniques like jaw-thrust, chin-lift, and bag-valve-mask ventilation, providers should have a good understanding of the pharmacology of agents administered, as well as their antagonists. All should be trained in ACLS [69].

When to Involve Anesthesia/Rescue Maneuvers in the Obese Patient

Most institutions identify risk factors that can serve as triggers for getting anesthesia providers involved early in the process. Table 3.9 provides a nonevidence-based list of potential factors that may increase the risk for moderate sedation in the obese [75].

Table 3.9 Possible risk factors for endoscopist-administered sedation in obese patients and triggers for using anesthesia providers (From Vargo [75], with permission)

American Society of Anesthesiologists physiologic classification IV or V
Sleep apnea requiring CPAP
Previous problems with procedural sedation or anesthesia
The use of sedatives and analgesics
Procedures that will require deep sedation (at a minimum), such as ERCP or EUS
Problematic or altered oropharyngeal anatomy
Mallampati grade III or IV
Dysmorphic facial features
Neck mass
Tracheal deviation
Micrognathia or retrognathia
Trismus
<3 cm mouth opening

CPAP continuous positive airway pressure, *ERCP* endoscopic retrograde cholangiopancreatography, *EUS* endoscopic ultrasound

Given that many studies have suggested that BMI is an independent risk factor for sedation-related adverse events [41–44], providers should be very familiar with airway/rescue techniques and management of complications (Table 3.10) [24, 76, 77]. All providers should be prepared to rescue patients from deeper levels of sedation than planned.

The most common complications during endoscopic sedation are hypoxemia and hypotension. Avoidance of these possible complications can be largely achieved by slow titration of sedation doses to the minimal depth of sedation needed to complete the procedure.

Hypotension during endoscopy very rarely results in permanent complications and can be reversed by a fluid bolus and possibly catecholamine infusion.

There are various airway management techniques. Nasal trumpet, or nasopharyngeal airway, is one of the most commonly used approaches, especially with the previously described difficulty to bag-mask ventilate obese patients; see "Inserting a Nasal Airway" in the online brochure from the American National Red Cross [78]. Nasal trumpet sizes range from 20 to 36 French on the internal diameter and 10–17 cm in length. Commonly used sizes are 24–28FR in females

Table 3.10 Useful countermeasures and rescue techniques for adverse events during sedation (From Da and Buxbaum [24], with permission)

Adverse effects associated with sedation	Countermeasure
Hypoxemia	Stop infusion of sedatives
	Increase oxygen supplementation
	Maintain airway
	Jaw-thrust maneuver
	Suctioning
	Mask ventilation
	Nasal airway
	Endotracheal intubation
	Advanced cardiac life support
Hypotension	Electrolyte solution
	Catecholamine infusion
Bradycardia	Atropine

and 28–32FR in males. The device should reach from the patient's nostril to the earlobe. A laryngeal mask airway is sometimes needed. Administration of propofol is at times required to facilitate tolerance of the laryngeal mask airway.

Measure the nasopharyngeal airway from the patient's earlobe to the tip of the nostril. Ensure that the diameter of the nasal trumpet is not larger than the nostril. Lubricate the nasal trumpet. Insert the trumpet with the bevel towards the septum (center of the nose) and advance it gently, along the floor of the nose. Try the other nostril if not advancing easily. The flange comes to rest on the nostril.

As the prevalence of obesity is increasing across the world, the exposure of clinicians to obese patients will continue to rise, especially as the obese population ages. With the potential for increased obesity associated cardiopulmonary comorbidities in them, especially OSA, it is imperative that endoscopists are familiar with nuances of sedation in the obese, its adverse effects and rescue manoeuvers.

References

1. Ogden CL, Carroll MD, Kit BK, Flegal KM. Prevalence of childhood and adult obesity the United States, 2011-2012. JAMA. 2014;311(8):806–14.
2. World Health Organization. Global status report on noncommunicable diseases. 2014. Geneva, Switzerland. http://www.who.int/nmh/publications/ncd-status-report-2014/en/. Accessed 2 Jun 2017.
3. Jirapinyo P, Thompson CC. Sedation challenges: obesity and sleep apnea. Gastrointest Endosc Clin N Am. 2016;26(3):527–37.
4. Harris ZP, Liu J, Saltzman JR. Quality assurance in the endoscopy suite: sedation and monitoring. Gastrointest Endosc Clin N Am. 2016;26(3):553–62.
5. 2017 UptoDate. The modified Mallampati classification for difficult laryngoscopy and intubation. Accessed 2 Jun 2017.
6. Samsoon GL, Young JR. Difficult tracheal intubation: a retrospective study. Anaesthesia. 1987;42(5):487–90.
7. Committee on Standards and Practice Parameters, Apfelbaum JL, Connis RT, Nickinovich DG, American Society of Anesthesiologists Task Force on Preanesthesia Evaluation, Pastnernak LR, et al. Practice advisory for preanesthesia evaluation: an updated report by the American Society of Anesthesiologists Task Force on Preanesthesia evaluation. Anesthesiology. 2012;116(3):522–38.
8. American Society of Anesthesiologists Task Force on Sedation and Analgesia by Non-Anesthesiologists. Practice guidelines for sedation and analgesia by non-anesthesiologists. Anesthesiology. 2002;96(4):1004–17.
9. Standards of Practice Committee of the American Society for Gastrointestinal Endoscopy, Lichtenstein DR, Jagannath S, Baron TH, Anderson MA, Banerjee S, Dominitz JA, et al. Sedation and anesthesia in GI endoscopy. Gastrointest Endosc. 2008;68(5):815–26.
10. Moller JT, Pedersen T, Rasmussen LS, Jensen PF, Pedersen BD, Ravlo O, et al. Randomized evaluation of pulse oximetry in 20,802 patients. I. Design, demography, pulse oximetry failure rate, and overall complication rate. Anesthesiology. 1993;78(3):436–44.
11. Pedersen T, Moller AM, Pedersen BD. Pulse oximetry for perioperative monitoring: systematic review of randomized, controlled trials. Anesth Analg. 2003;96(2):426–31.
12. Waring JP, Baron TH, Hirota WK, Goldstein JL, Jacobson BC, Leighton JA, et al. Guidelines for conscious sedation and monitoring during gastrointestinal endoscopy. Gastrointest Endosc. 2003;58(3):317–22.
13. Qadeer MA, Vargo JJ, Dumot JA, Zuccaro G, Stevens T, Parsi MA, et al. Capnography prevents hypoxemia during ERCP and EUS: a randomized controlled trial (abstract). Gastrointest Endosc. 2008;67(5):AB84.
14. Gross JB, Bachenberg KL, Benumof JL, Caplan RA, Connis RT, Coté CJ, et al. Practice guidelines for the perioperative management of patients with obstructive sleep apnea: a report by the American Society of Anesthesiologists Task Force on perioperative management of patients with obstructive sleep apnea. Anesthesiology. 2006;104(5):1081–93.
15. Cohen LB. Patient monitoring during gastrointestinal endoscopy: why, when, and how? Gastrointest Endoscopy Clin N Am. 2008;18(4):651–63.
16. Al-Sammak Z, Al-Falaki MM, Gamal HM. Predictor of sedation during endoscopic retrograde cholangiopancreatography—bispectral index vs clinical assessment. Middle East J Anesthesiol. 1891;2005:141–8.
17. Qadeer MA, Vargo JJ, Patel S, Dumot JA, Lopez AR, Trolli PA, et al. Bispectral index monitoring of conscious sedation with the combination of meperidine and midazolam during endoscopy. Clin Gastroenterol Hepatol. 2008;6(1):102–8.
18. Chen SC, Rex DK. An initial investigation of bispectral monitoring as an adjunct to nurse-administered propofol sedation for colonoscopy. Am J Gastroenterol. 2004;99(6):1081–6.
19. American Society of Anesthesiologists. Continuum of depth of sedation: definition of general anesthesia and levels of sedation/analgesia (15 Oct 2014). https://www.asahq.org/quality-and-practice-management/standards-and-guidelines/. Accessed 2 Jun 2017.
20. Nisbet AT, Mooney-Cotter F. Comparison of selected sedation scales for reporting opioid-induced sedation assessment. Pain Manag Nurs. 2009;10(3):154–64.

21. Consales G, Chelazzi C, Rinaldi S, De Gaudio AR. Bispectral index compared to Ramsay score for sedation monitoring in intensive care units. Minerva Anestesiol. 2006;72(5):329–36.
22. Drummond JC. Monitoring depth of anesthesia: with emphasis on the application of the bispectral index and the middle latency auditory evoked response to the prevention of recall. Anesthesiology. 2000;93(3):876–82.
23. Hasanein R, El-Sayed W. Ketamine/propofol versus fentanyl/propofol for sedating obese patients undergoing endoscopic retrograde cholangiopancretography (ERCP). Egyptian J Anesth. 2013;29(3):207–11.
24. Da B, Buxbaum J. Training and competency in sedation practice in gastrointestinal endoscopy. Gastrointest Endosc Clin N Am. 2016;26(3):443–62.
25. Nelson DB, Barkun AN, Block KP, Burdick JS, Ginsberg GG, Greenwald DA, et al. Propofol use during gastrointestinal endoscopy. Gastrointest Endosc. 2001;53(7):876–9.
26. Bryson HM, Fulton BR, Faulds D. Propofol. An update of its use in anesthesia and conscious sedation. Drugs. 1995;50(3):513–59.
27. AstraZeneca. Diprivan 1% (package insert). Wilmington: AstraZeneca; 2000.
28. Baxter Pharmaceutical Products. Propofol (package insert). New Providence; 2002.
29. Vuyk J. Pharmacokinetics and pharmacodynamic interactions between opioids and propofol. J Clin Anesth. 1997;9(6):23S–6S.
30. Marinella JA. Propofol for sedation in the intensive care unit: essentials for the clinician. Respir Med. 1997;91(9):505–10.
31. Kirkpatrick T, Cockshott ID, Douglas EJ, Nimmo WS. Pharmocokinetics of propofol (diprivan) in elderly patients. Br J Anaesth. 1988;60(2):146–50.
32. Walker JA, McIntyre RD, Schleinitz PF, Jacobson KN, Haulk AA, Adesman PW, et al. Nurse-administered propofol sedation without anesthesia specialists in 9152 endoscopic cases in an ambulatory surgery center. Am J Gastroenterol. 2003;98(8):1744–50.
33. Vargo JJ, Zuccaro G, Dumot JA, Shermock KM, Morrow JB, Conwell DL, et al. Gastroenterologist-administered propofol versus meperidine and midazolam for advanced upper endoscopy: a prospective, randomized trial. Gastroenterology. 2002;123(1):8–16.
34. Rex DK, Overley C, Kinser K, Coates M, Lee A, Goodwine BW, et al. Safety of propofol administered by registered nurses with gastroenterologists supervision in 2000 endoscopic cases. Am J Gastroenterol. 2002;97(5):1159–63.
35. Heuss LT, Schnieper P, Drewe J, Pflimlin E, Beglinger C. Risk stratification and safe administration of propofol by registered nurses supervised by the gastroenterologist: a prospective observational study of more than 2000 cases. Gastrointest Endosc. 2003;57(6):664–71.
36. Heuss LT, Drewe J, Schnieper P, Tapparelli CB, Pflimlin E, Beglinger C. Patient controlled versus nurse administered sedation for colonoscopy: a prospective randomized trial. Am J Gastroenterol. 2004;99(3):511–8.
37. Gillham MJ, Hutchinson RC, Carter R, Kenny GN. Patient-maintained sedation for ERCP with a target-controlled infusion of propofol: a pilot study. Gastrointest Endosc. 2001;54(1):14–7.
38. Fanti L, Agostoni M, Casta A, Guslandi M, Giollo P, Torri G, Testoni PA. Target-controlled propofol infusion during monitored anesthesia in patients undergoing ERCP. Gastrointest Endosc. 2004;60(3):361–6.
39. Stonell A, Leslie K, Absalom AR. Effect-site target targeted patient-controlled sedation with propofol: comparison with anaesthetist administration for colonoscopy. Anaesthesia. 2006;61(3):240–7.
40. Pambianco DJ, Vargo JJ, Pruitt RE, Hardi R, Martin JF. Computer-assisted personalized sedation for upper endoscopy and colonoscopy: a comparative, multicenter randomized study. Gastrointest Endosc. 2011;73(4):765–72.
41. Mehta PP, Kochhar G, Kalra S, Maurer W, Tetzlaff J, Singh G, et al. Can a validated sleep apnea scoring system predict cardiopulmonary events using propofol sedation for routine EGD or colonoscopy? A prospective cohort study. Gastrointest Endosc. 2014;79(3):436–44.
42. Wani S, Azar R, Hovis CE, Hovis RM, Coté GA, Hall M, Waldbaum L, et al. Obesity is a risk factor for sedation-related complications during propofol-mediated sedation advanced endoscopic procedures. Gastointest Endosc. 2001;74(6):1238–47.
43. Qadeer MA, Lopez AR, Dumot JA, Vargo JJ. Risk factors for hypoxemia during ambulatory gastrointestinal endoscopy in ASA I-II patients. Dig Dis Sci. 2009;54(5):1035–40.
44. Dhariwal A, Plevris JN, Lo NT, Finlayson ND, Heading RC, Hayes PC. Age, anemia, and obesity-associated oxygen desaturation during upper gastrointestinal endoscopy. Gastrointest Endosc. 1992;38(6):684–8.
45. National Heart, Lung, and Blood Institute. Health information for the public. Health topics. sleep apnea. What is sleep apnea? Updated 10 Jul 2012. https://www.nhlbi.nih.gov/health/health-topics/topics/sleepapnea. Accessed 3 Jun 2017.
46. American Academy of Sleep Medicine. Obstructive sleep apnea syndrome (780.53-0). The International Classification of Sleep Disorders, Revised: Diagnostic and coding manual. Westchester: American Academy of Sleep Medicine; 2001. p. 52–8.
47. Young T, Skatrud J, Peppard PE. Risk factors for obstructive sleep apnea in adults. JAMA. 2004;291(16):2013–6. Review
48. Chung F, Subramanyam R, Liao P, Sasaki E, Shapiro C, Sun Y. High STOP-BANG score indicates

a high probability of obstructive sleep apnoea. Br J Anaesth. 2012;108(5):768–75.

49. Kuruba R, Koche LS, Murr MM. Preoperative assessment and perioperative care of patients undergoing bariatric surgery. Med Clin North Am. 2007;91(3):339–51, ix.

50. Frey WC, Pilcher J. Obstructive sleep-related breathing disorders in patients evaluated for bariatric surgery. Obes Surg. 2003;13(5):676–83.

51. Chung F, Elsaid H. Screening for obstructive sleep apnea before surgery: why is it important? Curr Opin Anaesthesiol. 2009;22(3):405–11.

52. Coté GA, Hovis CE, Hovis RM, Waldbaum L, Early DS, Edmundowicz SA, et al. A screening instrument for sleep apnea predicts airway maneuvers in patients undergoing advanced endoscopic procedures. Clin Gastroenterol Hepatol. 2010;8(8):660–665.e1.

53. Chung F, Yegneswaran B, Liao P, Chung SA, Vairavanathan S, Islam S, et al. STOP questionnaire: a tool to screen patients for obstructive sleep apnea. Anesthesiology. 2008;108(5):812–21.

54. Chung F, Memtsoudis SG, Ramachandran SK, Nagappa M, Opperer M, Cozowicz C, et al. Society of Anesthesia and Sleep Medicine guidelines on preoperative screening and assessment of adult patients with obstructive sleep apnea. Anesth Analg. 2016;123(2):452–73.

55. Friedman SE, Andrus BW. Obesity and pulmonary hypertension: a review of pathophysiologic mechanisms. J Obes. 2012;2012:1. doi:10.1155/2012/505274.

56. Humbert M, Sitbon O, Chaouat A, Bertocchi M, Habib G, Gressin V, et al. Pulmonary arterial hypertension in France: results from a national registry. Am J Respir Crit Care Med. 2006;173(9):1023–30.

57. McQuillan BM, Picard MH, Leavitt M, Weyman AE. Clinical correlates and reference intervals for pulmonary artery systolic pressure among echocardiographically normal subjects. Circulation. 2001;104(23):2797–802.

58. Ramakrishna G, Sprung J, Ravi BS, Chandrasekaran K, McGoon MD. Impact of pulmonary hypertension on the outcomes of noncardiac surgery: predictors of perioperative morbidity and mortality. J Am Coll Cardiol. 2005;45(10):1691–9.

59. Kaw R, Pasupuleti V, Deshpande A, Hamieh T, Walker E, Minai OA. Pulmonary hypertension: an important predictor of outcomes in patients undergoing noncardiac surgery. Respir Med. 2011;105(4):619–24.

60. McLaughlin VV, Archer SL, Badesch DB, Barst RJ, Farber HW, Lindner JR, et al. ACCF/AHA 2009 expert consensus document on pulmonary hypertension a report of the ACCF task force on expert consensus documents and the AHA developed in collaboration with the ACCP; ATS; and the PHA. J Am Coll Cardiol. 2009;53(17):1573–619.

61. Fadell EJ, Richman AD, Ward WW, Hendon JR. Fatty infiltration of the respiratory muscles in the pickwickian syndrome. N Engl J Med. 1962;266:861–3.

62. Hillman DR, Walsh JH, Maddison KJ, Platt PR, Kirkness JP, Noffsinger WJ, Eastwood PR. Evolution of changes in upper airway collapsibility during slow induction of anesthesia with propofol. Anesthesiology. 2009;111(1):63–71.

63. Robinson RW, Zwillich CW, Bixler EO, Cadieux RJ, Kales A, White DP. Effects of oral narcotics on sleep-disordered breathing in healthy adults. Chest. 1987;91(2):197–203.

64. Shailaja S, Nichelle SM, Shetty AK, Hegde BR. Comparing ease of intubation in obese and lean patients using intubation difficulty scale. Anesth Essays Res. 2014;8(2):168–74.

65. Kheterpal S, Han R, Tremper KK, Shanks A, Tait AR, O'Reilly M, et al. Incidence and predictors of difficult and impossible mask ventilation. Anesthesiology. 2006;105(5):885–91.

66. Langeron O, Masso E, Huraux C, Guggiari M, Bianchi A, Coriat P, Riou B. Prediction of difficult mask ventilation. Anesthesiology. 2000;92(5):1229–36.

67. Dixon BJ, Dixon JB, Carden JR, Burn AJ, Schachter LM, Playfair JM, et al. Preoxygenation is more effective in the 25 degrees headup position than in the supine position in severely obese patients: a randomized controlled study. Anesthesiology. 2005;102(6):1110–5; discussion 5A.

68. Shiga T, Wajima Z, Inoue T, Sakamoto A. Predicting difficult intubation in apparently normal patients: a meta-analysis of bedside screening test performance. Anesthesiology. 2005;103(2):429–37.

69. Juvin P, Lavaut E, Dupont H, Lefevre P, Demetriou M, Dumoulin JL, Desmonts JM. Difficult tracheal intubation is more common in obese than in lean patients. Anesth Analg. 2003;97(2):595–600.

70. American Society of Anesthesiologists Task Force on Management of the Difficult Airway. Practice guidelines for management of the difficult airway: an updated report by the American Society of Anesthesiologists Task Force on Management of the Difficult Airway. Anesthesiology. 2003;98(5):1269–77.

71. Shah PN, Sundaram V. Incidence and predictors of difficult mask ventilation and intubation. J Anaesthesiol Clin Pharmacol. 2012;28(4):451–5.

72. Salimi A, Farzanegan B, Rastegarpour A, Kolahi AA. Comparison of the upper lip bite test with measurement of thyromental distance for prediction of difficult intubations. Acta Anaesthesiol Taiwan. 2008;46(2):61–5.

73. Singer AJ, Kahn SR, Thode HC Jr, Hollander JE. Comparison of forearm and upper arm blood pressures. Prehosp Emerg Care. 1999;3(2):123–6.

74. Hanley MJ, Abernethy DR, Greenblatt DJ. Effect of obesity on the pharmacokinetics of drugs in humans. Clinical Pharmacokinet. 2010;49(2):71–87.

75. Vargo JJ. Procedural sedation and obesity: waters left uncharted. Gastrointest Endosc. 2009;70(5):980–4.

76. American Association for Study of Liver Diseases, American College of Gastroenterology, American

Gastroenterological Association Institute, American Society for Gastrointestinal Endoscopy, Society for Gastroenterology Nurses and Associates, Vargo JJ, MH DL, Feld AD, Gerstenberger PD, Kwo PY, Lightdale JR, et al. Multisociety sedation curriculum for gastrointestinal endoscopy. Gastrointest Endosc. 2012;76(1):e1–25.

77. Lee T, Lee CK. Endoscopic sedation: from training to performance. Clin Endosc. 2014;47:141–50.
78. Administering emergency oxygen. Online resources. The American National Red Cross. 2011. https://www. redcross.org/images/MEDIA_CustomProductCatalog/ m4240191_AirwayAdjunctsFactandSkill.pdf. Accessed 3 Jun 2017.

Mojdeh S. Kappus, Natan Zundel,
and Diego R. Camacho

Jejunocolic Bypass

The jejunocolic bypass or shunt was first described by Payne, Dewind, and Commons in 1963 [1]. Using the knowledge they had gleaned from patients who had undergone major small bowel resections for various reasons as well as reports from Kremen, Linner, and Nelson in 1954 [2], who studied small intestinal bypass in dogs, Payne, Dewind, and Commons performed the first iteration of intestinal bypass for the treatment of morbid obesity in 1956. They hypothesized that in bypassing the majority of the small intestine fat absorption would decrease resulting in weight loss.

M.S. Kappus, M.D.
Department of Surgery, Montefiore Medical Center,
6285 Jockey Rd, Bronx, NY 10467, USA
e-mail: mojdeh.kappus@gmail.com

N. Zundel, M.D.
Department of General Surgery, Herbert Wertheim
College of Medicine, Florida International University,
17038 West Dixie Hwy #210, Miami,
FL 33160, USA
e-mail: drnazuma99@yahoo.com

D.R. Camacho, M.D., F.A.C.S. (✉)
Department of Surgery, Minimally Invasive and
Laparoscopic General Surgery, Montefiore Medical
Center, Montefiore Greene Medical Arts Pavilion,
3400 Bainbridge Ave, 4th Floor, Bronx,
NY 10467, USA
e-mail: dicamach@montefiore.org

In their landmark study in 1963, they describe the creation of a jejunocolic shunt in ten female patients with "uncontrolled obesity." Patient selection criteria were as follows: (1) patients must be at least 125 pounds overweight; (2) patients must have exhausted alternative weight loss methods without success; and (3) patients must have obesity-related comorbidities such as cardiopulmonary failure, diabetes, hypertension, or liver disease. Patients who met these criteria underwent various psychological and medical evaluations not unlike patients undergoing bariatric surgery today [1].

Surgical Procedure

Payne et al. describe entry into the abdomen via a transverse incision. In all cases, an exploratory laparotomy was first performed to detect any previously unidentified pathology. If the appendix was present, an appendectomy was performed, biopsies were taken of the liver, kidney, and jejunum, any noted umbilical hernias were repaired, and in some patients, a panniculectomy was performed. The jejunum was divided 15 in. from the ligament of Treitz (except in one case during which it was divided at 20 in. from the ligament of Treitz). The distal end of jejunum was closed and left as a blind end. The proximal end of jejunum was anastomosed to the proximal transverse colon in an end-to-side fashion. All procedures were performed using spinal anesthesia except one that was performed under a general anesthetic. After patients had achieved their calculated ideal body weight, they underwent a "revision" of their bypass. Six patients were restored to normal intestinal continuity, three received jejunoileal anastomoses, and one patient died of pulmonary embolism shortly after her initial operation. In two patients, intestinal continuity was re-established before ideal body weight could be achieved due to severe hypokalemia and hypocalcemia requiring prolonged hospitalization. Jejunocolic bypass was also described by Lewis et al. in 1966 [3]. In these procedures, the abdomen was entered via a right paramedian incision and the jejunum was divided either 20 or 30 in. from the ligament of Treitz. Once again the distal jejunum was closed and left as a blind end. The proximal jejunum was anastomosed to either the transverse colon or cecum in an end-to-side fashion. As Payne et al. had demonstrated that after reconstitution of intestinal continuity almost all patients had regained all of their previously lost weight, Lewis et al. elected not to restore intestinal continuity [1, 3]. Shibata et al. published a similar case series in which patients underwent end-to-side anastomosis of the proximal jejunum to the ascending colon with comparable results [4].

Outcomes

Across multiple early trials, patients experienced early weight loss in the first year following surgery. Additionally, they enjoyed resolution of multiple comorbidities including hypertension, hypercholesterolemia, diabetes, and cardiopulmonary failure. The majority of patients developed significant diarrhea and related anal discomfort and disease from their chronic diarrhea. Electrolyte and vitamin deficiencies were also demonstrated in all postoperative patients requiring continuous repletion. Vitamin B12, A, D, magnesium, potassium, and calcium were most notably depleted in these patients. Numerous additional complications have also been reported including chronic fatigue, joint disease [5], anemia, gall bladder disease, nephrolithiasis, fatty liver

disease, and cirrhosis. Ultimately, the jejunocolic bypass procedure was abandoned owing to these severe complications and many patients underwent revision to jejunoileal bypass [1, 3, 4].

Follow-Up

It is unlikely that an endoscopist today would encounter a postoperative patient with a jejunocolic bypass, although rare instances of pathologic jejunocolic or gastrojejunocolic fistulas have been reported [6]. Nevertheless, the invaluable lessons gained from this first foray into the world of intestinal bypass for the treatment of morbid obesity should not be forgotten.

Jejunoileal Bypass

The jejunoileal bypass procedure was first described by Payne and Dewind as a revisional procedure performed in patients who had previously undergone jejunocolic bypass [1]. Using the knowledge they had gleaned from their work on the jejunocolic bypass, they set out to perform the jejunoileal bypass as a primary procedure that would allow for more long-term weight loss with fewer detrimental side effects from severe malabsorption. In 1969, they published a case series of 70 patients on whom they had performed a jejunoileal bypass for the treatment of obesity [7]. Patients studied were both male and female, aged 21–56, greater than 100 lb overweight with associated comorbidities of obesity. Patients underwent an extensive preoperative medical and psychiatric evaluation. Interestingly, based on their experience with those patients who underwent jejunocolic bypass, Payne and Dewind made attempts to screen out patients who appeared "despondent" or "hostile" towards the physician as they felt that those patients would generally be unsuccessful in coping with the physical toll of such an extensive surgery on the body. Additionally, they felt that patients with a "reasonably successful education, employment, and marital history" would be more motivated and successful in maintaining their weight loss [7].

Surgical Procedure

Payne and Dewind describe entry into the abdomen via a supraumbilical transverse incision. When the liver was easily accessible, a biopsy was first taken. Attention was then placed on division of the jejunum. Although there were some early variations in the length of jejunum divided and bypassed, Payne and Dewind ultimately settled on dividing the jejunum 14 in. from the ligament of Treitz. The distal end of jejunum was closed and left as a blind end. It was then fixed to the mesentery so as to help prevent intussusception. The proximal end of jejunum was anastomosed to the ileum 4 in. proximal to the ileocecal valve in an end-to-side fashion (Fig. 4.1). Following this, the remainder of the abdomen was inspected and an appendectomy, cholecystectomy, hysterectomy, and umbilical herniorrhaphy were performed when indicated. All procedures were performed under general anesthesia [7].

In 1971, building on the experience of Payne and Dewind, Scott et al. described their successes with a slight variation on the original jejunoileal bypass [8]. A handful of patients who had undergone jejunoileal bypass suffered from a failure to lose a satisfactory amount of weight. Radiologic studies were undertaken that demonstrated "hypertrophy, dilation, and elongation" of the jejunoileal bypass, as well as reflux of barium into the bypassed ileum. With this in mind, Scott et al. determined that by completely dividing the ileum, reflux would no longer occur resulting in an adequate amount of malabsorption to allow for further weight loss. Thus the jejunum was divided 12 in. from the ligament of Treitz with the distal end of jejunum closed and left as a blind end. The ileum was then divided 12 in. proximal to the ileocecal valve. The proximal end of jejunum was anastomosed to the distal end of ileum in an end-to-end fashion. Finally, the proximal end of transected ileum was anastomosed to either the transverse or sigmoid colon to allow for drainage of the bypassed segment of small intestine (Fig. 4.2).

Fig. 4.1 Jejunoileal bypass (Payne technique). (Courtesy of Mojdeh S. Kappus, M.D.)

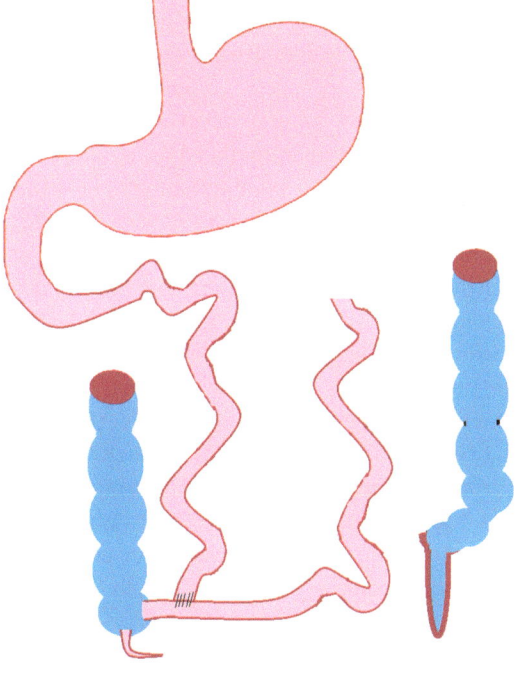

Fig. 4.2 Jejunoileal
bypass (Scott
technique). (Courtesy of
Mojdeh S. Kappus,
M.D.)

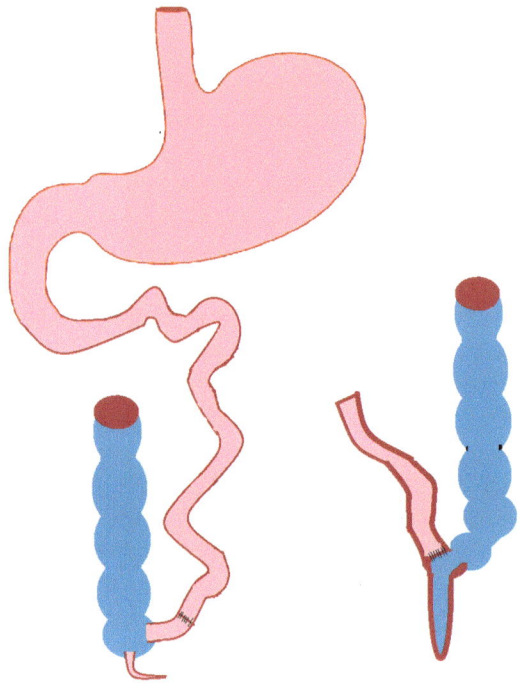

Outcomes

The jejunoileal bypass procedure was performed throughout the 1960s and 1970s for the treatment of morbid obesity with great success in helping patients achieve their ideal body weight and resolution of many comorbid conditions; however, many patients also suffered severe side effects. Similar to those who underwent jejunocolic bypass, patients suffered gastrointestinal symptoms including chronic diarrhea, anal excoriation, and flatulence [9–11]. They also suffered from electrolyte and vitamin deficiencies [12], dehydration, gall bladder disease, arthropathy, nephrolithiasis and in some cases renal failure secondary to hyperoxaluria and increased absorption of oxalate in the colon [13]. Patients also suffered from bacterial overgrowth or "bypass enteritis" in the long segment of bypassed small intestine [14]. Endotoxins released from these bacteria led to acute liver failure, cirrhosis, and even death in some patients [15].

Follow-Up

It is estimated that approximately 25,000 patients underwent jejunoileal bypass from the late 1960s to early 1980s [16]. Although many of these patients have had revisional surgery to restore intestinal continuity or to undergo gastric bypass, in rare circumstances, patients who have maintained their jejunoileal bypass may be encountered [17].

In a 20-year follow-up study of 141 patients who underwent jejunoileal bypass from 1973 to 1979, approximately 25% of patients had undergone reconstitution of bowel continuity due to various side effects and 5% had died. Of those remaining patients who had not been lost to follow-up the majority had maintained a relatively stable weight, typically having reached a plateau 2 years postoperatively. On average, patients who underwent jejunoileal bypass lost approximately 50 kg and maintained a weight of approximately 85 kg. Seventy percent of patients surveyed said they were satisfied with the results of their surgery [18].

Physicians caring for these patients must be aware of the numerous side effects of jejunoileal bypass [19]. Routine liver biopsy should be performed at regular intervals. Electrolytes and vitamin levels must be monitored and repleted as indicated. Patients should be monitored for signs of osteomalacia, nephrolithiasis, and renal failure. Chronic diarrhea may require pharmacologic treatment. Additionally, antibiotics may be administered intermittently for treatment of bypass enteritis or bacterial overgrowth.

It has been postulated that due to the increased exposure of the colonic mucosa to increased bile acids after jejunoileal bypass, risk of colorectal cancer may be increased in these patients. Animal models [20, 21] have demonstrated increased dysplasia and tumor formation in the colon following jejunoileal bypass; however, this has not been substantiated in follow-up of human subjects [22]. Interestingly, the jejunoileal bypass anatomy proved to be useful in one patient who on workup for anemia was unable to undergo a full colonoscopy due to tortuosity of the colon at the hepatic flexure. In this case, peroral small bowel enteroscopy was performed through the bypass, traversing the ileocecal valve and revealing an ulcerated mass in the cecum with biopsies consistent with adenocarcinoma [23].

Patients who have maintained their jejunoileal bypass should be counseled to consider revision to a safer procedure such as gastric bypass [24]. This however may also present challenges, especially in patients with severe malnutrition and electrolytes disturbances [25]. In one case report, a patient undergoing revision from jejunoileal bypass to sleeve gastrectomy was found to have brown bowel syndrome, a rare condition in which the bowel becomes atrophied and brown due to lipofuscin pigment deposition into the smooth muscle cells [26]. The likely pathogenesis of this condition is related to severe malnutrition. Reports such as this serve as a reminder of how little is truly known about the long-term effects of jejunoileal bypass and the implications for further surgical management of these patients.

Loop Gastric Bypass

The loop gastric bypass or loop gastrojejunostomy was first described by Mason and Ito in 1967 [27]. Using the knowledge they had gleaned from patients who had undergone hemigastrectomy and antral exclusions in the treatment of peptic ulcer disease, Mason and Ito determined that the "ideal operation" for obese patients should be restrictive but not as devastatingly malabsorptive as the alternatively described bariatric procedures of the time. They also found that by retaining the antrum and duodenum and either bypassing or excluding them rather than removing them from the body, they also maintained their inhibitory effects on gastric secretion. After confirming their suspicions with multiple animal studies, Mason and Ito performed the first loop gastrojejunostomy for morbid obesity in a 50-year-old woman with hypertension and a body mass index of 43. Notably, the operation was largely undertaken so as to reduce her body mass to improve her chances of eventually undergoing a successful hernia repair [27].

Surgical Procedure

Mason and Ito eventually performed a loop gastrojejunostomy on eight patients. They approached the abdominal cavity via either a midline or subcostal incision. They divided the gastric body horizontally leaving an estimated 20% of volume to accommodate food intake. A loop of jejunum was then brought up approximately 24 in. from the ligament of Treitz and anastomosed to the gastric pouch (Fig. 4.3). Over time, this procedure eventually evolved into the modern-day gastric bypass, now considered the gold standard of bariatric surgery [28, 29]. In 1997, a slight variation of this procedure was developed, known as the mini-gastric bypass or omega-loop gastric bypass [30]. In 2001, Rutledge reported a series of over a 1000 patients who had undergone the procedure with weight loss results comparable to the Roux-en-Y gastric bypass and sleeve gastrectomy. Entry into the

Fig. 4.3 Loop gastric bypass (Mason technique). (Courtesy of S. Mojdeh Kappus, M.D.)

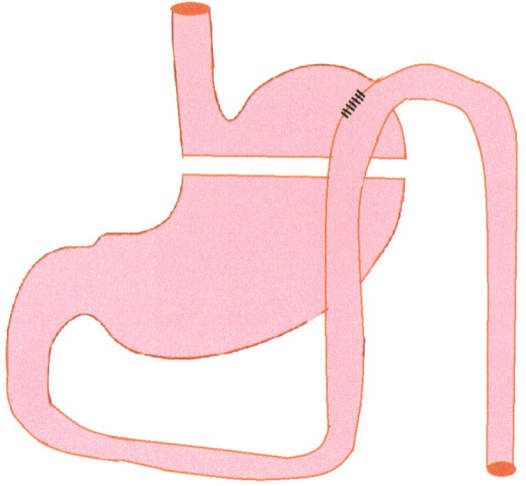

abdomen was gained laparoscopically after which the stomach was divided at the junction of the body and antrum. The stomach is then further divided vertically along an Ewald tube. Following this, the jejunum is measured approximately 200 cm from the ligament of Treitz. It is then brought up anterior to the colon and the side of the small bowel is anastomosed to the gastric pouch. In comparison to Mason and Ito's originally described loop gastrojejunostomy, the length of the biliopancreatic limb is greater in the mini-gastric bypass and the gastric pouch is stapled vertically rather than horizontally, thus excluding the fundus [27]. According to Rutledge, eliminating the fundus from the gastric pouch prevents future dilation and weight regain. Additionally, Rutledge felt that horizontal division of the stomach caused increased bile reflux through the gastroesophageal junction. This was thought to be lessened by vertical division of the stomach [30].

Outcomes

Mason's loop gastrojejunostomy has been revised over time and is considered the predecessor of the modern gastric bypass. This procedure has successfully helped hundreds of thousands morbidly obese patients lose weight with resolution of their comorbidities [31, 32]. Follow-up of mini-gastric bypass patients by Rutledge et al. has revealed similar early successes with the procedure. The mini-gastric bypass can now be performed at an average operating time of a little over 30 min, with a typical 1–2 day hospital length of stay. According to Rutledge, 30-day mortality and complications rates are nearly equivalent to the gastric bypass procedure. The most common complications following mini-gastric bypass were dyspepsia and ulcers at approximately 5% [33].

Follow-Up

There are now thousands of reported cases of patients who have undergone the mini-gastric bypass. The procedure is performed in some centers in the United States, but has gained more popularity in Europe [34]. Proponents of the mini-gastric bypass have noted that the risks are comparable to the Roux-en-Y gastric bypass and include vitamin deficiencies, pouch and stoma dilation leading to weight regain, internal hernia, anastomotic leak, and gall bladder disease. In terms of weight reduction, mini-gastric bypass may result in equal or more weight loss than the Roux-en-Y gastric bypass and has been successful in achieving resolution of many comorbid conditions [35]. One notable advantage of the mini-gastric bypass is that it only requires one anastomosis. Widespread implementation of the procedure has been slow due to concerns regarding bile reflux, afferent limb obstruction, potential for increased risk of gastritis, esophagitis, and possibly gastroesophageal cancer, marginal ulcer formation, and a higher degree of malabsorption than is seen in gastric bypass [36–38]. The majority of patients who have undergone this procedure, however, report success with their weight loss with few complications.

Horizontal Gastroplasty

Printen and Mason first described horizontal gastroplasty for the treatment of morbid obesity in 1973. Rather than achieving weight loss through malabsorption as in the jejunoileal bypass, gastroplasty restricted the intake of food by decreasing the functional size of the stomach without completely closing off the upper gastrointestinal tract.

Horizontal gastroplasty consisted of stapling across the upper portion of the stomach into a small pouch leaving only a small communicating stoma at the greater curvature (Fig. 4.4). Printen and Mason originally considered patients for horizontal gastroplasty who were under 40 years old

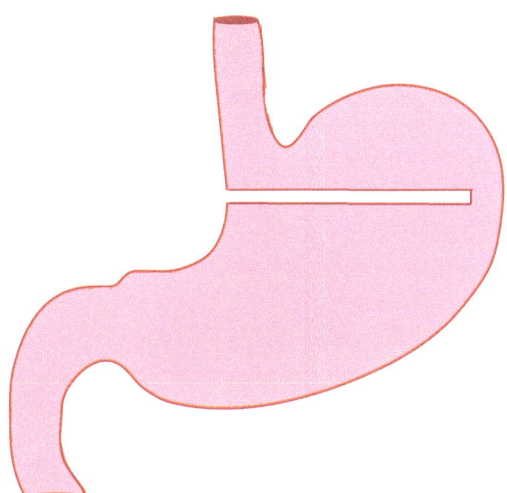

Fig. 4.4 Horizontal gastroplasty. (Courtesy of Mojdeh S. Kappus, M.D.)

with a weight that equaled or exceeded twice their ideal body weight. Patients must have attempted and failed weight loss with strict dietary control.

Surgical Procedure

The original horizontal gastroplasty involved division of the upper portion of the stomach from the lesser curvature towards the greater curvature leaving only a 1.0–1.5 cm channel between the upper and lower gastric pouches. A gastrostomy tube was placed in the antrum for feeding in case of postoperative edema causing obstruction.

Outcomes

Printen and Mason cited a lower mortality rate in their study group of 56 horizontal gastroplasties performed over a 7-year period in comparison to the gastric bypass, however, openly acknowledged inherent difficulties with the surgery and postoperative course [39]. Although designed to promote weight loss, the horizontal staple line was based on operations for peptic ulcer disease designed to facilitate postoperative weight gain. Accordingly, the fundal pouch was prone to stretching and many patients were ultimately able to regain weight by consuming high calorie beverages, emphasizing the importance of patient compliance and understanding with restrictive procedures. In 1987, Knol et al. reported less than a quarter of patients achieved a weight less than 50% above ideal body weight after 2–3 years. Twenty-five percent of patients experienced stomal dilatation resulting in no weight loss at all or even excess weight gain, and stomal stenosis was seen in four patients [40].

Follow-Up

Over the next decade, surgeons sought to improve the horizontal gastroplasty. Gomez proposed stabilizing the greater curvature stoma with circumferential nonabsorbable sutures to create a "pseudo-pylorus" [41]. This modification limited fundal distention, however led to early obstruction, suture migration, and difficulty visualizing the stoma via endoscopy. Long and Collins maintained the horizontal staple line, but placed the stoma along the lesser curvature [42]. Pace et al. described a "gastric partition" procedure with division of the stomach medially and laterally, leaving a central stoma [43] (Fig. 4.5).

Vertical Banded Gastroplasty

Experiences gleaned from the horizontal gastroplasty led to the realization that the fundus was too placid to achieve long-term restriction of food intake [44]. Tretbar and Sifers described a gastroplasty in which they migrated the staple line to the angle of His, extending inferiorly into the gastric body, a procedure described as a fundal exclusion [45]. In 1980, Mason introduced the vertical banded gastroplasty as it is known today. In addition to a vertical staple line, he placed a polypropylene mesh collar, traversing both stomach walls, around the outlet [46]. Later procedures replaced the mesh collar with an external silastic ring [47].

Surgical Procedure

After years of perfecting the vertical banded gastroplasty, Mason published a comprehensive review of the procedure and its evolution in 1998, 16 years after he had originally described it [48]. Ultimately, the procedure he recommended begins with folding the lesser curvature of the stomach around either a 28 French nasogastric tube or 32 French Ewald tube. The circular staple is then fired adjacent to the tube to create a window in the stomach, with careful attention paid to avoiding tension on the staple line or lesser curve. A linear staple is then used to create the gastric pouch. Although the original gastric pouch length was 9 cm, reflecting the full length of the linear stapler, Mason noted better outcomes with a staple line 4–6 cm in length, with a pouch volume of 20 mL. He found that the smaller, cylindrical pouch created less wall tension in accordance with the law of LaPlace. Mason preferred stapling in continuity rather than transecting the stomach, which, he felt, would increase the potential for infection of the Marlex mesh [49]. Others have argued however that transection of the stomach prevents staple line degradation that could subsequently lead to gastro-gastric fistula (GGF) [50]. After pouch construction, the Marlex

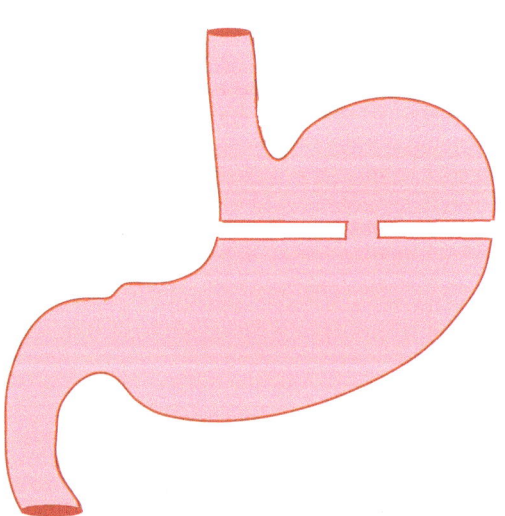

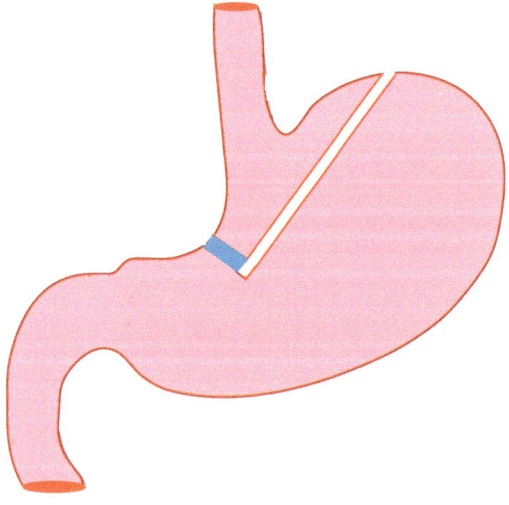

Fig. 4.5 Horizontal gastroplasty ("gastric partition"). (Courtesy of Mojdeh S. Kappus, M.D.)

Fig. 4.6 Vertical banded gastroplasty. (Courtesy of Mojdeh S. Kappus, M.D.)

mesh collar was placed, forming the outlet of the pouch (Fig. 4.6). Marlex mesh was chosen based on prior studies by Kroyer and Grace, who experimented with suture fixation on the greater curvature during the early years of the horizontal gastric bypass [51, 52]. Mason preferred Marlex mesh to silastic rings because he felt it to be less prone to slippage and obstruction [53, 54].

Outcomes

Initial outcomes of vertical gastroplasty varied greatly depending on surgical approach to pouch size and the material and technique chosen for outlet fixation. Mason emphasized the need to educate patients on proper eating habits and imparting on them and understanding of the size of their gastric pouch in increasing their chances of success [55]. Long-term follow-up of vertical banded gastroplasty patients revealed moderate to high success rates in helping morbidly obese patients achieve significant weight loss. At 2-year follow-up, approximately 70% of patients achieved at least 50% excess weight loss. Many patients, however, began to demonstrate slight increases in their weight at 5- and 10-year follow-up [55]. Side effects of gastroplasty in particular included vomiting, bezoar obstruction, outlet stenosis and obstruction, staple line breakdown, band erosion, mesh erosion or migration, mega-esophagus, and gastroesophageal reflux disease, in addition to staple line leaks, and fistula formation [56–59].

Follow-Up

Vertical banded gastroplasty faded from the armamentarium of the bariatric surgeon in the 1990s as patients with initially promising weight loss began to lose their momentum [60–62]. These patients may still be encountered and may require revisional bariatric surgery or therapeutic endoscopic procedures. Balsiger et al. described successful conversion from vertical banded gastroplasty to Roux-en-Y gastric bypass in 25 patients suffering from symptomatic gastro-esophageal reflux disease. Approximately 3 years later, 96% reported no reflux symptoms and achieved an average decrease in body mass index from 33 to 28 kg/m^2 [63]. Revisional procedures however must be performed with caution as complication rates have been reported to be as high as 40% [64]. In addition to gastroesophageal reflux, vertical banded gastroplasty patients may also present with outlet stenosis requiring endoscopic dilation [65]. Success of endoscopic dilation was temporary as the foreign body of the band still remained. Band erosion may also require endoscopic or laparoscopic removal.

Conclusion

The surgical treatment of morbid obesity has continued to evolve since the first jejunocolic bypass was described by Payne and Dewind [1] in 1963. It is important for physicians caring for patients that had undergone these early bariatric surgeries to understand their potential metabolic side effects and surgical complications. Although the majority of these procedures have been abandoned or revised, the principles on which they were developed have become the bedrock of the field of bariatric surgery.

References

1. Payne JH, DeWind LT, Commons RR. Metabolic observations in patients with jejunocolic shunts. Am J Surg. 1963;106:273–89.
2. Kremen AN, Linner JH, Nelson CH. Experimental evaluation of the nutritional importance of proximal and distal small intestine. Ann Surg. 1954;140(3):439–48.
3. Lewis LA, Turnbull RB, Page IH. Effects of jejunocolic shunt on obesity, serum lipoproteins, lipids, and electrolytes. Arch Intern Med. 1996;117(1):4–16.
4. Shibata HR, MacKenzie JR, Long RC. Metabolic effects of controlled jejunocolic bypass. Arch Surg. 1967;95(3):413–28.
5. Mir-Madjlessi SH, MacKenzie AH, Winkelman EL. Articular complications in obese patients after jejunocolic bypass. Cleve Clin Q. 1974;41(3):119–33.
6. Williams ER. Gastro-colic and gastro-jejuno-colic fistula. Br J Radiol. 2014;14(157):36–40.
7. Payne JH, DeWind LT. Surgical treatment of obesity. Am J Surg. 1969;118(2):141–7.

8. Scott HW, Sandstead HH, Brill AB, Burko H, Younger RK. Experience with a new technique of intestinal bypass in the treatment of morbid obesity. Ann Surg. 1971;147(4):560–71.

9. DeWind LT, Payne JH. Intestinal bypass surgery for morbid obesity: long term results. JAMA. 1976;236(20):2298–301.

10. Pi-Sunyer F. Jejunoileal bypass surgery for obesity. Am J Clin Nutr. 1976;29(4):409–16.

11. Kirkpatrick JR. Jejunoileal bypass. Arch Surg. 1987;122(5):610–4.

12. Halverson JD, Scheff RJ, Gentry K, Alpers DH. Jejunoileal bypass; late metabolic sequelae and weight gain. Am J Surg. 1980;140(3):347–50.

13. Mole DR, Tomson CR, Mortenson N, Winearls CG. Renal complications of jejuno-ileal bypass for obesity. Q J Med. 2001;94(2):69–77.

14. Requarth JA, Burchard KW, Colacchio TA, Stukel TA, Mott LA, Greenberg R, Weismann RE. Long-term morbidity following jejunoileal bypass. Arch Surg. 1995;130(3):318–25.

15. Lowell JA, Shenoy S, Ghalib R, Caldwell C, White FV, Peters M, et al. Liver transplantation after jejunoileal bypass for morbid obesity. J Am Coll Surg. 1997;185(2):123–7.

16. Deitel M, Shahi B, Anand PK, Deitel FH, Cardinell DL. Long term outcome in a series of jejunoileal bypass patients. Obes Surg. 1993;3(3):247–52.

17. Singh D, Laya AS, Clarkston Clarkston WK, Allen MJ. Jejunoileal bypass: a surgery of the past and a review of its complications. World J Gastroenterol. 2009;15(18):2277–9.

18. Jørgensen S, Olesen M, Gudman-Høyer E. A review of 20 years of jejunoileal bypass. Scand J Gastroenterol. 1997;32(4):334–9.

19. Herbert C. Intestinal bypass for obesity. Can Fam Physician. 1975;21(7):56–9.

20. Bristol JB, Wells M, Williamson RC. Adaptation to jejunoileal bypass promotes experimental colorectal carcinogenesis. Br J Surg. 1984;71(2):123–6.

21. McFarland RJ, Talbot RW, Woolf N, Gazet JC. Dysplasia of the colon after jejuno-ileal bypass. Br J Surg. 1987;74(1):21–2.

22. Sylvan A, Sjölund B, Janunger KG, Rutegård J, Stenling R, Roos G. Colorectal cancer risk after jejunoileal bypass: dysplasia and DNA content in long-time follow-up of patients operated on for morbid obesity. Dis Colon Rectum. 1992;35(3):245–8.

23. Burton JR, Katon R. Anterograde colonoscopy: per oral diagnosis of colon cancer with an enteroscope in a man with a jejunoileal bypass. Gastrointest Endosc. 2003;57(7):982–3.

24. Griffen WO, Young VL, Stevenson CC. A prospective comparison of gastric and jejunoileal bypass procedures for morbid obesity. Ann Surg. 1977;186(4):500–9.

25. Scott HW Jr, Dean RH, Harrison JS, Gluck FW. Metabolic complications of jejunoileal bypass operations for morbid obesity. Annu Rev Med. 1976;27:397–405.

26. Lee H, Carlin AM, Ormsby AH, Lee MW. Brown bowel syndrome secondary to jejunoileal bypass: the first case report. Obes Surg. 2009;19(8):1176–9.

27. Mason EE, Ito C. Gastric bypass in obesity. Obes Res. 1996;4(3):316–9.

28. Deitel M, Shikora SA. The development of the surgical treatment of morbid obesity. J Am Coll Nutr. 2002;21(5):365–71.

29. Fobi MA, Lee H, Holness R, Cabinda D. Gastric bypass operation for obesity. World J Surg. 1998;22(9):925–35.

30. Rutledge R. The mini gastric bypass: experience with the first 1,274 cases. Obes Surg. 2001;11(3):276–80.

31. Deitel M. Overview of operations for morbid obesity. World J Surg. 1998;22(9):913–8.

32. Moshiri M, Osman S, Robinson TJ, Khandelwal S, Bhargava P, Rohrmann CA. Evolution of bariatric surgery: a historical perspective. Am J Roentgenol. 2013;201(1):W40–8.

33. Rutledge R, Walsh TR. Continued excellent results with the mini-gastric bypass: six-year study in 2,410 patients. Obes Surg. 2005;15(9):1304–8.

34. Mahawar KK, Kumar P, Carr WR, Jennings N, Schroeder N, Balupuri S, et al. Current status of mini-gastric bypass. J Minim Access Surg. 2016;12(4):305–10.

35. Alden JF. Gastric and jejunoileal bypass: a comparison in treatment of morbid obesity. Arch Surg. 1977;112(7):799–806.

36. Mahawar K, Carr WR, Balupuri S, Small PK. Controversy surrounding 'mini' gastric bypass. Obes Surg. 2014;24(2):324–33.

37. Fisher BL, Buchwald H, Clark W, et al. Mini-gastric bypass controversy. Obes Surg. 2001;11(6):773–7.

38. McCarthy HB, Rucker RD, Chan EK, Rupp WM, Snover D, Goodale RL, et al. Gastritis after gastric bypass surgery. Surgery. 1985;98(1):68–71.

39. Printen KJ, Mason EE. Gastric surgery for relief of morbid obesity. Arch Surg. 1973;106(4):28–31.

40. Knol JA, Strodel WE, Eckhauser FE. Critical appraisal of horizontal gastroplasty. Am J Surg. 1987;153(3):256–61.

41. Gomez CA. Gastroplasty in the surgical treatment of morbid obesity. Am J Clin Nutr. 1980;33(2 Suppl):406–15.

42. Long M, Collins JP. The technique and early results of high gastric reduction for obesity. Aust N Z J Surg. 1980;50(2):146–9.

43. Pace WG, Martin EW, Tetirick T, Fabri PJ, Carey LC. Gastric partitioning for morbid obesity. Ann Surg. 1979;190(3):392–400.

44. Fabito DC. Gastric vertical stapling. Paper presented at: Bariatric Surgery Colloquim; 1 Jun 1981, Iowa City, IA, USA.

45. Tretbar LL, Sifers EC. Vertical stapling: a new type of gastroplasty (abstract). Int J Obes. 1981;5:538.

46. Mason EE. Vertical banded gastroplasty for obesity. Arch Surg. 1982;117(5):701–6.
47. Laws HL. Standardized gastroplasty orifice. Ann J Surg. 1981;141(3):393–4.
48. Mason EE, Doherty C, Cullen JJ, Scott D, Rodriguez EM, Maher JW. Vertical gastroplasty: evolution of vertical banded gastroplasty. World J Surg. 1998;22(9):919–24.
49. Fobi MA. Surgical treatment of obesity: a review. J Natl Med Assoc. 2004;96(1):61–75.
50. Kawamura I, Miyazawa Y, Yamazaki K, Chen CC, Bono K. Complications of vertical banded gastroplasty and its modified operative mode, K-gastroplasty: a preliminary report. Obes Surg. 1993;3(1):69–74.
51. Kroyer J. Horizontal gastroplasty with gastropexy for treatment of morbid obesity. Paper presented at: symposium on surgical treatment of obesity; 1984; Los Angeles, CA, USA.
52. Grace DM. Gastric restriction procedures for treating severe obesity. Am J Clin Nutr. 1992;55(2 Suppl):556S–9S.
53. Alper D, Ramadan E, Vishne T, Belavsky R, Avraham Z, Seror D, et al. Silastic ring vertical gastroplasty-long term results and complications. Obes Surg. 2000;10(3):250–4.
54. Eckhout GV, Willbanks OL. Vertical ring gastroplasty for morbid obesity: five year experience with 1,463 patients. Am J Surg. 1986;152(6):713–6.
55. Mason EE, Cullen JJ. Management of complications in vertical banded gastroplasty. Curr Surg. 2003;60(1):33–7.
56. Deitel M, Jones BA, Petrov I, Wlodarczyk SR, Basi S. Vertical banded gastroplasty: results in 233 patients. Can J Surg. 1986;29(5):322–4.
57. MacLean LD, Rhode BM, Samplin J, Forse RA. Results of the surgical treatment of obesity. Am J Surg. 1993;165(1):155–60; discussion 160–2.
58. Wynne-Jones G. Vertical ligated gastroplasty; ten years' follow-up in treatment of morbid obesity. Paper presented at: symposium on surgical treatment of obesity; 1990; Los Angeles, CA, USA.
59. Chua TY, Mendiola RM. Laparoscopic vertical banded gastroplasty: the Milwaukee experience. Obes Surg. 1995;5(1):77–80.
60. Fobi MA, Fleming AW. Vertical banded gastroplasty versus gastric bypass in treatment of obesity. J Natl Med Assoc. 1984;78:1092–8.
61. Sugarman HK, Laudrey GL, Kellum JM. Weight loss with vertical banded gastroplasty and roux-en-Y gastric bypass for morbid obesity with selective versus random assignment. Am J Surg. 1989;157:93–102.
62. Fobi MA. Vertical banded gastroplasty vs. gastric bypass: 10 years follow up. Obes Surg. 1993;3(2):161–4.
63. Balsiger BM. Gastroesophageal reflux after intact vertical banded gastroplasty: correction by conversion to roux-en-Y gastric bypass. J Gastrointest Surg. 2000;4(3):276–81.
64. Forse RA, Deitel M, Maclean LD. Revision of horizontal gastroplasty by vertical banded gastroplasty. Can J Surg. 1988;31(2):118–20.
65. Wayman CS, Nord HJ, Combs WM, Rosemurgy SR. The role of endoscopy after vertical banded gastroplasty. Gastrointest Endosc. 1992;38(1):44–6.

Anatomy of Commonly Performed Bariatric Procedures

Matthew T. Allemang and Kevin M. El-Hayek

Introduction

With the growing number of patients undergoing bariatric procedures, there is an added importance for the endoscopist to comprehend the complex issues surrounding this patient population. Endoscopy is a necessary tool for the evaluation and treatment of these patients and considerations must be made regarding safe sedation and expected findings in obese patients during the preoperative, intraoperative, and postoperative periods. Many bariatric patients have diagnosed and undiagnosed obstructive sleep apnea (OSA) for which there are a number of tools to help identify and modify periprocedural risks [1–4]. The current American Society for Gastrointestinal Endoscopy (ASGE) guidelines currently recommend consideration of anesthesia assistance for patients with obesity or OSA [5]. The use of preoperative endoscopic assessment of the bariatric surgery candidate has undergone a dramatic evolution. Many surgeons previously recommended routine preoperative upper endoscopy for all patients. However, studies over the years have revealed minimal benefit to this practice. Some societies, including the American Association of Clinical Endocrinologists (AACE), The Obesity Society (TOS), and American Society of Metabolic and Bariatric Surgery (ASMBS), recommend to perform preoperative upper endoscopy in the setting of significant gastrointestinal symptoms [6–8]. The remainder of this chapter will add to the endoscopists' understanding of this expanding population of patients in both the intraoperative and postoperative setting and cover the common anatomic findings of the adjustable gastric banding (AGB), Roux-en-Y gastric bypass (RYGB), vertical sleeve gastrectomy (VSG), and biliopancreatic diversion with duodenal switch (BPD-DS).

M.T. Allemang, M.D.
Section of Surgical Endoscopy, Department of General Surgery, Digestive Disease and Surgery Institute, Cleveland Clinic Foundation, 9500 Euclid Ave, Cleveland, OH 44195, USA
e-mail: alleman@ccf.org

K.M. El-Hayek, M.D. (✉)
Section of Surgical Endoscopy, Department of General Surgery, Digestive Disease and Surgery Institute, Cleveland Clinic Foundation, 9500 Euclid Ave, Cleveland, OH 44195, USA

Cleveland Clinic Lerner College of Medicine, Case Western Reserve University, 9500 Euclid Ave, Mail Code A-100, Cleveland, OH 44195, USA
e-mail: elhayek@ccf.org

Intraoperative Endoscopy

The evidence for intraoperative endoscopy, much like that for preoperative endoscopy in the obese patient population, consists mostly of cohort studies and personal experience in both RYGB and sleeve gastrectomy. The potential advantages for intraoperative endoscopy are as follows: direct inspection of anatomic configuration, ability to identify endoluminal bleeding or stenosis, and in some cases to perform endoscopic leak testing of the proximal intestinal reconstruction. There are a few studies encompassing the use of intraoperative endoscopy during bariatric surgery. Shin et al. reported a 326 consecutive laparoscopic RYGB (LRYGB) experience with intraoperative saline emersion and endoscopic pneumatic testing and reported no gastrojejunal (GJ) leaks [9]. Haddad et al. describe their experience with intraoperative endoscopic leak testing in 2311 patients undergoing LRYGB. A positive leak was detected in 80 patients (3.5%) though only 46 were reproducible or sustained air leak that required suture line reinforcement. Of these reinforced anastomoses, two patients went on to have clinical leaks that were managed conservatively. The cohort also resulted in two patients with false negative intraoperative leak tests that were discovered later [10]. This concept of non-reproducible air leaks was corroborated by Kligman at the University of Maryland, who reported a 257 consecutive LRYGB experience with 13 (5.1%) having persistent air leaks and 12 (4.7%) having non-reproducible air leaks during pneumatic endoscopic testing [11]. The difference between these two results was speculated to relate to laparoscopic air trapping behind loops of bowel or other organs that temporarily caused air bubbling during the endoscopic pneumatic leak testing. Finally amongst the LRYGB data, Al Hadad et al. had a positive intraoperative endoscopic air leak test in 1.75% of 342 LRYGB. Of these 46 underwent attempts at intraoperative location and reinforcement that still resulted in two postoperative leaks. They simultaneously reported two clinical leaks occurring in patients with negative intraoperative testing. This resulted in a 75% positive predictive value and 75% negative predictive value [12].

Intraoperative endoscopy during sleeve gastrectomy has been less well studied. Nimeri et al. looked at their experience with intraoperative endoscopy for laparoscopic sleeve gastrectomy and found a clinically significant stenosis in 3.2% requiring removal of imbricating sutures, though they did not report any long-term results of sleeve stenosis [13]. In 2008, Frezza et al. reported use of a 29Fr endoscope during construction of 20 laparoscopic sleeve gastrectomies [14]. A similar work by Diamantis et al. reported a series of 25 patients that had a sleeve gastrectomy with the aid of an endoscope instead of bougie [15].

Technical Considerations During Intraoperative Endoscopy

Intraoperative endoscopy is often more challenging than outpatient endoscopy for a number of reasons. First, patients will typically be in a supine position and intubated at the time of the evaluation, versus in a left lateral decubitus position when performed under moderate sedation in the preoperative setting. Also, depending on the severity of the obesity, esophageal intubation may be hindered at the cricopharyngeus due to obesity at the neck level. Several simple maneuvers will aid in the successful intraoperative evaluation during all bariatric operations. Initial consideration should be made to appropriately set up the room with the endoscopic tower or boom situated close to the patient's mouth. Typically a standard front-viewing endoscope is sufficient to perform the endoscopy and will give adequate detail during the evaluation. Excellent communication between the endoscopist and anesthesiologist is paramount. An initial request should be made to remove orogastric tubes, esophageal temperature probes, and other oral/ nasal devices. Following complete removal of all extra tubes, a bite block can be placed around the endotracheal tube. If an upper body-warming blanket is on, this should be turned off and the drapes around the patient's face loosened so the endoscopist can access the mouth easily. Finally, during initial passage of the endoscope, a generous jaw thrust and lubrication on the endoscope shaft is extremely helpful. Head and neck position should be in the neutral or somewhat extended position and avoidance of extensive neck flexion will aid in access to the oral cavity and passage through the upper esophageal sphincter. Performing endoscopy with the patient in a supine position may disorient the endoscopist who is more familiar with outpatient endoscopy, so it is critical to position the monitor in front of the proceduralist.

Postoperative Upper Endoscopy

Endoscopy after bariatric surgery should begin with a thorough history and physical and clinical evaluation, which is often augmented by a high quality upper gastrointestinal series. Routine upper endoscopy after surgery, much like preoperative endoscopy, is not indicated and should be dictated by the patient's symptoms. Several authors have shown that postoperative endoscopy is safe even in the first 30 days after the bariatric procedure [16]. Expected findings and possible interventions should be discussed with the patient such as biopsy, hemostasis, clipping, suturing, or balloon dilation in the event of positive findings. These therapeutic maneuvers are discussed in greater detail in later chapters.

Laparoscopic Adjustable Gastric Band (AGB)

The AGB is a fluid-filled adjustable band that is laparoscopically placed in the upper portion of the stomach as a restrictive procedure. An access port is secured to the anterior abdominal wall for adjustment of the band and can be accessed with any large caliber needle using proper sterile technique. Fluoroscopy is employed to aid in locating the port (Fig. 5.1). Previously popular, the long-term results of LAGB have caused this particular procedure to fall out of favor and therefore these are becoming less commonly encountered [17].

A patient with an AGB will have relatively normal endoscopic esophageal anatomy, though one should be aware that complications of pouch dilation or band slippage can occur and appear similar to a hiatal hernia [18]. Band slippage has also been hypothesized to share a common pathophysiology with that of band erosion [19]. The

normal and expected finding of a successfully placed AGB is extrinsic compression several centimeters distal to the Z-line. There may also be an anterior/lateral folding of the stomach seen in the retroflexed position due to the surgeon's anterior gastropexy of the band. This configuration looks much like what is seen in patients with prior Nissen fundoplication (see Fig. 5.1). The ability of the endoscopist to access the abdominal port with or without fluoroscopy is helpful for patients complaining of dysphagia in order to endoscopically prove whether a stenosis is alleviated with saline removal from the AGB system. Other findings specific to AGB include erosion of the band or buckle through the stomach or esophagus or herniation of the stomach through the band with migration or slippage that usually be seen on plain abdominal films prior to endoscopy. Foreign body erosions are described elsewhere in this book.

Roux-en-Y Gastric Bypass (RYGB)

The RYGB is a very popular restrictive and malabsorptive procedure that can be completed open or laparoscopically [20, 21]. The fundamental portions are a small gastric pouch with gastrojejunostomy (GJ) to the enteric (Roux) limb. This limb is passed anterior to the colon (antecolic) or through transverse colon mesentery (retrocolic) and then anastomosed to the biliopancreatic limb of jejunum to form a common channel where the bile and pancreatic enzymes meet the restricted oral intake (Fig. 5.2).

During endoscopic evaluation, a normal esophagus is encountered but once through the gastroesophageal junction (GEJ) a small gastric pouch is identified. The length of the gastric pouch is typically measured from the z-line to the GJ. The enteric anastomosis is carefully inspected for signs of inflammation, stenosis, or ulceration [22, 23]. A marginal ulceration is usually seen on the jejunal side of the anastomosis and can range from small and subtle (with the primary complaint of pain) to nearly circumferential causing stenosis and dysphagia. Because some marginal ulcers can be obscured by the anastomosis, it is

Fig. 5.1 Adjustable gastric band with retroflexed endoscopic view (reprinted with permission, Cleveland Clinic Center for Medical Art & Photography ©2005–2017. All rights reserved)

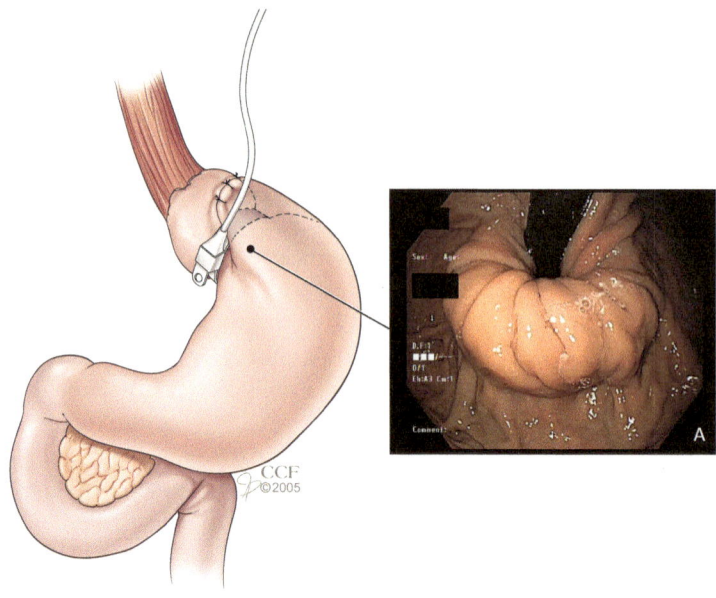

Fig. 5.2 Roux-en-Y gastric bypass with endoscopic view from (**a**) Z-line, (**b**) gastrojejunal anastomosis, (**c**) jejunojejunostomy (reprinted with permission, Cleveland Clinic Center for Medical Art & Photography ©2005–2017. All rights reserved)

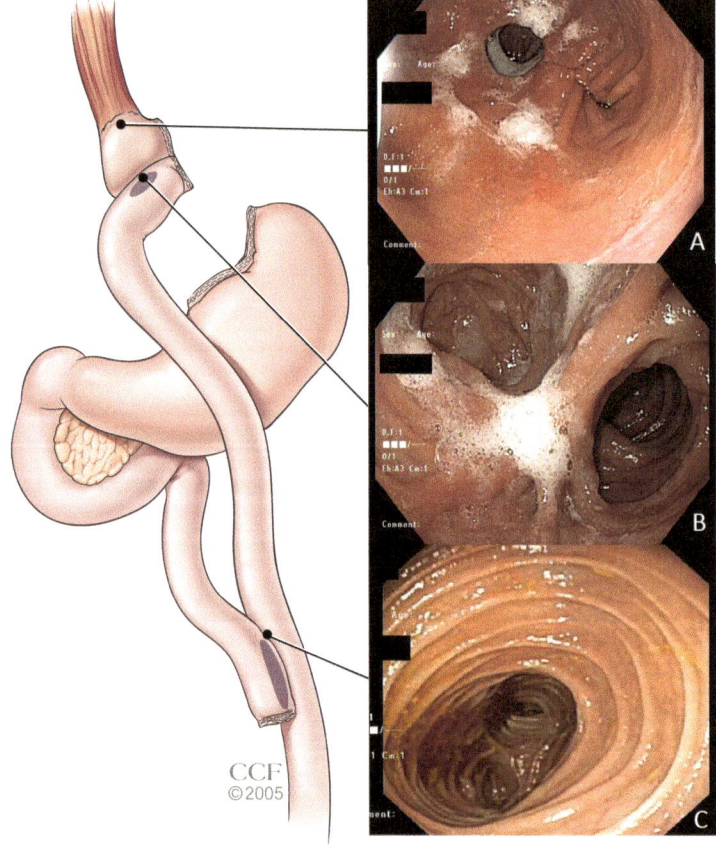

valuable to perform a retroflexion maneuver in the Roux limb to view the jejunum just distal to the anastomosis. The diameter and conformation of the GJ can vary slightly depending on the type of construction of the anastomosis (circular stapler, linear stapler, or hand sewn). The anastomotic stoma size can also change over time and should be clearly documented, as gastrojejunal stoma diameter has been implicated in weight regain for some patients [24]. Finally, a gastrogastric fistula may be encountered [25]. This abnormal connection between the gastric pouch and the remnant stomach was more common when an undivided stapling technique was used to create the gastric pouch. The size of the fistula can range from small and endoscopically undetectable to large enough for the endoscope to pass into the remnant stomach from the pouch. Hints of a fistula include bile within the gastric pouch. Common location of such a fistula is often at the angle of His. If suspected and not found, the upper endoscopy can be complimented with a contrasted upper gastrointestinal evaluation.

Due to the length of the Roux limb, the jejunojejunostomy is not routinely encountered on postoperative upper endoscopy without either push technique or through a remnant gastrostomy site (see Fig. 5.2), though one should always entertain the configuration of the Roux limb as it can be antecolic or retrocolic. In the latter configuration, the Roux limb is brought through mesentery of the transverse colon which has the possibility of an additional site for stenosis and herniation into the lesser sac that can be seen using a typical gastroscope [26].

Sleeve Gastrectomy

The laparoscopic vertical sleeve gastrectomy (VSG) has quickly gained in popularity for both patients and bariatric surgeons. This relatively short procedure offers fairly reliable and durable weight loss, as well as improvement in the related comorbidities [21, 27, 28]. The procedure consists of resecting the lateral portion of the proximal greater curve of the stomach to create a linear tube (Fig. 5.3).

The endoscopic evaluation will have normal esophageal anatomy and through the GEJ but immediately upon entering the stomach a linear, more restrictive stomach will be seen. It is important to assess the amount of fundus in the sleeve. Ideally this should be small to none. Further down the body of the stomach the interface of stomach incisura will be seen as the narrowest portion during the exam. This area is probably most important to evaluate as it can cause dysphagia and lead to gastroesophageal reflux disease in the postoperative patient. Once past the incisura, the endoscopist will enter a relatively normal antrum and pylorus. Again, in patients where a gastric twist is expected, this can often be seen well when the endoscope is retroflexed within the antrum. Mechanical obstructions and functional twists may lead to proximal dilation and stasis within the stomach and esophagus. Functional twists will often allow passage of the endoscope, but will certainly require the endoscopists to overexaggerate tip deflection and torque of the scope shaft. In addition to stenosis, the endoscopist should evaluate for linear staple line dehiscence with or without an associated abscess cavity.

Biliopancreatic Diversion with Duodenal Switch

The biliopancreatic diversion with duodenal switch (BPD-DS) is a much less common operation than those previously described but continues to be used at selected centers for patients with higher degrees of morbid obesity and many times is completed in two stages [29]. The weight loss is excellent but has a higher perioperative risk and long-term risk of protein–calorie malnutrition and vitamin deficiency. The first stage is often a vertical sleeve gastrectomy as previously described. The second stage proceeds with the dissection and division of the proximal duodenum. This is followed by creation of an alimentary limb constructed in similar fashion to the RYGB with a shorter common channel by measuring retrograde from the ileocecal valve.

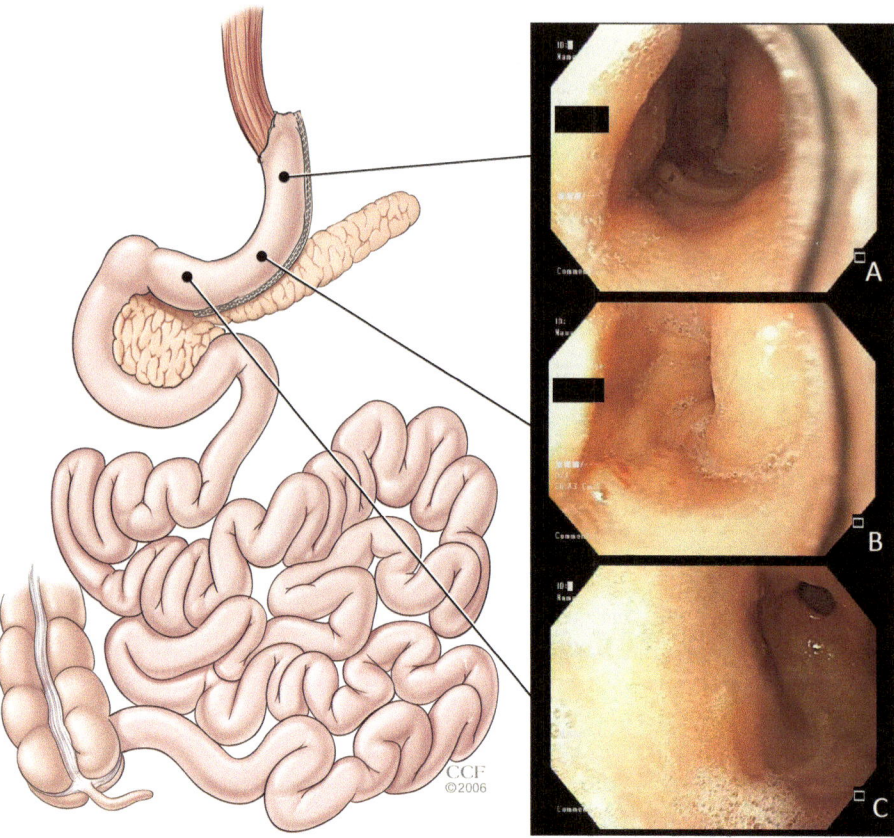

Fig. 5.3 Vertical sleeve gastrectomy with endoscopic view from (**a**) body, (**b**) incisura, (**c**) antrum (reprinted with permission, Cleveland Clinic Center for Medical Art & Photography ©2005–2017. All rights reserved)

Due to the similar proximal construction as the LSG, this endoscopic evaluation is the same and should emphasize inspection of the staple line and incisura. The difference on upper endoscopy is the duodenal-jejunal anastomosis created just past the pylorus (Fig. 5.4). Endoscopic evaluation is similar to that of the GJ in the RYGB evaluating for stenosis and ulceration. Finally, the enteroenterostomy is difficult to evaluate endoscopically without push techniques and is rarely necessary.

Conclusion

With the growing popularity of bariatric procedures, more and more endoscopists will encounter these patients and be asked to evaluate their postoperative anatomy. It is important to understand both the normal and pathologic evaluation of these patients. Further pathologic findings subsequent to therapeutic techniques are provided in later chapters.

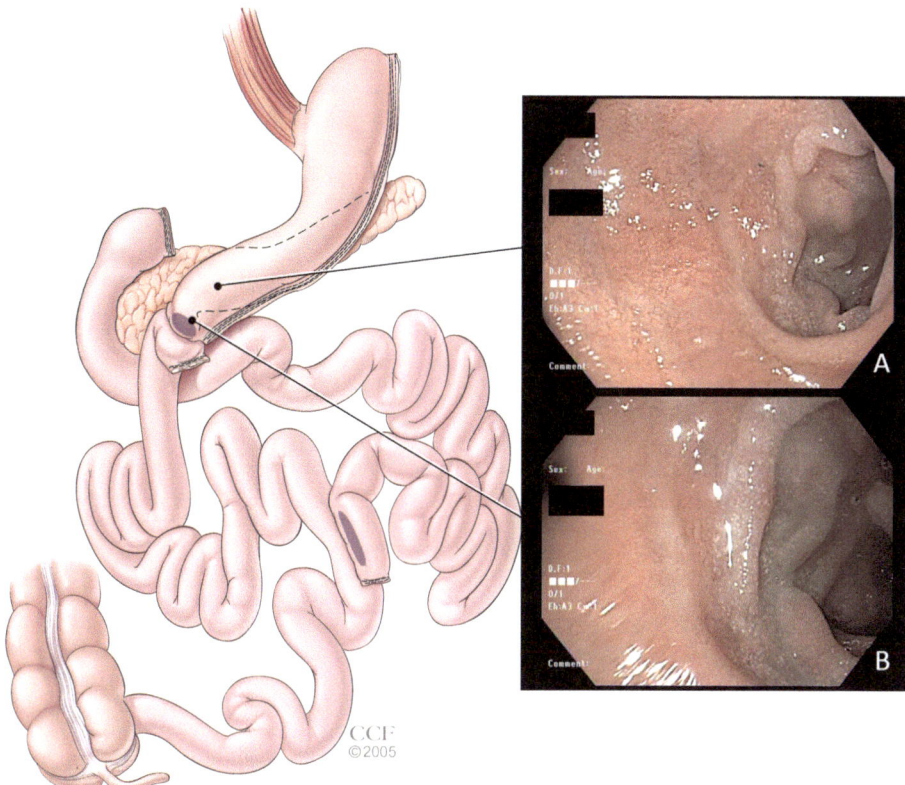

Fig. 5.4 (**a**) Proximal bulb view of duodenojejunostomy. (**b**) Close view of duodenojejunostomy anastomosis. Biliopancreatic diversion with duodenal switch with two endoscopic views of the duodeno-ileal anastomosis. The other endoscopic views are the same as a vertical sleeve gastrectomy (reprinted with permission, Cleveland Clinic Center for Medical Art & Photography ©2005–2017. All rights reserved)

References

1. Nagappa M, Wong J, Singh M, Wong DT, Chung F. An update on the various practical applications of the STOP-Bang questionnaire in anesthesia, surgery, and perioperative medicine. Curr Opin Anaesthesiol. 2017;20(1):118–25.
2. Chung F, Yang Y, Liao P. Predictive performance of the stop-bang score for identifying obstructive sleep apnea in obese patients. Obes Surg. 2013;23(12):2050–7.
3. Coté GA, Hovis CE, Hovis RM, Waldbaum L, Early DS, Edmundowicz SA, et al. A screening instrument for sleep apnea predicts airway maneuvers in patients undergoing advanced endoscopic procedures. Clin Gastroenterol Hepatol. 2010;8(8):660–665.e1.
4. Jirapinyo P, Abu Dayyeh BK, Thompson CC. Conscious sedation for upper endoscopy in the gastric bypass patient: prevalence of cardiopulmonary adverse events and predictors of sedation requirement. Dig Dis Sci. 2014;59(9):2173–7.
5. Standards of Practice Committee of the American Society for Gastrointestinal Endoscopy, Lichtenstein DR, Jagannath S, Baron TH, Anderson MA, Banerjee S, Dominitz JA, et al. Sedation and anesthesia in GI endoscopy. Gastrointest Endosc. 2008;68(5):815–26.
6. Schigt A, Coblijn U, Lagarde S, Kuiken S, Scholten P, Van Wagensveld B. Is esophagogastroduodenoscopy before Roux-en-Y gastric bypass or sleeve gastrectomy mandatory? Surg Obes Relat Dis. 2014;10(3):411–7.
7. Abd Ellatif ME, Alfalah H, Asker WA, El Nakeeb AE, Magdy A, Thabet W, et al. Place of upper endoscopy before and after bariatric surgery: a multicenter experience with 3219 patients. World J Gastrointest Endosc. 2016;8(10):409–17.
8. Mechanick JI, Youdim A, Jones DB, Garvey WT, Hurley DL, McMahon MM, et al. Clinical practice guidelines for the perioperative nutritional, meta-

bolic, and nonsurgical support of the bariatric surgery patient--2013 update: cosponsored by American Association of Clinical Endocrinologists, The Obesity Society, and American Society for Metabolic & Bariatric Surgery. Obesity (Silver Spring). 2013;21(Suppl 1):S1–27.

9. Shin RB. Intraoperative endoscopic test resulting in no postoperative leaks from the gastric pouch and gastrojejunal anastomosis in 366 laparoscopic Roux-en-Y gastric bypasses. Obes Surg. 2004;14(8):1067–9.

10. Haddad A, Tapazoglou N, Singh K, Averbach A. Role of intraoperative esophagogastroenteroscopy in minimizing gastrojejunostomy-related morbidity: Experience with 2,311 laparoscopic gastric bypasses with linear stapler anastomosis. Obes Surg. 2012;22(12):1928–33.

11. Kligman MD. Intraoperative endoscopic pneumatic testing for gastrojejunal anastomotic integrity during laparoscopic Roux-en-Y gastric bypass. Surg Endosc Other Interv Tech. 2007;21(8):1403–5.

12. Al Hadad M, Dehni N, Elamin D, Ibrahim M, Ghabra S, Nimeri A. Intraoperative endoscopy decreases postoperative complications in laparoscopic roux-en-y gastric bypass. Obes Surg. 2015;25(9):1711–5.

13. Nimeri A, Maasher A, Salim E, Ibrahim M, Al HM. The use of intraoperative endoscopy may decrease postoperative stenosis in laparoscopic sleeve gastrectomy. Obes Surg. 2016;26(7):1398–401.

14. Frezza EE, Barton A, Herbert H, Wachtel MS. Laparoscopic sleeve gastrectomy with endoscopic guidance in morbid obesity. Surg Obes Relat Dis. 2008;4(5):575–9.

15. Diamantis T, Alexandrou A, Pikoulis E, Diamantis D, Griniatsos J, Felekouras E, et al. Laparoscopic sleeve gastrectomy for morbid obesity with intra-operative endoscopic guidance. Immediate peri-operative and 1-year results after 25 patients. Obes Surg. 2010;20(8):1164–70.

16. Sharma G, Ardila-Gatas J, Boules M, Davis M, Villamere J, Rodriguez J, et al. Upper gastrointestinal endoscopy is safe and feasible in the early postoperative period after Roux-en-Y gastric bypass. Surgery. 2016;160:885–91.

17. Colquitt JL, Pickett K, Loveman E, Frampton GK. Surgery for weight loss in adults. Cochrane Database Syst Rev. 2014;(8):CD003641.

18. Brown WA, Burton PR, Anderson M, Korin A, Dixon JB, Hebbard G, et al. Symmetrical pouch dilatation after laparoscopic adjustable gastric banding: incidence and management. Obes Surg. 2008;18(9):1104–8.

19. Singhal R, Bryant C, Kitchen M, Khan KS, Deeks J, Guo B, et al. Band slippage and erosion after laparoscopic gastric banding: a meta-analysis. Surg Endosc. 2010;24(12):2980–6.

20. Nguyen NT, Goldman C, Rosenquist CJ, Arango A, Cole CJ, Lee SJ, et al. Laparoscopic versus open gastric bypass: a randomized study of outcomes, quality of life, and costs. Ann Surg. 2001;234(3):279–91.

21. Schauer PR, Bhatt DL, Kirwan JP, Wolski K, Aminian A, Brethauer SA, et al. Bariatric surgery versus intensive medical therapy for diabetes — 5-year outcomes. N Engl J Med. 2017;376(7):641–51.

22. Csendes A, Burgos AM, Altuve J, Bonacic S. Incidence of marginal ulcer 1 month and 1 to 2 years after gastric bypass: a prospective consecutive endoscopic evaluation of 442 patients with morbid obesity. Obes Surg. 2009;19(2):135–8.

23. Csendes A, Burgos AM, Burdiles P. Incidence of anastomotic strictures after gastric bypass: a prospective consecutive routine endoscopic study 1 month and 17 months after surgery in 441 patients with morbid obesity. Obes Surg. 2009;19(3):269–73.

24. Abu Dayyeh BK, Lautz DB, Thompson CC. Gastrojejunal stoma diameter predicts weight regain after Roux-en-Y gastric bypass. Clin Gastroenterol Hepatol. 2011;9(3):228–33.

25. Carrodeguas L, Szomstein S, Soto F, Whipple O, Simpfendorfer C, Gonzalvo JP, et al. Management of gastrogastric fistulas after divided Roux-en-Y gastric bypass surgery for morbid obesity: analysis of 1292 consecutive patients and review of literature. Surg Obes Relat Dis. 2005;1(5):467–74.

26. Ahmed AR, Rickards G, Messing S, Husain S, Johnson J, Boss T, et al. Roux limb obstruction secondary to constriction at transverse mesocolon rent after laparoscopic Roux-en-Y gastric bypass. Surg Obes Relat Dis. 2009;5(2):194–8.

27. Himpens J, Dobbeleir J, Peeters G. Long-term results of laparoscopic sleeve gastrectomy for obesity. Ann Surg. 2010;252(2):319–24.

28. ASMBS Clinical Issues Committee. Updated position statement on sleeve gastrectomy as a bariatric procedure. Surg Obes Relat Dis. 2012;8:e21–6.

29. Hess DS, Hess DW. Biliopancreatic diversion with a duodenal switch. Obes Surg. 1998;8(3):267–82.

Management of Acute Bleeding After Bariatric Surgery

Adil Haleem Khan and Leena Khaitan

Introduction

Gastrointestinal bleeding after bariatric surgery is a rare but potentially devastating complication of the weight loss surgery [1–10]. With improvement in technique and introduction of newer materials and methods, the incidence of bleeding has decreased, but continues to be clinically relevant. Most bleeding cases respond to conservative management. The altered anatomy and different possible sources of bleeding can make diagnosis and management of these bleeds a challenging task. Both bariatric surgeons and general surgeons need to be familiar with these sources of bleeding, and also with the acute management of this complication. Delay in diagnosis and management can have serious consequences in these patients.

Epidemiology

Bleeding after bariatric surgery is divided into luminal and intra-abdominal bleeds. Studies have shown that the majority of these postoperative bleeds are intra-abdominal bleeds. The incidence of postoperative bleeding varies among different bariatric surgical procedures and different techniques used. Incidence of bleeding after Roux-en-Y gastric bypass (RYGB) is 1–5% [6–10]. The incidence is reported to be higher in laparoscopic compared to open procedures. Also the circular stapler technique has been described to have a higher incidence of bleeding compared with linear stapler anastomoses (2.9% vs. 1.2%) [11].

The incidence of acute bleeding after laparoscopic sleeve gastrectomy (SG) is about 1–2% [1–3]. Laparoscopic gastric banding has the lowest incidence of bleeding and is reported to be 0.1% [12].

Risk Factors

Various risk factors for postoperative bleeding have been assessed. These include advanced age, use of anti-inflammatories (NSAIDs), history of antiplatelet medication use, and patient comorbidities. Rabl et al. looked at their experience and found that the only statistically significant factor indicating a higher bleeding risk was presence of diabetes [13]. Some other studies report advanced age as a risk factor for higher bleeding risk. Laparoscopic procedures have also been shown to have higher rate of bleeding compared to open procedures. Janik et al. recently published a predictive model of bleeding after sleeve gastrectomy and attributed obstructive sleep apnea, hypertension, surgeon expertise, and staple line reinforcement as important contributors

A.H. Khan, M.D. • L. Khaitan, M.D., M.P.H (✉)
Department of Surgery, University Hospitals
Cleveland Medical Center, 11100 Euclid Avenue,
Cleveland, OH 44106, USA
e-mail: adilhaleemkhan@gmail.com;
leena.khaitan@uhhospitals.org

© Springer International Publishing AG 2018
B. Chand (ed.), *Endoscopy in Obesity Management*, DOI 10.1007/978-3-319-63528-6_6

to risk of postoperative bleeding [14]. Use of heparin or lovenox postoperatively, to reduce risk of DVT, has shown variable risk for bleeding after bariatric surgery with no consensus as to choice of anticoagulation. Ketorolac is commonly used for pain control after bariatric procedures. No strong clinical data exists to show that it increases the risk of bleeding postoperatively in bariatric patients.

Clinical Presentation and Diagnosis

The clinical presentation of a patient's bleeding depends on the source and degree. Patients will have hematemesis if the source of bleeding is the gastro-jejunostomy or luminal bleeding after sleeve gastrectomy. On the other hand if the patient has bleeding from the remnant stomach or jejuno-jejunostomy, the patient will more likely present with melanotic stools and minimal nausea or pain symptoms. With free intra-abdominal bleeding, nonspecific abdominal distention, hypotension, and/or pain can be the presenting symptoms. If a surgical drain was left in place, a large amount of sanguinous drainage can be seen, if the drain is in vicinity to the source. However, the drainage can also be minimal if the patient is clotting well or the bleed is slow. In all these bleeding scenarios, patients will likely exhibit signs of shock with tachycardia, hypotension, pallor, and a drop in hematocrit. Imaging has a limited role in patients with acute bleeding. CT scan can be performed in patients if cause of tachycardia is not certain and patient is otherwise hemodynamically stable. Tagged red blood cell scan can be helpful if the source is not clear. However, the anastomoses and staple lines should always be the first concern early in the postoperative period (Table 6.1).

Management

Initial Stabilization

Most cases of postoperative bariatric surgery bleeding are self-limiting and respond to conservative measures. Studies have shown a success

Table 6.1 Sources of bleeding after bariatric surgery

Procedure	Intraluminal sources	Extraluminal sources
Sleeve gastrectomy	Internal bleeding from staple line	External bleeding from staple line Omental bleeding Abdominal wall trocar site bleeding
Roux-en-Y gastric bypass	Gastro-jejunostomy Pouch staple line internally Jejuno-jejunostomy Remnant stomach	Pouch staple line externally Gastric remnant staple line Small bowel mesentery Omental bleeding Abdominal wall trocar site bleeding

rate of more than 80% in managing these bleeds non-operatively. The initial approach to all these scenarios is similar to any patient who presents with acute gastrointestinal hemorrhage [15]. Two large bore IVs must be placed if not already done during the initial operation. Fluid boluses should be given to help restore loss of intravascular volume. Labs including hematocrit, electrolytes and renal panel, type and cross and coagulation profile should be sent. Patient should be placed on continuous monitoring to ensure prompt recognition of any change in vital signs. Patients may require a higher level of care, and be transferred to an intensive care unit. All blood thinners should be stopped. In case of large volume hematemesis, airway protection is of paramount importance to protect the airway.

The next step is to locate the site of bleeding. If the patient has hematemesis, bleeding from gastric pouch or internal bleeding from the sleeve gastrectomy is suspected. These patients should be taken promptly to the operating room for management as discussed later. If the patient has melena, bleeding is suspected to be from jejuno-jejunostomy or excluded stomach. These patients should be managed non-operatively if clinically stable and bleeding is not profuse. If the patient is not responding to fluid resuscitation or continues to require blood transfusion, strong consideration needs to be given to take the patient back to operating room for intervention. In some of these cases, imaging may be helpful to localize bleeding. Most of the time early operative intervention works best. Finally, patients with intraperitoneal bleeding are managed conservatively as patients with melena if clinically stable. If the patient continues to show signs of hemodynamic instability or requires more than 6 units in 24 h, they need to return to the operating room.

Bleeding from Sleeve Gastrectomy or Gastro-jejunostomy

Once a patient with hematemesis is suspected to have bleeding from the gastric pouch or gastrojejunal anastomosis, the patient is taken back to the operating room. We prefer to perform simultaneous endoscopy and laparoscopy using the same trocar sites as the initial operation. Anesthesia is advised to keep patient well resuscitated to ensure stable blood pressure on initiating pneumoperitoneum; however, some patients will require initiation of vasopressor therapy. Once all trocars are in place and pneumoperitoneum established, the Roux limb or distal stomach is clamped so that insufflation does not obscure visualization. Then upper endoscopy is performed with carbon dioxide to avoid prolonged bowel distention. All clots are suctioned out or flushed with sterile saline flushes. The site of bleeding is recognized. The bleeding can be managed endoscopically or with externally placed sutures. For external repair with sutures, a blunt grasper is used to locate the exact site of bleeding by pushing on the stomach externally. Once the bleeding site is recognized, it is oversewn with full thickness sutures around the area. Blood is suctioned again to ensure hemostasis. It is important to ensure that the patient's blood pressure is adequate at this point and that bleeding sites are not obscured due to vasoconstriction resulting from hypotension. The bleeding site can also be managed with clips placed endoscopically or injection with epinephrine. In a fresh anastomosis, injection and cautery are discouraged.

Role of Endoscopy

Endoscopic only control of bleeding from gastrojejunal anastomosis has been described in the literature [16–22]. Initial concerns were about the safety of endoscopy and endoscopic interventions in the immediate postoperative period in a fresh staple line. Jamil et al. described 80% success rate of control of bleeding using heater probe, endoclips, and epinephrine injection. However, a significant number of patients (17%) required re-intervention due to a second bleeding episode [23]. One patient died due to aspiration in this study. Therefore it is suggested that endoscopy should be performed after airway control to prevent this complication. Most commonly, early in the postoperative period, a combined endoscopic and laparoscopic approach is recommended.

Bleeding from Remnant Stomach

In patients presenting with melena with continued hemodynamic instability or requirement of 6 or more units of blood in less than 24 h, operative exploration is warranted. If the bleeding is in the remnant, distention in the left upper quadrant may be seen on physical exam. Patients should be adequately resuscitated to ensure hemodynamic stability with initiation of pneumoperitoneum. The previous port sites can be reused for entry into the abdomen. When bleeding is from the remnant stomach, it will often be distended with retained clots. A gastrotomy should be made along the greater curvature. All of the clots should be evacuated. Once decompression is accomplished, the gastrotomy can be closed with stapling or suturing. The causative staple line should be oversewn. The gastrotomy site can also be used for placement of a gastrostomy tube that is held in place with a balloon and purse-string suture. We prefer to leave a gastrostomy tube in the remnant to monitor for ongoing bleeding and for decompression if the patient develops a postoperative ileus. This tube also allows feeding access to ensure adequate nutrition in the postoperative period if needed to supplement the oral intake.

Role of Endoscopy

RYGB changes the intestinal anatomy, making the remnant stomach inaccessible to routine endoscopy. Hence endoscopic management of these bleeds has been a challenging task. While intraoperative endoscopy can be performed by making a gastrostomy for access, this is associated with additional morbidity. Double balloon endoscopy (DBE) is a technique that can be utilized to manage these cases. While performing this procedure requires expertise, successful management of gastric remnant bleeds using DBE has been described in literature [24–26]. Caution must be taken in early postoperative period as excessive insufflation can lead to anastomotic dehiscence and result in a leak. If bleeding is not controlled with these measures, completion gastrectomy can be considered.

Bleeding from Jejuno-jejunostomy

Clinically these patients are indistinguishable from patients with bleeding from the remnant stomach as both will present with melena. Attempts at conservative measures with resuscitation and transfusion are successful in the majority of patients. Imaging can be used for bleeding localization. If patients are taken back to the operating room, it still may not be clear if the source of bleeding is the remnant stomach or jejunojejunal anastomosis. The jejuno-jejunostomy is best accessed through the blind end of the biliopancreatic limb or at the common channel suture line. The blood can be evacuated and staple lines can be oversewn or undergo mechanical clipping to stop the bleeding. A revision of the entire anastomosis can be considered in extreme cases, but rarely required. Case reports of bowel obstruction from clots at this distal anastomosis have also been described and therefore complete evacuation of the clot and possible gastric remnant tube placement be considered.

Role of Endoscopy

While data is lacking, double balloon enteroscopy or other form of deep bowel enteroscopy can be utilized in diagnosis and management of bleeding from the jejuno-jejunostomy.

Free Intraperitoneal Bleeding

If the patient with postoperative bleeding has no melena or hematemesis, and shows signs of bleeding with tachycardia and dropping hematocrit and/or sanguinous output from an intraperitoneal drain, intra-abdominal bleeding should be suspected. Initial attempt is made with close monitoring and resuscitation, as most bleeding will stop spontaneously. In case of ongoing blood transfusion requirement or hemodynamic instability, the patient will be taken to the operating room for exploration. All clots will be evacuated. All staple lines, mesenteric edges, and omental edges will be inspected. All trocar sites should be investigated. Abdomen will be washed and two large drains left in place to monitor for ongoing bleeding. Conversion to open should be considered if not manageable laparoscopically.

Prevention

Use of buttress material has been an area of great interest. Multiple trials have shown its benefit in reducing bleeding rate. Angrisani et al. showed that bleeding from gastric pouch was lower if bovine pericardium was used to buttress the staple line [27]. Dapri et al. compared buttressing with oversewing and no reinforcement. The results showed that blood loss using bioabsorbable buttressing material was significantly lower compared to oversewing or using no reinforcement [28]. D'ugo et al. showed reduction in bleeding with staple line reinforcement (SLR) but no difference in bleeding rates among the various methods of reinforcement used [29]. Shikora et al. also showed a benefit of staple line reinforcement in reducing bleeding risk. His study showed differences in outcome with the various reinforcement materials with bovine pericardium having the best results [30]. A recent report from the Metabolic and Bariatric Surgery

Accreditation and Quality Improvement Program showed decreased rate of bleeding with SLR [31]. However, the overall bleeding rate was low in all groups accounting for clinically small difference in outcomes. Table 6.2 summarizes results showing the effects of SLR on the risk of bleeding [31].

Staple height has been another factor shown to effect rate of bleeding. Nguyen et al. published a randomized controlled multicenter trial that showed that rate of bleeding was significantly lower with 3.5 mm staple height compared to 4.8 mm when constructing the gastro-jejunostomy [32].

Fibrin glue is another method described as a method to reduce bleeding. Different types of fibrin glue products have been studied yet none have shown significant promise in reducing the incidence of bleeding complications. Sroka et al. showed higher bleeding rates with the use of fibrin glue when compared to suturing the staple line [33]. However, more recently, Coskun et al. reported on 1000 consecutive sleeve gastrectomy patients. In all these patients, fibrin glue was used. He reported a very low bleeding rate of 0.3% with no patient developing a leak or stricture suggesting possible benefit of using fibrin glue [34].

Perioperative blood pressure control is also an easily ignored but very important step in decreasing incidence of postoperative bleeding. While low blood pressure is not desired, maintaining systolic blood pressure in the range of 110–160 mmHg helps decrease risk of bleeding from fresh staple lines. Patient should be closely monitored and adequate pain control provided to help prevent rise in blood pressure. If the blood pressure continues

to remain high despite good pain control, adequate antihypertensive medications should be used to control blood pressure.

Role of Endoscopy

Intraoperative endoscopy plays a very important role in preventing postoperative intraluminal bleeds in sleeve gastrectomy and in RYGB. We recommend the routine use of endoscopy at the end of the bariatric procedure to rule out bleeding from these sources. Endoscopy will provide the added benefit of viewing the anatomy internally and performing the leak test. If bleeding is seen, it can be easily controlled by placing a suture under laparoscopic and endoscopic guidance. This can help prevent a trip back to the operating room from bleeding resulting from these sources.

Figure 6.1 shows our proposed protocol to manage bleeding after bariatric surgery.

Conclusion

Extensive literature has described chronic gastrointestinal bleeding after bariatric surgery mostly resulting from marginal ulceration or peptic ulcer disease. Acute gastrointestinal hemorrhage after laparoscopic bariatric surgery is a potentially rare complication. While newer techniques are being devised to decrease this complication, it continues to be clinically relevant with associated significant morbidity and mortality if not promptly diagnosed and managed. Clinicians should be aware of signs and symptoms that indicate bleeding. Prompt resuscitation and close monitoring are key in all patients with bleeding. Timing of intervention will be based on potential site of bleeding and clinical status of the patient. In most patients, intraluminal bleeding can be identified endoscopically and controlled laparoscopically. If the particular site of bleeding is not recognized, clot evacuation and oversewing of staple lines can be accomplished surgically. Endoscopy plays an important role in localizing and controlling upper gastrointestinal bleeds in this population.

Table 6.2 Effect of surgical technique on bleeding risk after sleeve gastrectomy

Technique used	Frequency of bleeding (%)
No SLR	0.95
Routine oversew	0.89
Selective oversew	1.29
SLR	0.78
Routine SLR	0.75
Selective SLR	0.96

SLR Staple line reinforcement

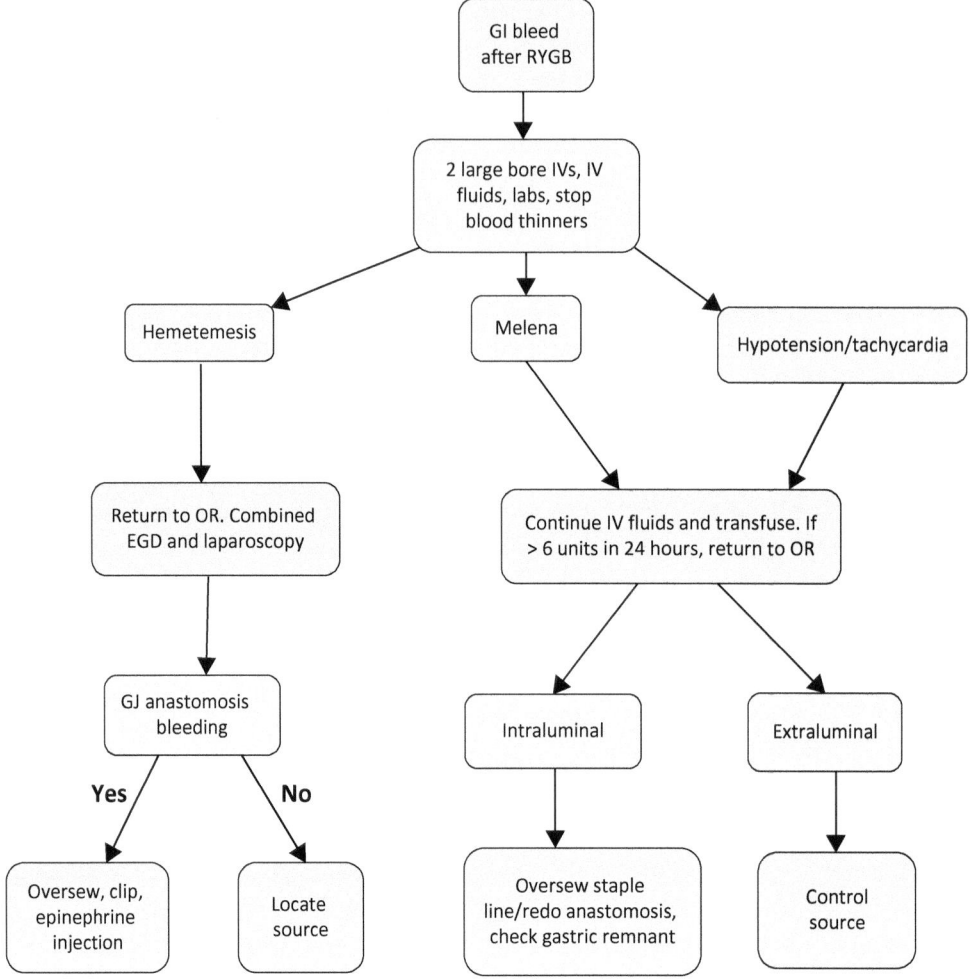

Fig. 6.1 Algorithm for management of bleeding after bariatric surgery. *GI* gastrointestinal, *RYGB* Roux-en-Y gastric bypass, *IV* intravenous, *OR* operating room, *EGD* esophagogastroduodenoscopy, *GJ* gastro-jejunostomy

References

1. De Angelis F, Abdelgawad M, Rizzello M, Mattia C, Silecchia G. Perioperative hemorrhagic complications after laparoscopic sleeve gastrectomy: four-year experience of a bariatric center of excellence. Surg Endosc. 2016; doi:10.1007/s00464-016-5383-y.
2. Kassir R, Bouviez N, Gugenheim J, Tiffet O, Boutet C. Postoperative bleeding and leakage after sleeve gastrectomy: a single-center experience. Obes Surg. 2016 Oct;26(10):2488–9.
3. Khoursheed M, Al-Bader I, Mouzannar A, Ashraf A, Bahzad Y, Al-Haddad A, et al. Postoperative bleeding and leakage after sleeve gastrectomy: a single-center experience. Obes Surg. 2016;26(12):3007.
4. Heneghan HM, Meron-Eldar S, Yenumula P, Rogula T, Brethauer SA, Schauer PR. Incidence and manage-

ment of bleeding complications after gastric bypass surgery in the morbidly obese. Surg Obes Relat Dis. 2012;8(6):729–35.
5. Ferreira LE, Song LM, Baron TH. Management of acute postoperative hemorrhage in the bariatric patient. Gastrointest Endosc Clin N Am. 2011;21(2):287–94.
6. Nguyen NT, Longoria M, Chalifoux S, Wilson SE. Gastrointestinal hemorrhage in the bariatric patient. Gastrointest Endosc Clin N Am. 2011;21(2):287–94.
7. Nguyen NT, Rivers R, Wolfe BM. Early gastrointestinal hemorrhage after laparoscopic gastric bypass. Obes Surg. 2003;13(1):62–5.
8. Podnos YD, Jimenez JC, Wilson SE, Stevens CM, Nguyen NT. Complications after laparoscopic gastric bypass: a review of 3464 cases. Arch Surg. 2003;138(9):957–61.
9. Steffen R. Early gastrointestinal hemorrhage after laparoscopic gastric bypass. Obes Surg. 2003;13(3):466.

10. Bakhos C, Alkhoury F, Kyriakides T, Reinhold R, Nadzam G. Early postoperative hemorrhage after open and laparoscopic Roux-en-Y gastric bypass. Obes Surg. 2009;19(2):153–7.

11. Finks JF, Carlin A, Share D, O'Reilly A, Fan Z, Birkmeyer J, Birkmeyer N. Effect of surgical techniques on clinical outcomes after laparoscopic gastric bypass--results from the Michigan Bariatric Surgery Collaborative. Surg Obes Relat Dis. 2011;7(3):284–9.

12. Belachew M, Belva PH, Desaive C. Long-term results of laparoscopic adjustable gastric banding for the treatment of morbid obesity. Obes Surg. 2002;12(4):564–8.

13. Rabl C, Peeva S, Prado K, James AW, Rogers SJ, Posselt A, Campos GM. Early and late abdominal bleeding after Roux-en-Y gastric bypass: sources and tailored therapeutic strategies. Obes Surg. 2011;21(4):413–20.

14. Janik MR, Walędziak M, Brągoszewski J, Kwiatkowski A, Paśnik K. Prediction model for hemorrhagic complications after laparoscopic sleeve gastrectomy: development of SLEEVE BLEED calculator. Obes Surg. 2017;27(4):968–72.

15. Feinman M, Haut ER. Upper gastrointestinal bleeding. Surg Clin North Am. 2014;94(1):43–53.

16. Valli PV, Gubler C. Review article including treatment algorithm: endoscopic treatment of luminal complications after bariatric surgery. Clin Obes. 2017;7(2):115–22.

17. Abd Ellatif ME, Alfalah H, Asker WA, El Nakeeb AE, Magdy A, Thabet W, et al. Place of upper endoscopy before and after bariatric surgery: a multicenter experience with 3219 patients. World J Gastrointest Endosc. 2016;8(10):409–17.

18. Gomberawalla A, Lutfi R. Benefits of intraoperative endoscopy: case report and review of 300 sleeves gastrectomies. Ann Surg Innov Res. 2015;9:13. doi:10.1186/s13022-015-0023-0.

19. Eisendrath P, Deviere J. Major complications of bariatric surgery: endoscopy as first-line treatment. Nat Rev Gastroenterol Hepatol. 2015;12(12):701–10.

20. Campos JM, Moon R, Teixeira A, Ferraz AA, Ferreria F, Kumbhari V. Endoscopic management of massive hemorrhage 12 h post laparoscopic Roux-en-Y gastric bypass. Obes Surg. 2015;25(10):1981–3.

21. García-García ML, Martín-Lorenzo JG, Torralba-Martínez JA, Lirón-Ruiz R, Miguel Perelló J, Flores Pastor B, et al. Emergency endoscopy for gastrointestinal bleeding after bariatric surgery. Therapeutic algorithm. Cir Esp. 2015;93(2):97–104.

22. Fernández-Esparrach G, Bordas JM, Pellisé M, Gimeno-García AZ, Lacy A, Delgado S, et al. Endoscopic management of early GI hemorrhage after laparoscopic gastric bypass. Gastrointest Endosc. 2008;67(3):552–5.

23. Jamil LH, Krause KR, Chengelis DL, Jury RP, Jackson CM, Cannon ME, Duffy MC. Endoscopic management of early upper gastrointestinal hemorrhage following laparoscopic Roux-en-Y gastric bypass. Am J Gastroenterol. 2008;103(1):86–91.

24. Chacón S, Esteban P, Campillo-Soto A, Del Pozo P, Torrella E, Shanabo J, Pérez CE. Endoscopic approach to bariatric surgery. The role of double-balloon enteroscopy. Rev Esp Enferm Dig. 2008;100(6):365–6.

25. Moretto M, Mottin CC, Padoin AV, Berleze D, Repetto G. Endoscopic management of bleeding after gastric bypass - a therapeutic alternative. Obes Surg. 2004;14(5):706.

26. Puri V, Alagappan A, Rubin M, Merola S. Management of bleeding from gastric remnant after gastric bypass. Surg Obes Relat Dis. 2012;8(1):e3–5.

27. Angrisani L, Lorenzo M, Borrelli V, Ciannella M, Bassi UA, Scarano P. The use of bovine pericardial strips on linear stapler to reduce extraluminal bleeding during laparoscopic gastric bypass: prospective randomized clinical trial. Obes Surg. 2004;14(9):1198–202.

28. Dapri G, Cadière GB, Himpens J. Reinforcing the staple line during laparoscopic sleeve gastrectomy: prospective randomized clinical study comparing three different techniques. Obes Surg. 2010;20(4):462–7.

29. D'Ugo S, Gentileschi P, Benavoli D, Cerci M, Gaspari A, Berta RD, et al. Comparative use of different techniques for leak and bleeding prevention during laparoscopic sleeve gastrectomy: a multicenter study. Surg Obes Relat Dis. 2014;10(3):450–4.

30. Shikora SA, Mahoney CB. Clinical benefit of gastric staple line reinforcement (SLR) in gastrointestinal surgery: a meta-analysis. Obes Surg. 2015;25(7):1133–41.

31. Berger ER, Clements RH, Morton JM, Huffman KM, Wolfe BM, Nguyen NT, et al. The impact of different surgical techniques on outcomes in laparoscopic sleeve gastrectomies: the first report from the Metabolic and Bariatric Surgery Accreditation and Quality Improvement Program (MBSAQIP). Ann Surg. 2016;264(3):464–73.

32. Nguyen NT, Dakin G, Needleman B, Pomp A, Mikami D, Provost DA, et al. Effect of staple height on gastrojejunostomy during laparoscopic gastric bypass: a multicenter prospective randomized trial. Surg Obes Relat Dis. 2010;6(5):477–82.

33. Sroka G, Milevski D, Shteinberg D, Mady H, Matter I. Minimizing hemorrhagic complications in laparoscopic sleeve gastrectomy--a randomized controlled trial. Obes Surg. 2015;25(9):1577–83.

34. Coskun H, Yardimci E. Effects and results of fibrin sealant use in 1000 laparoscopic sleeve gastrectomy cases. Surg Endosc. 2017;31(5):2174–9.

Management of Leaks with Endoluminal Stents

Salvatore Docimo, Jr. and Aurora D. Pryor

Introduction

Obesity is the second leading cause of preventable death in the United States, second only to smoking [1]. Surgery has demonstrated better long-term results compared to lifestyle modifications [2]. Laparoscopic sleeve gastrectomy (LSG) and laparoscopic Roux-en-Y gastric bypass (RYGB) are the most frequently performed bariatric procedures today [3]. With an increase in the volume of bariatric surgery being performed over the last decades, the incidence of complications, such as anastomotic and staple line leaks, has increased [4]. The occurrence of anastomotic leakage, a major morbidity, is 1.6–4.8% after LRYGB and 1.7–2.4% after LSG, respectively [5–8].

Options for management of bariatric leaks include a combination of surgical or percutaneous drainage and leak repair. Surgical options for leak management include anastomotic revision, primary repair, and bowel, gastric or omental patching [9]. Considering surgical re-exploration for bariatric leaks carries an increased morbidity

(15–50%) and mortality (2–10%) [10, 11], less invasive treatment modalities have gained popularity. Flexible endoscopy has emerged as both a diagnostic and therapeutic option due to its lower morbidity and mortality [9]. This chapter focuses on the use of endoscopically placed stents as a means to treat bariatric leak.

Laparoscopic Sleeve Gastrectomy Leak

A variety of causes are believed to be the source of anastomotic or staple line leaks: wrong staple size for tissue thickness, staple line malformation, tissue trauma, and tissue ischemia [12]. Most LSG leaks appear in the proximal third of the stomach (75–89%) near the gastroesophageal junction [5], carry a mortality rate of 0.11–9% and occur at a mean of 7 days postoperatively [13, 14]. Leaks after LSG can be classified based on observed occurrence following an index procedure. Table 7.1 demonstrates the classification system put forth by an international sleeve gastrectomy expert panel [15]. Sleeve gastrectomy leaks are also often associated with distal stricture, usually narrowing at the angularis, or "functional twist" of the stomach. This distal narrowing can create a proximal high-pressure zone, potentially causing leak, or impairing leak healing. Diagnostic modalities for LSG leaks include an upper gastrointestinal contrast study with a water-soluble contrast material or a computed

S. Docimo, Jr. D.O., M.Sc (✉) • A.D. Pryor, M.D.
Division of Bariatric, Foregut, and Advanced Gastrointestinal Surgery, Department of Surgery, Health Sciences Center T18-040, Stony Brook School of Medicine, Stony Brook, NY 11794-8191, USA
e-mail: Salvatore.Docimo@stonybrookmedicine.edu; aurora.pryor@sbumed.org; aurora.pryor@stonybrookmedicine.edu

© Springer International Publishing AG 2018
B. Chand (ed.), *Endoscopy in Obesity Management*, DOI 10.1007/978-3-319-63528-6_7

Table 7.1 Classification system for sleeve gastrectomy leaks (from Rosenthal [15], with permission)

Classification	Time from index procedure
Acute leak	≤7 days
Early leak	Within 1–6 weeks
Late leak	≥6 weeks
Chronic leak	≥12 weeks

tomography (CT) scan with oral and intravenous contrast. Computed tomography offers improved sensitivity and additional radiographic information, such as fluid collections in left upper quadrant or free intraperitoneal air [16].

Treatment strategies for LSG leaks include CT guided drainage, endoscopic stenting, and operative exploration, which may include drainage, repair of the acute perforation, or Roux-en-Y reconstruction [17]. The most common leak site is at the angle of His or the gastroesophageal junction. Risk factors for a leak include ischemia at the proximal portion of the staple line, previous gastric surgery (gastric banding), or an area of stenosis within the gastric sleeve which results in an increase of proximal intraluminal pressure [18]. Ligation of the short gastric arteries further increases susceptibility to ischemia and perforation at the former angle of His.

An increased pressure gradient found within a newly created tubular stomach also plays a role in leak formation. A functional pylorus may contribute to leaks by creating a large pressure gradient within the newly created tubular stomach [19]. An assessment of the volume and intraluminal pressure of the stomach after LSG demonstrated the volume of the sleeve to be less than 10% of a whole stomach. The mean intraluminal pressure of a sleeve gastrectomy was noted to be higher compared to a whole stomach (43 ± 8 mmHg vs. 34 ± 6 mmHg, $P < 0.005$) [20].

Any patient suspected of having a LSG leak should undergo radiographic evaluation with an UGI or CT scan of the abdomen and pelvis with oral and intravenous contrast. Any LSG leak patient undergoing endoscopic stent management should have any abscess or intra-abdominal collection drained (either surgically or percutaneous) prior to or soon thereafter stent placement

[17, 21]. Peritonitis or septic shock excludes stent management and warrants surgical exploration, drainage, and enteral access. Leaks located in the proximal or mid-portion of the sleeve are the most amenable to treatment with stents [15, 22–24]. Distal staple line leaks are often not amenable to stent treatments due to the stent's smaller diameter, which limits its ability to adequately seal the defect [25].

Laparoscopic Roux-En-Y Gastric Bypass Leaks

The development of a leak following a RYGB can lead to significant morbidity and mortality [26]. A higher incidence of leaks have been associated with risk factors, such as male sex, BMI > 50, age > 55 years of age, and revisional procedures [27]. Approximately 70–80% of leaks occur at the gastrojejunal anastomosis, 10–15% at the gastric pouch, 5% at the jejuno-jejunal anastomosis, and 3–5% at the gastric remnant [28]. Technical factors during surgery that may lead to anastomotic breakdown include excess tension, staple line malformation, inappropriate staple height for tissue thickness, and ischemia. Ischemia, or inadequate oxygenation of the anastomosis, may be a direct result of tension, excessive dissection leading to poor blood flow, or comorbidities such as atherosclerosis, diabetes mellitus, or coronary artery disease that limit oxygenation of the anastomotic site [29].

Csendes et al. [30] evaluated 60 leaks following 1762 RYGB surgeries and proposed a classification system based on the postoperative day of occurrence, severity of the leaks based on two types, and location. Classification of leaks aims to improve description and treatment planning. Table 7.2 provides the classification system for RYGB leaks.

Diagnostic modalities for the evaluation of a leak following a RYGB include an upper gastrointestinal series or a CT scan. Upper gastrointestinal contrast studies have demonstrated a sensitivity of 79.4% and a specificity of 95% in the setting of leak [31]. Whereas, a contrast CT scan in the same setting has dem-

Table 7.2 Classification system for Roux-en-Y gastric bypass leaks (from Csendes et al. [30], with permission)

Classification Criteria	Type	Description
Timing	Early	1–4 days post-op
	Intermediate	5–9 days post-op
	Late	≥10 days post-op
Severity	Type I	Small localized leak; amenable to percutaneous drainage
	Type II	Systemic repercussion; need for aggressive surgical drainage
Leak location	Type I	Gastric pouch
	Type II	Gastrojejunal anastomosis
	Type III	Jejunal stump
	Type IV	Jejuno-jejunal anastomosis
	Type V	Excluded stomach
	Type VI	Duodenal stump (resectional bypass)
	Type VII	Blind end biliary jejunal limb after laparoscopic surgery

onstrated a sensitivity of 95% and a specificity of 100% [31]. A CT scan also offers additional information beyond contrast extravasation, such as fluid collection, inflammatory changes, intraperitoneal free air, and pleural effusions [28].

Evolution of Endoluminal Stents and Bariatric Leaks

In 1885, Sir Charles James Symonds (1852–1932) successfully placed the first esophageal stent at Guy's Hospital in London [32]. The stent, a 6-in., rigid, esophageal tube was placed across a malignant stricture via a conical bougie or copper wire introducer. To prevent migration, a silk suture was attached to the proximal end of the tube, brought out of the patient's mouth and tied to the patient's ear. Enteral feeding consisting of a liquid diet was allowed. The tube was removed every 10 days for cleaning and then replaced [33]. Frimberger [34] later developed and deployed the first self-expandable metal stent (SEMS) for gastrointestinal strictures. The Frimberger stent consisted of a metal spiral coil that was tightly wound around a pediatric gastroscope. The pediatric gastroscope was inserted distal to the stricture site and the stent deployed. Radial expansion of the stent and tumor expansion in-between the metal coil held the stent in place. However, a 30% migration was also noted in this early stent design [33, 34].

In 1993, Knyrim et al. [35] published results of his randomized controlled trial comparing the use of SEMS to rigid prostheses for the palliation of malignant dysphagia. Significantly higher complications related to stent insertion were noted among the rigid prosthesis group. These findings led to the replacement of rigid prosthesis with SEMS for palliation of malignant dysphagia [35].

Historically, SEMS were designed and FDA approved for use in the palliation of obstructive lesions, such as esophageal and colorectal masses. The application of SEMS was later expanded to include esophageal leak. The earliest published data regarding the use of endoscopically placed stents across an anastomotic leak was described in thoracic patients who underwent esophageal resections [12]. In 1990, Domschke et al. [36] placed a 20-mm uncovered SEMS in a patient with unresectable esophageal cancer. In 1991, Song et al. [37] first described the placement of a covered SEMS for malignant esophageal strictures. Song further improved SEMS by allowing for removability of the stent via two drawstrings attached to the upper, inner margin of the stent [38].

Considering the complication rates for laparoscopic revisional bariatric surgery are reported to be 39%, [39] with a conversion rate of 47.6%, [40] the need for less invasive methods of intervention is evident. Conservative management of bariatric leaks, prior to the introduction of endoluminal stents, included percutaneous drainage, nil-per-os, and parenteral feeding. Although not approved by the FDA for gastrojejunal or gastric leak, endoluminal stents became a hallmark of conservative management for bariatric leaks considering it offered both diversion of enteric contents and the option for early enteral feeding. The stent itself does not heal the dehiscence, but allows local sepsis diversion and hopefully allows the body to heal the defect.

The treatment of anastomotic leak in bariatric surgery with SEMS has increased in the past decade in conjunction with advancements in endoscopic technology [41]. Due to the low frequency of bariatric leaks, much of the published data consists of low volume case series, which inhibits our ability to draw significant conclusions regarding the most appropriate indications for SEMS in bariatric leak.

The treatment of leak in the setting of bariatric surgery should be determined by the clinical status upon presentation. Current consensus states an unstable patient with a contained or uncon-

tained leak should undergo immediate surgical intervention [15]. Therefore, patients who present with peritonitis and signs of sepsis will benefit from immediate surgical intervention with laparoscopic washout, drain placement, and feeding access, as needed [42]. In hemodynamically stable patients, treatment with nonsurgical drainage (CT or ultrasound [US] guided) and stent placement is an option. Intra-abdominal collections noted on previous radiography should be drained, whether via CT or US guidance or laparoscopic intervention, prior to placement of a stent [21]. Figure 7.1 demonstrates an algorithm for decision-making regarding the use of SEMS after a bariatric leak.

A meta-analysis of seven studies demonstrated a radiographically confirmed closure rate of 87.7% (95% CI: 79.4–94.2%) [43] post-bariatric leaks. The benefit of deploying stents to treat leaks is twofold: they act as a barrier between the intraperitoneal cavity and the endoluminal bacteria and they allow for anastomotic patency

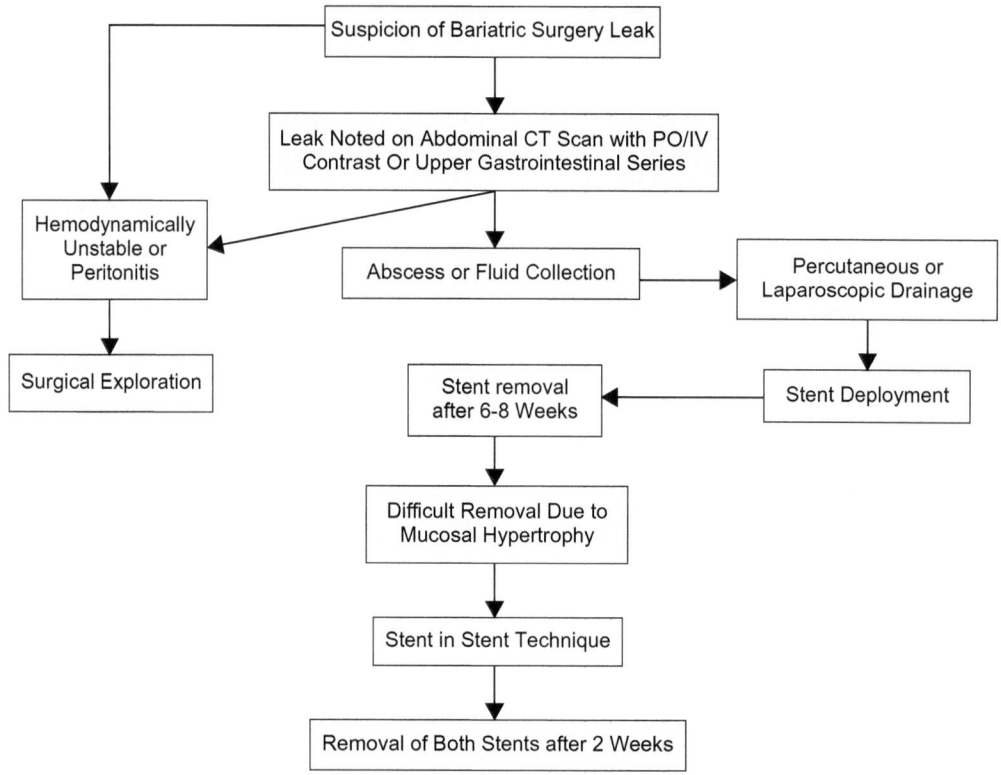

Fig. 7.1 Algorithm for self-expanding stent placement after bariatric surgery leak

to prevent stenosis [12]. Early enteral feeding is also an advantage of stent placement. We typically begin enteral feeds consisting of a liquid diet following confirmation of successful stent placement, usually with an upper gastrointestinal series (UGI) as early as post-procedure day 1. The UGI should confirm no continued leakage from the area of dehiscence. Early enteral feeding reduces the need for parenteral nutrition and the potential morbidity associated with it, thus improving recovery times and shortening length of stay [43].

Types of Endoluminal Stents

The most common types of stents are self-expandable plastic stents (SEPS) and self-expandable metal stents (SEMS). Covered SEMS (C-SEMS) are typically the most utilized in the setting of post-bariatric surgery leak. A few of the more commonly available stents include the WallFlex esophageal stent (Boston Scientific, Marlborough, MA, USA), the Mega esophageal stent (Taewoong Medical Industries, Gyeonggi-do, South Korea), and EndoMaXX stent (Merit Medical Endotek, South Jordan, UT, USA) and the Evolution stent (Cook Medical). Table 7.3 (need to add Cook to table) describes characteristics of commonly used stents.

Most metal stents are produced from NiTiNOL (Nickel Titanium Naval Ordinance Laboratory), an alloy developed by the United States Navy [44]. Nitinol exhibits two unique properties: Shape memory and Super-Elasticity. Shape memory allows a particular atomic structure (austenite shape) to be imprinted on nitinol by having it heated to 500 °C. After cooling, the nitinol can be deformed (compressed for deployment) into a more complex atomic structure (martensite shape). On rewarming to body temperature, the atoms attempt to regain the original austenite structure. Medical grade nitinol can be rewarmed at body temperature. Nitinol's super-elasticity allows for deformation of the metal 20–30 times more than most other metals before a permanent change occurs [45]. Figure 7.2 demonstrates commonly used SEMS. Most plastic stents are pro-

Table 7.3 Commonly utilized stents for the treatment of bariatric leaks

Name	Type	Coverage	Length (mm)	Stent flare diameter (OD) mm
WallFlex stent	SEMS	Partially	150	23
Mega stent	SEMS	Fully	230	24–28
EndoMaXX stent	SEMS	Fully	150	24
Evolution esophageal stent	SEMS	Fully	120	23–25

SEMS self-expanding metal stent, *OD* outside diameter

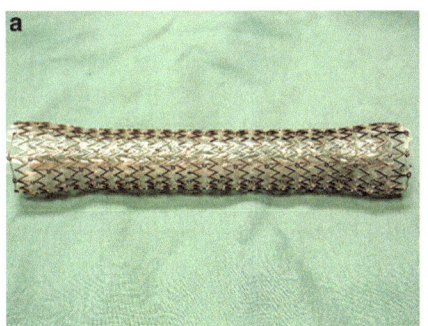
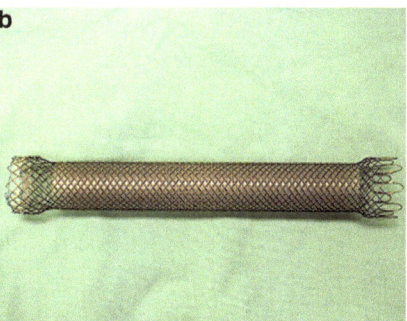

Fig. 7.2 (**a**) Fully covered Endomaxx stent (Merit Medical Endotek, South Jordan, UT, USA) and (**b**) partially covered WallFlex esophageal stent (Boston Scientific, Marlborough, MA, USA)

duced from polyester. Regardless of construction, most stents have some design element to help minimize post-deployment migration as well.

Stents used for leak management are either fully or partially covered. Partially covered SEMS offer the luxury of less migration compared to fully covered SEMS and SEPS [46]. The uncovered ends allow for mucosal proliferation into the stent matrix, which provides an anchoring effect. Fully covered SEMS won't allow for mucosal ingrowth and anchoring, allowing for less difficulty during stent removal. However, fully covered SEMS are more prone to migration [47, 48]. We generally prefer the use of fully covered stents in our practice.

The endoscopist should also be aware of the variability in stent delivery systems. Some delivery systems allow for either proximal or distal stent deployment, with several SEMS having the ability to be recaptured if the initial position of the stent is not correct [9]. Delivery systems of SEPS tend to be the larger and stiffer, making SEPS more ideal for proximal leaks, which tend to have less angulation of the distal landing sites. Self-expanding metal stent delivery systems are more flexible with smaller diameters, making SEMS ideal for leaks found in more angulated lumens, such as in the setting of a sleeve gastrectomy leak [9]. Figure 7.3 demonstrates an undeployed SEMS and the delivery system.

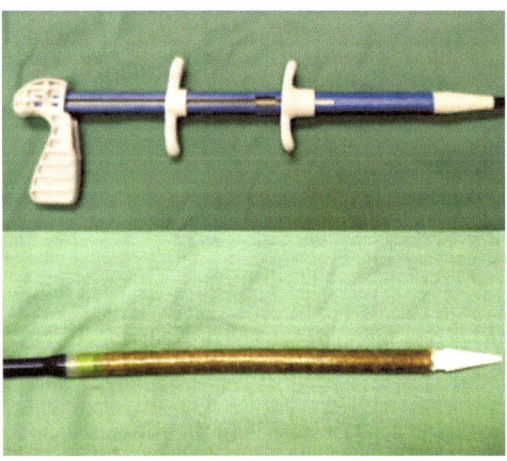

Fig. 7.3 Stent deployment system: a deployment system handle (*top*) and an undeployed Endomaxx Stent (*bottom*) (Merit Medical Endotek, South Jordan, UT, USA)

Typically, an upper gastrointestinal endoscope is used to evaluate and confirm a leak if not done previously with radiographic modalities. Intraoperative fluoroscopy with intraluminal injection of water-soluble contrast via the upper gastrointestinal endoscope may be utilized to confirm the area of leak. A Multi-3 V Plus extraction balloon (Olympus, Center Valley, PA, USA) catheter may be used for definitive localization and injection of contrast within the perforation. Adequate landing zones above and below the leak must be confirmed endoscopically. Obstructions (strictures or postoperative intraluminal twists) at the distal landing zone must be dealt with accordingly prior to deployment of the stent. Failure to recognize a distal obstruction will inhibit healing of the leak due to a buildup of intraluminal pressure distal to the stent.

Endoluminal Stent Deployment

In most instances, esophageal stents can be placed with moderate sedation. Patients with multiple medical comorbidities (ASA III and IV) or presenting with an acute perforation or anastomotic breakdown (following bariatric surgery) may be better suited to undergo endotracheal intubation [49] in order to protect the airway. An upper endoscopy to determine the proximal and distal landing zones of the stent is required. Placement of intraluminal clips or radiopaque markers on the patient (such as a paper clip or clamp) can help define these sites for radiographic deployment. Fig. 7.4 demonstrates a deployed endoluminal stent and radiographic evaluation.

Stent deployment may occur under fluoroscopic or endoscopic guidance. Endoscopic guidance requires the positioning of a guidewire well beyond the leak site. The endoscope is removed (leaving the guidewire in place) and the stent deployment system is inserted over the guidewire. The endoscope is reinserted down to the level of the proximal landing zone alongside the guidewire and stent system. Deployment occurs under direct endoscopic visualization to ensure

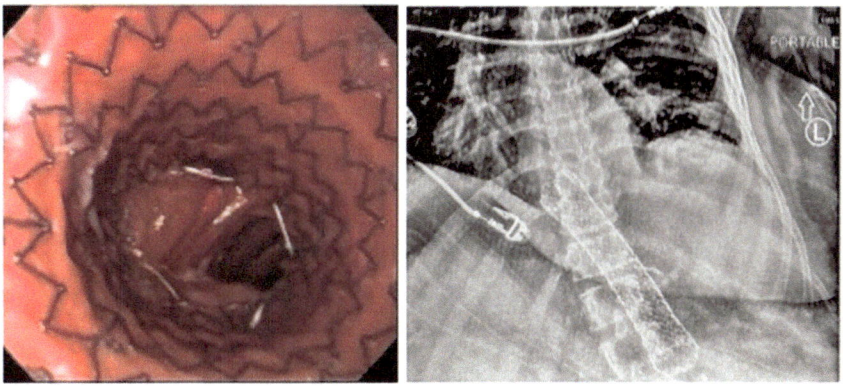

Fig. 7.4 Endoscopic view of a deployed esophageal stent and radiographic evaluation

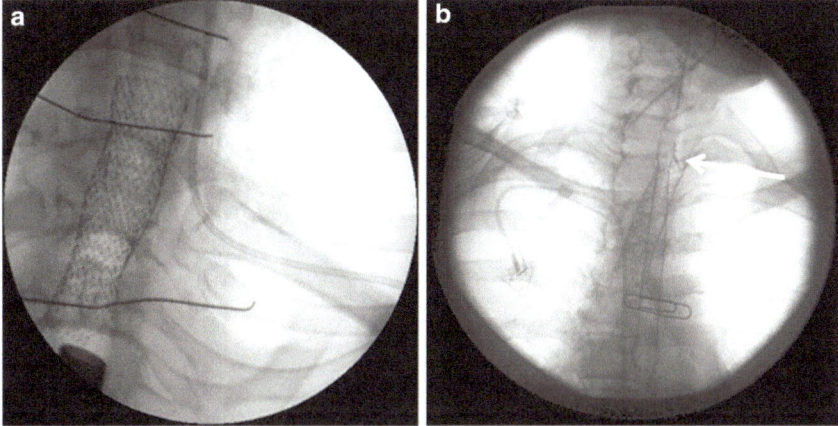

Fig. 7.5 (**a**) Fluoroscopy demonstrating radiographic positioning using various radiopaque markers; (**b**) paperclip and (*arrow*) endoscopic clip (from Ross and Kozarek [49], with permission)

proper proximal landing zone positioning. This can be aided with fluoroscopy as well.

For radiologic placement, radiopaque endoscopic clips or external markers, such as a paperclip, are utilized to identify the location of the leak and landing zones (Fig. 7.5) [49]. A guidewire is endoscopically placed distal to the leak and its position is confirmed with fluoroscopy. The endoscope is removed. The stent deployment system is then passed over the guidewire, utilizing the external radiopaque markers and those found on the stent itself for proper positioning. The stent is then deployed under fluoroscopic guidance. Post-deployment repositioning of the stent to its final resting position with the aid of the endoscope may be necessary. Water-soluble

contrast injected via the endoscope through the stent may be used to confirm the correct position, patency, and diversion of fluids from the site of the leak.

Regardless of deployment technique, the chosen stent should be long enough to cover the defect. Braided or knitted SEMS foreshorten by 30–40% with deployment [49]. Foreshortening typically occurs at the distal end of the stent. For most bariatric cases, the endoscopist should err on the side of a longer stent in order to ensure adequate proximal and distal coverage. Figure 7.6 [44] demonstrates foreshortening of braided/knitted stents.

It is essential that any area of distal narrowing be treated with a stent as well. We prefer larger

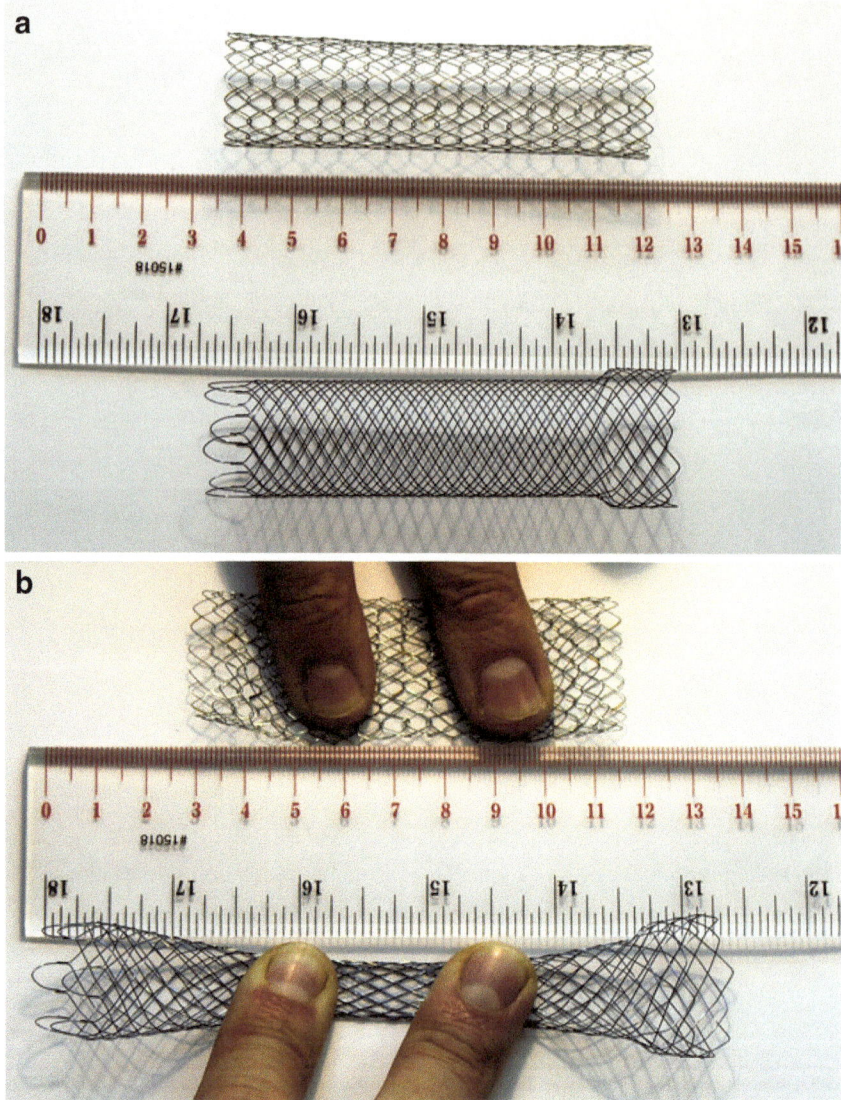

Fig. 7.6 Demonstration of stent lengthening and foreshortening (from Laasch [44], with permission)

diameter stents to minimize any post-removal stricture. Full coverage (leak site and distal obstruction) will occasionally require placement of nested stents to maximize coverage. For these cases the distal stent is placed first, and subsequently the more proximal stent. For most sleeve leaks, stents should begin in the esophagus and terminate just proximal to the pylorus. For bypass leaks, the entire pouch is usually excluded with the stent extending from esophagus to jejunum. To minimize post-deployment migration, there are several techniques that have been employed.

Stents are designed with antimigration struts or ribs, and many endoscopists find these adequate. Options to limit stent migration include securing the proximal end with through the scope clips or with an endoluminal suturing device, such as the Overstitch device (Apollo Endosurgery, Austin, TX, USA). Wilcox et al. [50] evaluated the pull-out force of SEMS in a porcine explant model in which SEMS were secured with an endoscopic suturing device fixation and through the scope clips. Self-expanding metal stent fixation with an endoscopic suturing device resulted in a statistically significant change in pullout force. Self-expanding metal stent fixation with clips did not demonstrate a significantly increased pullout force compared to no fixation [50]. When a distal stricture is present, we have found that most stents do not require additional fixation. However, if repositioning is required for early migration we then augment fixation.

Post-Placement Management

We typically start patients on a liquid diet following upper gastrointestinal series confirming no leak. Stents are left in place for at least 2 weeks and replaced if necessary. If the patient has a change in symptoms while the stent is indwelling, a radiograph should be obtained to confirm that the stent has not migrated. Migration can typically be managed with endoscopic repositioning. Occasionally, surgical retrieval may be indicated. A dedicated post-stent protocol should be in place to prevent complications from stent placement. This may include weekly plain films to assess location of the stent and comparison to prior images.

Removal of endoluminal stents is facilitated by design which includes a drawstring along the proximal edge of the stent. Figure 7.7 demonstrates a retrievable WallFlex stent. Grasping and pulling of the drawstring causes a collapse and decrease in the diameter of the stent, facilitating its removal. The interval between stent placement and removal is not well defined. A longer duration of stent placement leads to an increased level

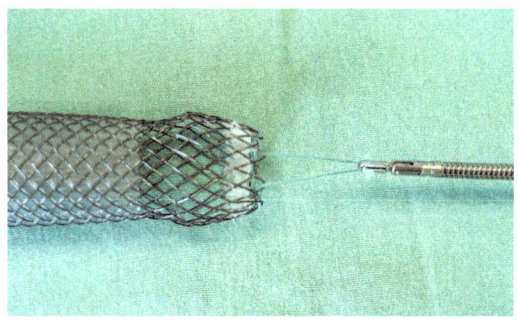

Fig. 7.7 Demonstration of a retrievable WallFlex esophageal stent (Boston Scientific, Marlborough, MA, USA)

of difficulty during removal. A short stent placement period may be not allow for adequate healing of the leak, but a second stent can be placed if necessary. A meta-analysis by Puli et al. [43] demonstrated the majority of studies removed the stents 1–2 months after placement. The authors proposed 6–8 weeks as the ideal timeframe for leak closure and avoidance of mucosal hypertrophy, which may lead to increased difficulty during stent removal [43]. We have had excellent results with 2–4 weeks stent duration time.

Complications of Endoluminal Stents and their Management

A meta-analysis by Puli et al. found stents are overall well tolerated with reported symptoms being nausea, dysphagia, and retrosternal discomfort that resolves within a few days [43]. Stent migration is a common complication often noted in published data with an occurrence rate of 5–62% [51–55]. Stent migration has been attributed to failure of direct contact between the mucosa of the esophagus, gastric pouch or sleeve and stent design which was intended for esophageal leaks [43]. Stent migration can add to increased hospital costs by delaying recovery, or requiring additional endoscopic or surgical procedures. Migration may even cause intestinal obstruction or even transmural erosion [50, 56]. One study described the need for surgical removal of three stents due to migration into the small bowel with failure to pass the stent via the rectum [57]. Therefore a stent protocol must be in place in order to quickly identify a potential migration and allow for endoscopic repositioning.

Complications during stent removal can also occur. Embedding of both ends of a partially covered SEMS may present a challenging removal depending on the amount of granulation tissue formation. Granulation tissue formation depends on the type and size of the stent, radial and axial forces, and the duration of stent placement [58]. Self-expanding metal stent removal can be associated with both bleeding and mucosal tears [59].

Options for removal of a well-embedded stent include argon plasma coagulation (APC) and a "stent-in-stent" technique. Argon plasma coagu-lation of the hyperplastic mucosa can be technically difficult and time consuming [46]. The *stent-in-stent* technique involves placement of a new stent with the same diameter and length within the lumen of an embedded stent. The radial force of the second stent against the first stent causes pressure ischemia, necrosis of the hyperplastic granulation tissue, and improved mobilization and removal of both stents [58]. Aiolfi et al. [58] described a 100% success rate of removal using the stent-in-stent technique for SEMS left in place for a median of 40 days after placement of a second stent for a median of 9 days. Vasilikostas et al. [60] described their experience with the stent-in-stent technique for successful removal of partially covered SEMS with fully covered SEMS in the setting of five sleeve gastrectomy leaks. The initial stents remained in place for 1 month with the second stent remaining in position for 2 weeks prior to successful removal of both stents. We suggest leaving the second stent in place for at least 5 days. See the algorithm in Fig. 7.1 describing options for a difficult stent removal.

Endoluminal Stents and Sleeve Gastrectomy Leaks

In a study of 17 LSG leaks with endoscopic placement of SEMS, the median duration of stent placement was 42 days with a successful closure in 13 (76%) of 17 cases [61]. Garofalo et al. [62] described the successful closure of 90.9% (10/11) of LSG leaks with the average time for closure being 9.9 (range: 4–24) weeks. Treatment with a Wallstent failed in three of five patients with these three patients undergoing successful re-stenting with a Mega stent [62]. Southwell et al. [53] described their experience with management of 21 LSG leaks. An average of 1.6 therapeutic stents per patient were required with an average of five upper endoscopies. Primary resolution was noted in 15/21 (71%) patients with con-firmed leak closure after a mean of 55 days. For the remaining six patients, five achieved leak resolution at a mean of 128 days. Overall, 20/21 (95%) patients achieved leak resolution with a mean duration of 128 days [53]. Table 7.4 dem-onstrates recent data on stents and LSG leaks, specifically [14, 53, 61–63].

Table 7.4 Success rate of stent management in laparoscopic sleeve gastrectomy leaks

Study (year)	n (received stents)	Time from surgery to leak presentation	Type of stent	Indwelling stent time (days)	Success rate (%)	Migration (%)	Average time for closure (weeks)
Garofalo (2016) [62]	11	2 acute leak, 8 early leak, 1 late leak	Wallstent and mega stent	n/a	90.9	n/a	9.9
Southwell (2016) [53]	21	6 acute (29%), 12 early (57%), 1 late leak (5%), 2 chronic leak (9%)	Niti-S; Ultraflex	n/a	95	n/a	10.7
Moon (2015) [63]	6	27.2 days	23 × 100 and 23 × 150 mm	n/a	66.6	50	n/a
Alazmi (2014) [61]	17	n/a	UltraFlex (SEMS) + polyFlex 18 × 150 mm SEPS	42	76	UGI 1 week post-stent removal	n/a
Sakran (2013) [14]	9	7 days	n/a	n/a	55	n/a	n/a

n/a Not applicable

Endoluminal Stents and Roux-En-Y Gastric Bypass Leaks

The data evaluating the use of stents in the RYGB leaks, specifically, is limited. In a retrospective review of 69 of gastrojejunal anastomosis leaks occurring in 2214 patients, 35 patients received stents. Eight patients required additional endoscopic repositioning of their stent. The stent was removed at approximately 14 days or less in 80% of cases, with four patients requiring 4 weeks and three patients requiring 6 weeks of stent placement. Thirty patients were considered completely healed or had a shallow blind fistula on contrast studies. The remaining five patients were noted to have a "thin fistula in the drain tract" from previously placed drains [52].

Edwards et al. described their experience with six leaks after Roux-en-Y gastric bypass. Their leaks were managed with endoscopic SEPS placement. Three patients received a stent following surgical control of their intra-abdominal collection. The stents remained in place for a mean of 35 days. Stent migration was noted in 5 (83%) of the patients. Successful closure was confirmed with an UGI study in 5 (83%) patients. One patient developed a chronic fistula which failed several episodes of stent placement and Tisseel fibrin glue (Baxter, Deerfield, IL, USA) injections and required surgical intervention [64]. Table 7.5 demonstrates recent data on stents and RYGB leaks, specifically.

Meta-Analysis of Leaks and Endoluminal Stents

Due to the low frequency of leaks following bariatric surgery, meta-analyses of previously published data have been performed. Puli et al. [43] included seven studies and evaluated 67 patients with leaks due to a variety of bariatric surgeries: RYGB, sleeve gastrectomy, duodenal switch alone, biliopancreatic diversion, sleeve gastrectomy with duodenal switch, and vertical banded gastroplasty. The pooled proportion of successful leak closures with SESs was 87.77% (95% CI, 79.39–94.19%). Stent migration was noted in 16.94% (95 CI, 9.32–26.27%). However, no information regarding the type of stent used or duration of stent placement was provided [43].

An analysis of 91 patients who developed a leak following a Roux-en-Y gastric bypass or a sleeve gastrectomy was performed by Murino et al. [55]. A partially covered Ultraflex stent (Boston Scientific Corp, Marlborough, MA, USA) or partially covered Cremer nitinol stent (Endoflex GmbH, Voerde, Germany) was placed. The median delay between bariatric surgery and placement of a SEMS was 25 days (range 2–308) with a duration of stenting for 69.5 days (range 5–346). Complete closure was noted in 74 (81%) patients using SEMS. Stent-related complications were noted in 23 patients: 5 (5%) hemorrhages, 2 (2%) perforations, 7 (8%) SEMS migrations, and 13 (14%) esophageal strictures [55].

Table 7.5 Success rate of stent management in Roux-en-Y gastric bypass leaks

Study (year)	n	Time from surgery to leak presentation (days)	Type of stent	Indwelling stent time (days)	Success rate (%)	Migration (%)
Freedman (2013) [52]	35	n/a	Danis (ELLA-CS, s.r.o., Czech Republic)	14	85.5	23
Edwards (2008) [64]	6	20	PolyFlex (Boston Scientific, Marlborough MA, USA)	35	83	83

Conclusion

Endoscopic management of bariatric leaks utilizing endoluminal stents currently remains a promising option. Patient stability is critical when determining patient selection for stent management. In stable, non-septic patients, endoluminal stents remain a viable treatment option in the endoscopic surgeon's armamentarium. However, determining methods of best practice for bariatric leaks remains difficult due to their low incidence rates. Definitive conclusions regarding the length of insertion time for endoluminal stents and options for preventing stent migration remain elusive. Once stents are deployed, a stent surveillance protocol must be in place to prevent complications including early migration and inadvertent long-term dwell times.

References

1. Mokdad AH, Marks JS, Stroup DF, Gerberding JL. Actual causes of death in the United States, 2000. JAMA. 2004;291(10):1238–45.
2. Sjöström L, Lindroos AK, Peltonen M, Torgerson J, Bouchard C, Carlsson B, et al, Swedish Obese Subjects Study Scientific Group. Lifestyle, diabetes, and cardiovascular risk factors 10 years after bariatric surgery. N Engl J Med. 2004;351(26):2683–93.
3. Buchwald H, Oien DM. Metabolic/bariatric surgery worldwide 2011. Obes Surg. 2013;23(4):427–36.
4. Alaedeen D, Madan AK, Ro CY, Khan KA, Martinez JM, Tichansky DS. Intraoperative endoscopy and leaks after laparoscopic roux-en-Y gastric bypass. Am Surg. 2009;75(6):485–8; discussion 488.
5. Aurora AR, Khaitan L, Saber AA. Sleeve gastrectomy and the risk of leak: a systematic analysis of 4,888 patients. Surg Endosc. 2012;26(6):1509–15.
6. Whitlock KA, Gill RS, Ali T, Shi X, Birch DW, Karmali S. Early outcomes of roux-en-Y gastric bypass in a publically funded obesity program. ISRN Obes. 2013;2013:296597.
7. van Rutte PW, Smulders JF, de Zoete JP, Nienhuijs SW. Outcome of sleeve gastrectomy as a primary bariatric procedure. Br J Surg. 2014;101(6):661–8.
8. Weiner RA, El-Sayes IA, Theodoridou S, Weiner SR, Scheffel O. Early post operative complications: incidence, management, and impact on length of hospital stay. A retrospective comparison between laparoscopic gastric bypass and sleeve gastrectomy. Obes Surg. 2013;23(12):2004–12.
9. Andrade JE, Martinez JM. Management of postsurgical leaks and fistulae. In: Thompson C, Ryan MB, editors. Bariatric endoscopy. New York: Springer; 2013. p. 91–101.
10. Gonzalez R, Sarr MG, Smith CD, Baghai M, Kendrick M, Szomstein S, et al. Diagnosis and contemporary management of anastomotic leaks after gastric bypass for obesity. J Am Coll Surg. 2007;204(1):47–55.
11. Madan AK, Lanier B, Tichansky DS. Laparoscopic repair of gastrointestinal leaks after laparoscopic gastric bypass. Am Surg. 2006;72(7):586–90.
12. Walsh C, Karmali S. Endoscopic management of bariatric complications: a review and update. World J Gastrointest Endosc. 2015;7(5):518–23.
13. Parikh M, Issa R, McCrillis A, Saunders JK, Ude-Welcome A, Gagner M. Surgical strategies that may decrease leak after laparoscopic sleeve gastrectomy: a systematic review and meta-analysis of 9991 cases. Ann Surg. 2013;257(2):231–7.
14. Sakran N, Goitein D, Raziel A, Keidar A, Beglaibter N, Grinbaum R, et al. Gastric leaks after sleeve gastrectomy: a multicenter experience with 2,834 patients. Surg Endosc. 2013;27(1):240–5.
15. Rosenthal RJ, International Sleeve Gastrectomy Expert Panel, Diaz AA, Arvidsson D, Baker RS, Basso N, et al. International sleeve gastrectomy expert panel consensus statement: best practice guidelines based on experience of >12,000 cases. Surg Obes Relat Dis. 2012;8(1):8–19.
16. Prathanvanich P, Chand B. Laparoscopic sleeve gatrectomy: management of complications. In: Brethauer SA, Schauer PR, Schirmer BD, editors. Minimally invasive bariatric surgery. New York: Springer; 2015. p. 151–71.
17. Nimeri A, Ibrahim M, Maasher A, Al HM. Management algorithm for leaks following laparoscopic sleeve gastrectomy. Obes Surg. 2016;26(1):21–5.
18. Kim J, Azagury D, Eisenberg D, DeMaria E, Campos GM. ASMBS position statement on prevention, detection, and treatment of gastrointestinal leak after gastric bypass and sleeve gastrectomy, including the roles of imaging, surgical exploration, and nonoperative management. Surg Obes Relat Dis. 2015;11(4):739–48.
19. Deitel M, Gagner M, Erickson AL, Crosby RD. Third international summit: current status of sleeve gastrectomy. Surg Obes Relat Dis. 2011;7(6):749–59.
20. Yehoshua RT, Eidelman LA, Stein M, Fichman S, Mazor A, Chen J, et al. Laparoscopic sleeve gastrectomy—volume and pressure assessment. Obes Surg. 2008;18(9):1083–8.
21. Márquez MF, Ayza MF, Lozano RB, Morales Mdel M, Díez JM, Poujoulet RB. Gastric leak after laparoscopic sleeve gastrectomy. Obes Surg. 2010;20(9):1306–11.
22. Jurowich C, Thalheimer A, Seyfried F, Fein M, Bender G, Germer CT, Wichelmann C. Gastric leakage after sleeve gastrectomyclinical presentation and therapeutic options. Langenbeck's Arch Surg. 2011;396(7):981–7.
23. de Aretxabala X, Leon J, Wiedmaier G, Turu I, Ovalle C, Maluenda F, et al. Gastric leak after sleeve gastrectomy: analysis of its management. Obes Surg. 2011;21(8):1232–7.

24. Martin-Malagon A, Rodriguez-Ballester L, Arteaga-Gonzalez I. Total gastrectomy for failed treatment with endotherapy of chronic gastrocutaneous fistula after sleeve gastrectomy. Surg Obes Relat Dis. 2011;7(2):240–2.

25. El-Ghazaly T, Prathanvanich P, Chand B. Endoscopic stent placement and suturing: management of gastrointestinal anastomotic leaks. In: Kroh M, Reavis KM, editors. The SAGES manual operating through the endoscope. New York: Springer; 2016. p. 127–50.

26. Hamilton EC, Sims TL, Hamilton TT, et al. Clinical predictors of leak after laparoscopic roux-en-Y gastric bypass for morbid obesity. Surg Endosc. 2003;17(5):679–84.

27. O'Brien PE, MacDonald L, Anderson M, Brennan L, Brown WA. Long-term outcomes after bariatric surgery: fifteen-year follow-up of adjustable gastric banding and a systematic review of the bariatric surgical literature. Ann Surg. 2013;257(1):87–94.

28. Lo Menzo E, Szomstein S, Rosenthal RJ. Laparoscopic gastric bypass: management of complications. In: Brethauer SA, Schauer PR, Schirmer BD, editors. Minimally invasive bariatric surgery. 2nd ed. New York: Springer; 2015. p. 261–9.

29. Afaneh C, Dakin GF. Enteric leaks after gastric bypass: prevention and management. In: Herron DM, editor. Bariatric surgery complications and emergencies. Cham: Springer International; 2016. p. 81–90.

30. Csendes A, Burgos AM, Braghetto I. Classification and management of leaks after gastric bypass for patients with morbid obesity: a prospective study of 60 patients. Obes Surg. 2012;22(6):855–62.

31. Bingham J, Shawhan R, Parker R, Wigboldy J, Sohn V. Computed tomography scan versus upper gastrointestinal fluoroscopy for diagnosis of staple line leak following bariatric surgery. Am J Surg. 2015;209(5):810–4. discussion 814

32. Symonds CJ. The treatment of malignant stricture of the oesophagus by tubage or permanent catheterism. Br Med J. 1887;1(1373):870–3.

33. Irani S, Kozarek RA. History of GI stenting: rigid prostheses in the esophagus. In: Kozarek R, Baron T, Song HY, editors. Self-expandable stents in the gastroinstestinal tract. New York: Springer; 2013. p. 3–13.

34. Frimberger E. Expanding spiral – a new type of prosthesis for the palliative treatment of malignant esophageal stenoses. Endoscopy. 1983;15(S 1):213–4.

35. Knyrim K, Wagner HJ, Bethge N, Keymling M, Vakil N. A controlled trial of an expansile metal stent for palliation of esophageal obstruction due to inoperable cancer. N Engl J Med. 1993;329(18):1302–7.

36. Domschke W, Foerster EC, Matek W, Rödl W. Self expanding mesh stent for esophageal cancer stenosis. Endoscopy. 1990;22(03):134–6.

37. Song HY, Choi KC, Cho BH, Ahn DS, Kim KS. Esophagogastric neoplasms: palliation with a modified gianturco stent. Radiology. 1991;180(2):349–54.

38. Song HY, Park SI, Jung HY, Kim SB, Kim JH, Huh SJ, et al. Benign and malignant esophageal strictures: treatment with a polyurethane-covered retrievable expandable metallic stent. Radiology. 1997;203(3):747–52.

39. Shimizu H, Annaberdyev S, Motamarry I, Kroh M, Schauer PR, Brethauer SA. Revisional bariatric surgery for unsuccessful weight loss and complications. Obes Surg. 2013;23(11):1766–73.

40. Khaitan L, Van Sickle K, Gonzalez R, Lin E, Ramshaw B, Smith CD. Laparoscopic revision of bariatric procedures: is it feasible? Surg Endosc. 2005;19(6):822–5.

41. Aryaie AH, Singer JL, Fayezizadeh M, Lash J, Marks JM. Efficacy of endoscopic management of leak after foregut surgery with endoscopic covered self-expanding metal stents (SEMS). Surg Endosc. 2017;31(2):612–7.

42. Sethi M, Parikh M. Enteric leaks after sleeve gastrectomy: prevention and management. In: Herronr DM, editor. Bariatric surgery complications emergencies. Cham: Springer International; 2016. p. 91–105.

43. Puli SR, Spofford IS, Thompson CC. Use of self-expandable stents in the treatment of bariatric surgery leaks: a systematic review and meta-analysis. Gastrointest Endosc. 2012;75(2):287–93.

44. Laasch H. Current designs of self-expanding stents. In: Kozarek R, Baron T, Song H, editors. Self-expandable stents in the gastrointestinal tract. New York: Springer; 2013. p. 51–69.

45. Kauffman GB, Mayo I. The story of Nitinol: the serendipitous discovery of the memory metal and its applications. Chem Educ. 1996;2(2):1–12.

46. Eisendrath P, Cremer M, Himpens J, Cadière GB, Le Moine O, Devière J. Endotherapy including temporary stenting of fistulas of the upper gastrointestinal tract after laparoscopic bariatric surgery. Endoscopy. 2007;39(07):625–30.

47. Efthimiou E, Stein L, Szego P, Court O, Christou N. Stent migration causing alimentary limb obstruction necessitating laparotomy and surgical stent extraction. Surg Obes Relat Dis. 2009;5(3):375–7.

48. van Boeckel PG, Sijbring A, Vleggaar FP, Siersema PD. Systematic review: temporary stent placement for benign rupture or anastomotic leak of the oesophagus. Aliment Pharmacol Ther. 2011;33(12):1292–301.

49. Ross AS, Kozarek RA. Esophageal stents: indications and placement techniques. In: Kozarek R, Baron T, Song HY, editors. Self-expandable stents in the gastrointestinal tract. New York: Springer; 2013. p. 129–40.

50. Wilcox VT, Huang AY, Tariq N, Dunkin BJ. Endoscopic suture fixation of self-expanding metallic stents with and without submucosal injection. Surg Endosc. 2015;29(1):24–9.

51. Salinas A, Baptista A, Santiago E, Antor M, Salinas H. Self-expandable metal stents to treat gastric leaks. Surg Obes Relat Dis. 2006;2(5):570–2.

52. Freedman J, Jonas E, Näslund E, Nilsson H, Marsk R, Stockeld D. Treatment of leaking gastrojejunostomy after gastric bypass surgery with special emphasis on stenting. Surg Obes Relat Dis. 2013;9(4):554–8.

53. Southwell T, Lim TH, Ogra R. Endoscopic therapy for treatment of staple line leaks post-laparoscopic sleeve gastrectomy (LSG): experience from a large bariatric surgery centre in New Zealand. Obes Surg. 2016;26(6):1155–62.

54. El Mourad H, Himpens J, Verhofstadt J. Stent treatment for fistula after obesity surgery: results in 47 consecutive patients. Surg Endosc. 2013;27(3):808–16.

55. Murino A, Arvanitakis M, Le Moine O, Blero D, Devière J, Eisendrath P. Effectiveness of endoscopic management using self-expandable metal stents in a large cohort of patients with post-bariatric leaks. Obes Surg. 2015;25(9):1569–76.

56. Ko HK, Song HY, Shin JH, Lee GH, Jung HY, Park SI. Fate of migrated esophageal and gastroduodenal stents: experience in 70 patients. J Vasc Interv Radiol. 2007;18(6):725–32.

57. Eubanks S, Edwards CA, Fearing NM, Ramaswamy A, de la Torre RA, Thaler KJ, et al. Use of endoscopic stents to treat anastomotic complications after bariatric surgery. J Am Coll Surg. 2008;206(5):935–8. discussion 938–9

58. Aiolfi A, Bona D, Ceriani C, Porro M, Bonavina L. Stent-in-stent, a safe and effective technique to remove fully embedded esophageal metal stents: case series and literature review. Endosc Int Open. 2015;3(4):E296–9.

59. Siersema PD, Hirdes MM. What is the optimal duration of stent placement for refractory, benign esophageal strictures? Nat Clin Pract Gastroenterol Hepatol. 2009;6(3):146–7.

60. Vasilikostas G, Sanmugalingam N, Khan O, Reddy M, Groves C, Wan A. 'stent in a stent'–an alternative technique for removing partially covered stents following sleeve gastrectomy complications. Obes Surg. 2014;24(3):430–2.

61. Alazmi W, Al-Sabah S, Ali DA, Almazeedi S. Treating sleeve gastrectomy leak with endoscopic stenting: the Kuwaiti experience and review of recent literature. Surg Endosc. 2014;28(12):3425–8.

62. Garofalo F, Noreau-Nguyen M, Denis R, Atlas H, Garneau P, Pescarus R. Evolution of endoscopic treatment of sleeve gastrectomy leaks: from partially covered to long, fully covered stents. Surg Obes Relat Dis. 2016;13:925. doi:10.1016/j.soard.2016.12.019. [Epub ahead of print].

63. Moon RC, Shah N, Teixeira AF, Jawad MA. Management of staple line leaks following sleeve gastrectomy. Surg Obes Relat Dis. 2015;11(1):54–9.

64. Edwards CA, Bui TP, Astudillo JA, de la Torre RA, Miedema BW, Ramaswamy A, et al. Management of anastomotic leaks after roux-en-Y bypass using self-expanding polyester stents. Surg Obes Relat Dis. 2008;4(5):594–9.

Treatment of Obstructions and Strictures with Balloons and Bougies

Amanda M. Johner and Kevin M. Reavis

Introduction

The development of an anastomotic stricture is one of the most frequent complications of bariatric surgery and is associated with substantial morbidity. Although both Roux-en-y gastric bypass (RYGB) and sleeve gastrectomy may result in stenosis, this complication is more commonly observed after RYGB. In the bariatric surgery patient, gastrojejunostomy strictures are the most common gastric anastomotic strictures seen by general surgeons and gastroenterologists and will become increasingly more common with the rise of bariatric surgery (Fig. 8.1) [1, 2]. Recently, the incidence of anastomotic gastrojejunostomy strictures post gastric bypass has been reported as 3.7–7.8% at the gastrojejunal anastomosis site [3–6] with no difference between open versus laparoscopic approaches [1, 2, 7]. However, several previous studies that included the early period of RYGB surgery cases (2000–2005)

A.M. Johner, B.Sc., M.D., M.H.Sc., F.R.C.S.C.
General Surgery, Lions Gate Hospital,
231 15th St E, North Vancouver, BC,
Canada, V7L 2L7
e-mail: amanda.johner@gmail.com

K.M. Reavis, M.D., F.A.C.S. (✉)
Foregut and Bariatric Surgery, Department of
Gastrointestinal and Minimally Invasive Surgery,
The Oregon Clinic, 4805 NE Glisan Street, Ste 6N60,
Portland, OR 97213, USA
e-mail: kreavis@orclinic.com

reported a relatively high incidence of postoperative stricture, ranging from 11% to 17% [8, 9]. Less frequent stricture locations include the jejunojejunal anastomosis and sites of passage through the mesocolon or intestinal adhesions. Although obstruction at the jejunojejunal anastomosis is occasionally referred to as a "distal stricture," these obstructions are most likely due to kinking of the anastomosis or excessive narrowing of the common enterotomy closure due to technical error. True stricture formation along a stapled small bowel anastomosis is uncommon.

Etiology

The etiology of gastrojejunal strictures is not well understood. These strictures are thought to be the result of fibrosis and an inflammatory response secondary to a number of plausible factors including those related to the patient (female gender [1], healing capacity [2], presence of diabetes, chronic ingestion of non-steroidal anti-inflammatory drugs (NSAIDs), alcohol, or smoking), surgical technique (type of anastomosis [1, 2, 3], anastomotic tension [2], suture materials or staples, large volume gastric pouch [7], surgeon inexperience [10]), and postoperative complications (anastomotic ischemia [1, 2], anastomotic leak [3, 7], gastric acid secretion from the neopouch [3, 7], marginal ulcerations [3, 7]). The development of a stricture seems to be related to the initial size of the anastomosis; a 2003 study

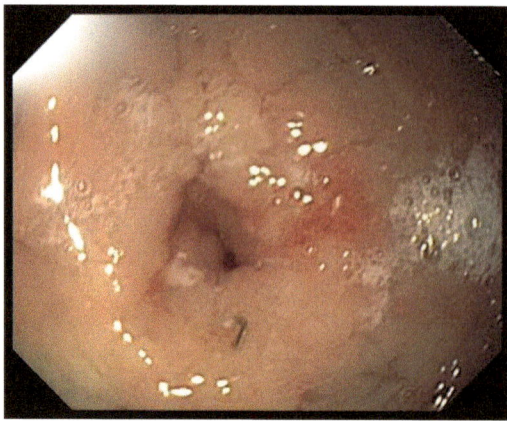

Fig. 8.1 Gastrojejunal anastomotic stricture (photo courtesy of Kevin Reavis, MD)

showed that switching from a 21-mm circular stapler to a 25-mm circular stapler reduced the rate of stricture formation by a factor of 3, from 27 to 9% [2]. For stapled anastomosis, firm apposition or compression of the tissue edges may be helpful in reducing stricture rate. A recent study demonstrated that a circular stapler with 3.5-mm stapler height resulted in a lower stricture rate than one with 4.5-mm staples [11]. The use of staple line reinforcement materials has also been shown to reduce stricture rate [12]. Some surgeons feel that hand-sewn anastomoses are less likely to stricture, while others prefer linear stapled or circular anastomosis; no single study has convincingly supported one of these approaches as superior.

Gastric stenosis is also seen following sleeve gastrectomy. Although laparoscopic sleeve gastrectomy is generally considered a straightforward procedure, surgical technique is one of the major determinants of postoperative complications. The incisura angularis in sleeve gastrectomy is most vulnerable to postoperative stricture, and its incidence has been reported as 3–3.5% [13, 14]. A 2011 review of 230 sleeve patients from University of Texas San Antonio revealed symptomatic stenosis in eight patients (3.5%) [13]. When a stenosis occurs, it is usually one of two types: functional (the passage of the endoscope is possible, but the sleeve is twisted with various degrees of rotation needed to pass the

scope through the gastric lumen) or mechanical (the passage of the endoscope is very difficult or impossible). The mechanisms of stenosis after laparoscopic sleeve gastrectomy could involve either a misalignment of the staple line or result from an anatomic stricture of the gastric sleeve.

Diagnosis

The diagnosis of a post-bariatric surgery gastrointestinal stricture can usually be made based on history alone. Stomal stenosis should be suspected in patients who present with nausea, vomiting, and/or dysphagia [15–17]. However, the positive predictive value of these symptoms for stomal stenosis is only 40% [15]. The absence of these symptoms essentially rules out the diagnosis. While a significant majority of gastrojejunal strictures present between 3 and 6 months following surgery [4, 8, 16, 18, 19], some patients may present much later, even a year or more postoperatively [20]. The time course was illustrated in a prospective study of 400 RYGB patients who underwent routine endoscopy (i.e., regardless of symptoms) following surgery at 1 month and again after a mean of 17 months [21]. Stomal stenosis were diagnosed and treated in 25% of patients at 1 month and in none of the patients at the second examination. The majority of stenosis were mild (stomal diameter of 7–9 mm), and nearly 30% of patients with stomal stenosis were asymptomatic. The typical stricture patient presents with solid food intolerance progressing to liquid intolerance as the stricture narrows. In severe cases, the patients may be unable to swallow their own oral secretions. Radiographic contrast studies are not usually helpful; they are not very sensitive in detecting strictures and pose the risk of contrast aspiration. Upper endoscopy is the primary diagnostic modality of choice. It is difficult to precisely measure a stricture and no formal definition of stricture exists, but most endoscopists consider an anastomosis that is too narrow to permit passage of a standard upper endoscope (approximately 9.5 mm in diameter) to represent a stricture. This is also in the setting of dysphagic symptoms.

Dilation Therapy

After being diagnosed endoscopically, and ideally, once the root cause of the stricture has been resolved, this complication can be treated endoscopically with dilation. Dilation is accomplished by application of expansible forces against a lumenal stenosis. Dilation can be performed with fixed-diameter push-type dilators (bougie dilators) or radial expanding balloon dilators, with or without a guide wire to help positioning, and with or without endoscopy or fluoroscopy. The optimal technique remains to be determined.

Rigid Dilators

Rigid dilators have been the traditional treatment for esophageal strictures, applying both axial and radial forces as they are advanced through a stenosis [15]. Bougie dilators come in a variety of designs, calibers, and lengths. Hurts and Maloney dilators are flexible push-type dilators that do not accommodate a guide wire (Fig. 8.2). They are internally weighted with tungsten for gravity assistance when passed with the patient in the upright position. Wire-guided bougie dilators, like the Savary-Gilliard dilators, do have a central channel to accommodate a guide wire, which is typically placed through the endoscope's instrument channel and advanced beyond the stricture site. The endoscope is then withdrawn and the wire position maintained. The wire is grasped at the patient's mouth and its length noted. The initial choice of dilator depends on the estimated diameter of the stricture. A general rule is that a 24 Fr, 30 Fr, and 36 Fr are trialed for strictures <6 mm, 7–10 mm, and >10 mm, respectively. The dilator is lubricated and loaded onto the guide wire and passed with a fingertip grasp through the stricture and then subsequently removed. The guide wire length at the patient's mouth is then noted again and further dilation can take place with larger diameter bougies. The first dilator to be used is estimated endoscopically by comparing the lumen with the diameter of the endoscope. The "Rules of Threes" should be employed, stating that: during any one dilation session, a maximum of three consecutive dilators of progressively increasing size (a total of 3 mm) should be passed after the first one that meets moderate resistance [1]. Endoscopic evaluation after dilation can be performed to assess any damage to the mucosa. Fluoroscopy is an aid to help determine that the bougie has passed the strictured segment, being advantageous in situations where direct visualization with the endoscope cannot be performed. Direct visualization throughout the procedure is possible with newer, transparent bougies that fit over a standard endoscope. Fluoroscopy can also be used with these dilators, as there is a radiopaque marker often on the dilators.

Fig. 8.2 (**a**) Tapered tip, blunt tip and wire-guided dilators, and (**b**) close up (photos courtesy of Kevin Reavis, MD)

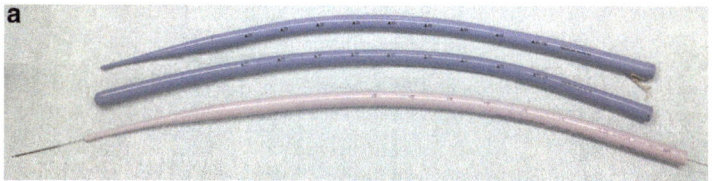

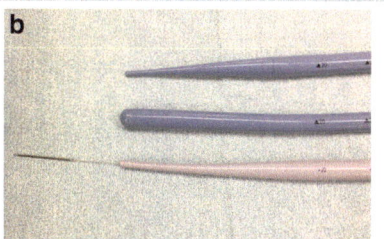

Through-the-Scope Dilators

While rigid dilators have been reported to be successful after gastric bypass surgery [6, 16], through-the-scope (TTS) balloon dilation generally is the preferred method due to the long distance from the mouth to the anastomosis and the presence of a potentially difficult curvature of the roux limb (Fig. 8.3) [1, 6]. First introduced by London et al. in 1981 for two patients who failed the conventional, bougie rigid dilator technique [17], balloon dilation has gained widespread popularity in anastomotic strictures for its less traumatic effect on tissue. Contrary to rigid dilators, balloon dilators exert only radial forces when expanded within a stenosis. There is tremendous variability in the type of balloon dilators that exist, such as single diameter, multi-diameter, and hydrostatic or pneumatic balloons [18]. At this time, through-the-scope balloon dilators are generally preferred to rigid dilators given their ease of use, safety, and the ability to perform multiple dilations under direct endoscopic visualization without the need to repeatedly intubate the esophagus.

TTS balloon dilation, as a procedure, begins with an initial evaluation of the stricture via endoscopy or a barium study. The balloon diameter used is dependent on the diameter size of the stricture [1]. A general rule is that 10-mm, 12-mm, and 15-mm balloons are used for strictures of <6 mm, 7–10 mm, and >10 mm, respectively. The endoscope is placed in the stomach, distal to the stricture if possible, and the balloon is passed through the scope to the end of the endoscope. The endoscope is then withdrawn through the stricture and the balloon is inflated with radio-contrast or water for 30–60 s. The endoscope remains in the esophagus allowing the operator to directly visualize the dilation through the balloon, an advantage of balloon dilators over nontransparent bougies. If fluoroscopy is used, the balloon is inflated until the waste deformity from the stricture disappears. Fluoroscopic control has the advantages of visualizing both the proximal and distal ends of the stricture, not simply the entrance as in endoscopy, and allows visual control of the whole balloon catheter. The

goal of dilation is to achieve a diameter at least 2.5 times the original stricture diameter or at least 12 mm, with repeated dilations as necessary with progressively larger balloon sizes and repeated sessions reserved for recurrences [1, 6].

The primary goal of dilation therapy is symptom resolution, which can usually be attained at a stomal diameter of 10–12 mm [19]. The size of the balloon or bougie used to perform dilation therapy should be guided by factors such as the severity of the stenosis, the time since surgery, the size of the initial anastomosis, and the presence of marginal ulceration. Most recent studies describing the use of balloon dilators in this setting have utilized balloons ranging from 10 to 18 mm [4, 5, 8, 19–23], with some suggesting an optimal goal of 15 mm [4, 21, 24].

Very tight stenosis should be gradually dilated over multiple sessions using progressively larger dilators and generally adhering to the "rule of threes" (i.e., dilating no more than 3 mm sizes in a single session) [1]. Endoscopists should exercise caution when attempting to pass a balloon dilator beyond a tight stenosis after RYGB because of the short blind stump of jejunum immediately (and sometimes directly) beyond the gastrojejunal anastomosis. In these situations, guide wire assisted dilation under fluoroscopic guidance may be necessary.

Gastrojejunal strictures respond favorably to dilation with efficacy rates reaching 100% and require less dilation sessions compared to esophageal anastomotic strictures, with 55–90% of patients requiring only one session [2, 6, 25]. While most patients respond to a single dilation, some will require a second or third; up to 13% may require four to five treatments with or without the addition of directly injected steroids to reduce post-dilation fibrosis [5]. Extrapolating for the esophageal stricture data, predictive factors that determine the success of dilation include stricture diameter >13 mm [26], stricture length <12 mm [27], and strictures without prior history of leakage [27]. Predictors of failure of dilation include interval from surgery to the first initial intervention <90 days [26] and balloon dilation to 12 mm or less [26]. Through-the-scope balloon dilation has very few complications and an

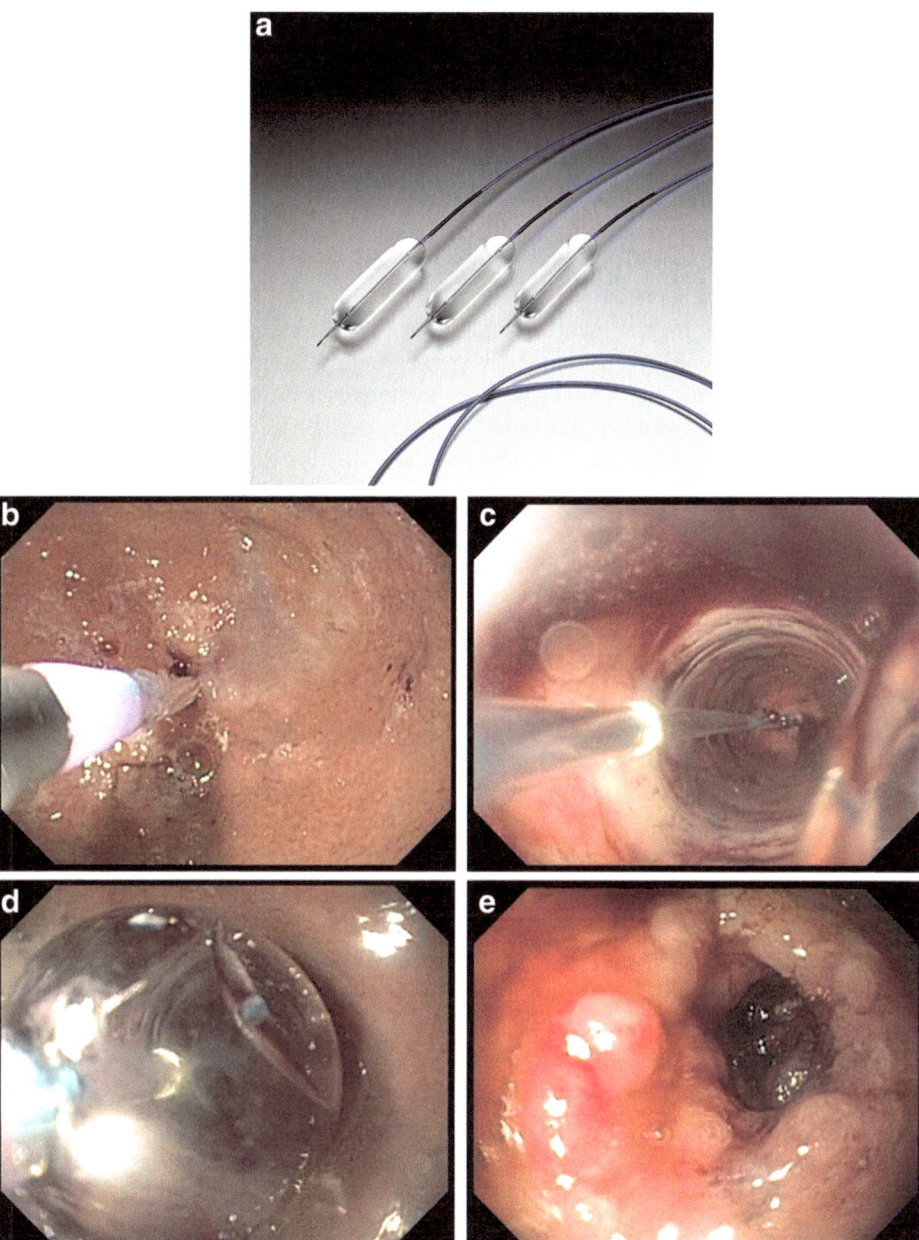

Fig. 8.3 (**a**) CRE™ Balloon dilatation catheters (photo courtesy of Boston Scientific, Marlborough MA, USA, with permission). (**b**) Balloon dilator insertion through a stricture, with "through the balloon" view (**c**), "outside the balloon" view (**d**), and post-dilation view (**e**) (latter photos courtesy of Kevin Reavis, MD)

acceptable perforation rate of 2–3% of patients undergoing dilation for stomal stenosis [5, 6, 23]. In a 2008 study of 61 patients who underwent 128 dilations, 3 patients experienced radiographic evidence of perforation afterwards [28]. These patients were immediately taken to the operating room for laparoscopic exploration; although the site of the perforation was not found in any of the 3, all of the patients in this series responded well to surgical drainage, bowel rest, and intravenous antibiotics. Alternative strategies including the use of endoscopically placed fully covered esophageal stents to allow for nonsurgical management of the perforation can also be considered. Recent data have indicated that the number of dilation session and ischemic segments in the stricture are significant risk factors for perforation, while the ischemic segment and fistula have been positively associated with dilation failure [29]. The risk can be minimized by starting with a dilator that is only slightly larger than the diameter of the stoma and increasing the size gradually. Avoidance of overly aggressive dilation will also reduce the risk of creating an excessively large stoma, which can potentially contribute to weight regain and dumping syndrome.

Strictures can also occur following sleeve gastrectomy. When obstructive symptoms are present post-sleeve gastrectomy, and if an upper GI series demonstrates true stricture, endoscopic or surgical intervention is required. A 2011 review of 230 sleeve patients from University of Texas San Antonio revealed symptomatic stenosis in eight patients (3.5%) [13]. The location of the stenosis in all but one of these patients was the mid-body of the sleeve near the incisura angularis. Patients in this cohort were all treated with endoscopic balloon dilatation with a 15–18 mm balloon. All patients were successfully treated with one or two balloon dilatations (mean 1.6) and were ultimately able to tolerate a regular diet by 50 days after first treatment. Scheffel and Weiner reported three cases of sleeve obstruction managed with different approaches [30]. One patient was found to have kinking of her sleeve due to adhesions and was successfully treated with laparoscopic adhesiolysis. A second patient required conversion to gastric bypass. A third patient presented with long-segment stenosis and required laparoscopic adhesiolysis coupled with stent implantation for 3 weeks. Ogra et al. reported successful treatment of fixed stenosis at the incisor angularis after sleeve gastrectomy with conventional balloon dilation followed by use of a 30-mm achalasia balloon [14]. According to Shnell et al. [31], balloon dilation has an overall modest success rate of 44%; they used either TTS balloon dilation (3 cases) or pneumatic balloon dilations (14 cases) for treatment of sleeve

stenosis. More often than not, a stricture at the mid-body of the sleeve gastrectomy has both a mechanical and rotational technical failure. Conventional balloons are not successful and larger diameter achalasia balloons are required.

Additional Techniques

For symptomatic strictures following either sleeve gastrectomy or RYGB, the role for other treatments is usually reserved for refractory strictures, defined as clinical dysphagia despite dilation, in strictures that are unable to be mechanically dilated to 14 mm or to remain at least 14 mm dilated [20, 32] despite 3–5 balloon dilation attempts [6, 33]. Additional techniques that may improve the effectiveness and durability of dilation therapy for stomal stenosis include glucocorticoid injection and the removal of suture material at the site of the stenosis, although the benefit of these maneuvers has not been studied rigorously [19, 34]. Occasionally, serial dilation every couple of weeks for a period of time is necessary. Short-term stenting has also been used to successfully treat stomal stenosis that is refractory to repeated dilation sessions, but complications such as pain and stent migration are common [33]. In rare instances, needle-knife electrocautery incision can be used to cut open a completely obstructed stoma [20]. When endoscopic management of strictures fails, operative revision of the anastomosis or stricturoplasty is appropriate. The enteroenterostomy, when strictured, is more difficult to manage endoscopically due to its location. A stricture in this location often requires surgical revision.

Conclusions

Endoscopic management is generally one of the best methods to identify the characteristics of a stenosis and simultaneously treat this complication. The majority of bariatric centers recommend early management of stenosis using EGD balloon dilation as the first therapeutic option. Since the introduction of through-the-scope technology, endoscopic balloon dilation of post-operative strictures has become generally accepted as an effective and safe therapeutic tool. The clinical success rate of balloon dilation, which indicates resolution of obstructive symptoms and passage of the endoscope without disturbance, exceeds 90%. Clearly, endoscopy plays a pivotal role in the management of post-bariatric strictures, and close cooperation between bariatric interventionalists of medical and surgical backgrounds may further increase the success rate of endoscopic procedures.

References

1. Stangl JR, Gould J, Pfau PR. Endoscopic treatment of luminal anastomotic strictures. Tech Gatrointest Endosc. 2006;8(2):72–80.
2. Nguyen NT, Stevens CM, Wolfe BM. Incidence and outcome of anastomotic structure after laparoscopic gastric bypass. J Gastrointest Surg. 2003;7(8):997–1003. discussion 1003
3. Carrodeguas L, Szomstein S, Zundel N, Lo Menzo E, Rosenthal R. Gastrojejunal anastomotic strictures following laparoscopic Roux-en-Y gastric bypass surgery: analysis of 1291 patients. Surg Obes Relat Dis. 2006;2(2):92–7.
4. Peifer KJ, Shiels AJ, Azar R, Rivera RE, Eagon JC, Jonnalagadda S. Successful endoscopic management of gastrojejunal anastomotic strictures after Roux-en-Y gastric bypass. Gastrointest Endosc. 2007;66(2):248–52.
5. Ukleja A, Afonso BB, Pimentel R, Szomstein S, Rosenthal R. Outcome of endoscopic balloon dilation of strictures after laparoscopic gastric bypass. Surg Endosc. 2008;22(8):1746–50.
6. Da Costa M, Mata A, Espinós J, Vila V, Roca JM, Turró J, Ballesta C. Endoscopic dilation of gastrojejunal anastomotic strictures after laparoscopic gastric bypass. Predictors of initial failure. Obes Surg. 2011;21(1):36–41.
7. Cusati D, Sarr M, Kendrick M, Que F, Swain JM. Refractory strictures after Roux-en-Y gastric bypass: operative management. Surg Obes Relat Dis. 2011;7(2):165–9.
8. Barba CA, Butensky MS, Lorenzo M, Newman R. Endoscopic dilation of gastroesophageal anastomosis stricture after gastric bypass. Surg Endosc. 2003;17(3):416–20.
9. Rossi TR, Dynda DI, Estes NC, Marshall JS. Stricture dilation after laparoscopic Roux-en-Y gastric bypass. Am J Surg. 2005;189(3):357–60.
10. Carter JT, Tafreshian S, Campos GM, Tiwari U, Herbella F, Cello JP, et al. Routine upper GI series

after gastric bypass does not reliably identify anastomotic leaks or predict stricture formation. Surg Endosc. 2007;21(12):2172–7.
11. Hanna K, Seder CW, Chengelis D, McCullough PA, Krause K. Shorter circular staple height is associated with lower anastomotic stricture rate in laparoscopic gastric bypass. Surg Obes Relat Dis. 2012;8(2):181–4.
12. Scott JD, Cobb WS, Corbonell AM, Traxler B, Bour ES. Reduction in anastomotic strictures using bioabsorbable circular staple line reinforcement in laparoscopic gastric bypass. Surg Obes Relat Dis. 2011;7(5):637–43.
13. Parikh A, Alley JB, Peterson RM, Harnisch MC, Pfluke JM, Tapper DM, Fenton SJ. Management options for symptomatic stenosis after laparoscopic vertical sleeve gastrectomy in the morbidly obese. Surg Endosc. 2012;26(3):738–46.
14. Ogra R, Kini GP. Evolving endoscopic management options for symptomatic stenosis post-laparoscopic sleeve gastrectomy for morbid obesity: experience at a large bariatric surgery unit in New Zealand. Obes Surg. 2015;25(2):242–8.
15. Abele JE. The physics of esophageal dilatation. Hepatogastroenterology. 1992;39(6):486–9.
16. Csendes A, Burgos AM, Burdiles P. Incidence of anastomotic strictures after gastric bypass: a prospective consecutive routine endoscopic study 1 month and 17 months after surgery in 441 patients with morbid obesity. Obes Surg. 2009;19(3):269–73.
17. London RL, Trotman BW, DiMarino AJ Jr, Oleaga JA, Freiman DB, Ring EJ, et al. Dilatation of severe esophageal strictures by an inflatable balloon catheter. Gastroenterology. 1981;80(1):173–5.
18. Lin SC, Sy E, Lin BW, Lee JC. Management of colorectal anastomotic strictures using multidiameter balloon dilation. J Soc Colon Rectal Surgeon (Taiwan). 2009;20:62–8.
19. Catalano M, Chua T, Rudig G. Endoscopic balloon dilation of stomal stenosis following gastric bypass. Obes Surg. 2007;17(3):298–303.
20. Lee JK, Van Dam J, Morton JM, Curet M, Banerjee S. Endoscopy is accurate, safe, and effective in the assessment and management of complications following gastric bypass surgery. Am J Gastroenterol. 2009;104(3):575–82.
21. Ahmad J, Martin J, Ikramuddin S, Schauer P, Slivka A. Endoscopic balloon dilation of gastroenteric anastomotic stricture after laparoscopic gastric bypass. Endoscopy. 2003;35(9):725–8.
22. Ryskina KL, Miller KM, Aisenberg J, Herron DM, Kini SU. Routine management of stricture after gastric bypass and predictors of subsequent weight loss. Surg Endosc. 2010;24(3):554–60.
23. Go MR, Muscarella P II, Needleman BJ, Cook CH, Melvin WS. Endoscopic management of stomal stenosis after roux-en-Y gastric bypass. Surg Endosc. 2004;18(1):5–9.
24. American Society for Gastrointestinal Endoscopy Standards of Practice Committee, Evans JA,

Muthusamy VR, Acosta RD, Bruining DH, Chandrasekhara V, Chathadi KV, et al. The role of endoscopy in the bariatric surgery patient. Gastrointest Endosc. 2015;81(5):1063–72.

25. Caro L, Sanchez C, Rodriguez P, Bosch J. Endoscopic balloon dilation of anastomotic strictures occurring after laparoscopic gastric bypass for morbid obesity. Dig Dis. 2008;26(4):314–7.

26. Chung WC, Paik CN, Lee JM, Jung SH, Chang UI, Yang JM. The findings influencing restenosis is esophageal anastomotic stricture after endoscopic balloon dilation: restenosis in esophageal anastomotic stricture. Surg Laparosc Endosc Percutan Tech. 2009;19(4):293–7.

27. Ikeya T, Ohwada S, Ogawa T, Tanahashi Y, Takeyoshi I, Koyama T, et al. Endoscopic balloon dilation for benign esophageal stricture: factors influencing its effectiveness. Hepato-Gastroenterology. 1999;46(26):959–66.

28. Gill RS, Whitlock KA, Mohamed R, Sarkhoush K, Birch DW, Karmali S. The role of upper endoscopy in treating postoperative complications in bariatric surgery. J Interv Gastroenterol. 2012;2(1):37–41.

29. de Moura EG, Orso IR, Aurélio EF, de Moura ET, de Moura DT, Santo MA. Factors associated with complications or failure of endoscopic balloon dilation of anastomotic stricture secondary to roux-en-Y gastric bypass surgery. Surg Obes Relat Dis. 2016;12(3):582–6.

30. Scheffel O, Weiner RA. Therapy of stenosis after sleeve gastrectomy: stent and surgery as alternatives therapy of stenosis after sleeve gastrectomy: stent and surgery as alternatives—case reports. Case reports. Obes Facts. 2011;4 Suppl 1:47–9.

31. Shnell M, Fishman S, Eldar S, Goitein D, Santo E. Balloon dilatation for symptomatic gastric sleeve stricture. Gastrointest Endosc. 2014;79(3):521–4.

32. Kochhar R, Poornachandra KS. Intralesional steroid injection therapy in the management of resistant gastrointestinal strictures. World J Gastrointest Endosc. 2010;2(2):61–8.

33. Marcotte E, Comeau E, Meziat-Burdin A, Menard C, Rateb G. Early migration of fully covered double-layered metallic stents for post-gastric bypass anastomotic strictures. Int J Surg Case Rep. 2012;3(7):283–6.

34. Obstein KL, Thompson CC. Endoscopy after bariatric surgery (with videos). Gastrointest Endosc. 2009;70(6):1161–6.

Andrew T. Strong and Matthew D. Kroh

Introduction

Chapter 8 "Management of Leaks with Endoluminal Stents" serves as a prologue to this chapter. Numerous techniques and studies point to the advantage of endoscopic stenting as a salvage or rescue procedure in the setting of a perioperative leak or perforation [1, 2]. Some leaks that fail endoscopic management continue to be amenable to early surgical revision, though evidence points to this being most effective in the first 120 days after an operation [3]. Failure of these techniques sets the stage for a chronic fistula, and indeed perioperative leak is the most common underlying pathology of chronic fistulae (Fig. 9.1). The other two common underlying conditions to chronic fistulae are foreign body erosions and chronic

A.T. Strong, M.D.
Section of Surgical Endoscopy, Department of General Surgery, Digestive Disease and Surgery Institute, Cleveland Clinic, Cleveland Clinic Lerner College of Medicine, 9500 Euclid Avenue, Cleveland, OH 44195, USA
e-mail: stronga@ccf.org

M.D. Kroh, M.D. (✉)
Section of Surgical Endoscopy, Department of General Surgery, Digestive Disease and Surgery Institute, Cleveland Clinic, Cleveland Clinic Lerner College of Medicine, 9500 Euclid Avenue, Cleveland, OH 44195, USA

Digestive Disease Institute, Cleveland Clinic Abu Dhabi, PO Box 112412, Abu Dhabi, United Arab Emirates
e-mail: Mkroh@ClevelandClinicAbuDhabi.ae

ulceration. Endoscopic identification and management of all types of fistulae will be the focus of this chapter.

There is no consensus definition of a fistula following bariatric surgery. In particular, there is no clear differentiation between a postoperative leak and a chronic fistula [4]. As such, accurate estimates of the incidence of postoperative fistula is challenging, beyond stating it is an uncommon, but frustrating complication of bariatric surgery. In most published literature, the term fistula is used more commonly >12 weeks after the index operation, though this is inconsistently applied [5]. Traditionally the term fistula refers to an abnormal connection between two tubular epithelialized structures [6, 7]. A temporal element is implicit in this definition, as it is clearly differentiated from a gastrointestinal perforation [7]. Naming of fistulae is typically from the origin to the terminus, which in general is from the higher pressure organ to the lower pressure organ [6, 7]. A simple fistula generally refers to a single outlet, whereas a complex fistula contains multiple outlets [8].

Principles of Endoscopic Management of Gastrointestinal Fistulae

When considering endoscopic intervention following bariatric surgery, the therapeutic endoscopist must be prepared, and some key points are worth bearing in mind. The length of time

© Springer International Publishing AG 2018
B. Chand (ed.), *Endoscopy in Obesity Management*, DOI 10.1007/978-3-319-63528-6_9

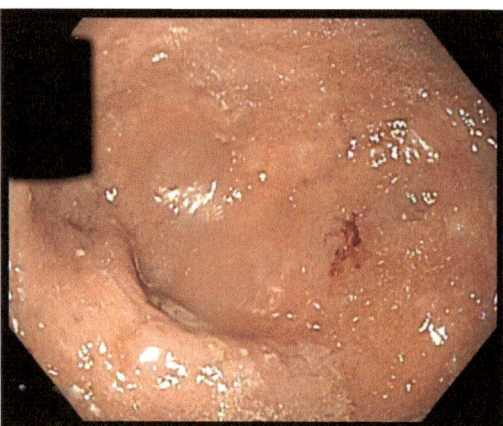

Fig. 9.1 Endoscopic appearance of a chronic gastrointestinal fistula, communicating from the gastric pouch after Roux-en-Y gastric bypass to abscess cavity. Note the fibrotic rim of tissue that surrounds the fistula

between a bariatric operation and endoscopic evaluation is an important factor. Suspicion for anastomotic leak, and/or tenuous anastomoses in the first 28 days after an operation should warrant careful evaluation, and should be done in consultation with the bariatric surgeon, if the endoscopist is not the surgeon. Prior to attempting endoscopic management, having a bariatric surgeon experienced in surgically treating the expected pathology should be available, and if not available, consideration should be made to transfer to a center where these capabilities exist.

Indications for Endoscopy

Dysphagia, persistent nausea and vomiting, or abdominal pain are common indications for endoscopy after bariatric surgery, and often, strictures and ulceration are common underlying pathophysiology. Presentations of fistulae can range from relatively insidious, such as unexplained weight loss after a period of weight stabilization or unexplained weight regain in the absence of increased caloric intake, but also can present as profuse upper gastrointestinal bleeding, empyema, or pneumomediastinum. In general, the anatomical endpoint of the fistula will dictate the presentation.

Expected Appearance of Altered Gastrointestinal Anatomy and Correlation with Radiographic Studies

Bariatric surgery alters the appearance of the upper gastrointestinal tract, and the therapeutic endoscopist must be cognizant of the expected endoscopic appearance of post-bariatric anatomy to identify abnormalities (see Chaps. 5 and 6 for expected anatomy) [9–11]. Given that fistulae may develop years after bariatric operations, even familiarity with historic operations is required [10, 11]. Correlation of endoscopic appearance with radiographic studies can be helpful, including use of contrast-enhanced fluoroscopy during endoscopic procedures. If leaks and/or fistulae are expected, water-soluble contrast radiography may be a better initial test and can help guide a subsequent endoscopic evaluation [12].

Limitations of Endoscopy in the Bariatric Surgery Population

Prior to attempting endoscopic management, limitations of endoscopic technology as related to post-bariatric surgery anatomy should be considered. Most pathology originates in the stomach; however, a small gastric pouch and/or narrow gastric sleeve precludes retroflexion in many cases. For more distal pathologies, the lengths of intestinal limbs may dictate use of deep endoscopic techniques, including push endoscopy or balloon-assisted devices. Some small intestinal pathology may be inaccessible per os and therefore may prevent attempted endoscopic intervention entirely.

Characteristics of an Ideal Endoscopic Therapy

While specifics of management will be further discussed below, no consensus exists about the best approach to chronic fistulae. While this perhaps correctly forces the endoscopist to individually consider each patient and their respective fistulae, creating a treatment algorithm is challenging. Regardless of the endoscope, adjuncts, or devices used, an ideal endoscopic therapy would have the following characteristics: able to be performed under conscious or deep sedation, have a short procedure time, utilize safe and efficacious devices, be relatively simple to perform with reproducible outcomes, and have a durable clinical effect.

The Endoscopic Armamentarium for Management of Chronic Fistulae

A number of endoscopic tools are at the disposal of the therapeutic endoscopist, though availability and technical expertise may vary. Endoscopic interventions that have been described include endoscopic stenting, endoscopic clipping, endoscopic suturing, mechanical debridement, thermal debridement/de-granulation, placement of various occlusive devices, placement of sealing or glue agents, endoscopic vacuum-assisted wound closure, and endoscopic dilation and internal drainage. Specific studies involving use of these devices will be discussed below, but the technologies will be briefly introduced here.

Endoscopic Stents

Endoscopic stents have been applied to palliate or treat chronic strictures, as well as to seal gastrointestinal perforations [13]. Stent technology has been reviewed elsewhere, as well as detailed in Chap. 8 [14, 15]. In general, enteral stents are self-expanding designs crafted with either metal (self-expanding metal stent, SEMS) or plastic struts (self-expanding plastic stents; SEPS). The struts may be covered with polyester or silicone for the full length, or partially covered leaving the struts exposed as the ends. The ends are typically flared to increase the holding power and to prevent migration. Deployment mechanisms are available through the scope, and over a guidewire, necessitating fluoroscopic guidance. Prior to embarking on stent therapy, the patient must be

counseled that repeat interventions for exchange will occur at regularly scheduled intervals as needed, and additional interventions may be necessary to address stent-related complications. A strong body of evidence exists for the use of stents to treat acute leaks after bariatric surgery (see Chap. 8); however, literature supporting use of stents to treat chronic fistulae is limited [1, 16]. Use of enteral stents as a stand-alone therapy is less successful in the management of chronic fistulae, but stent use may prevent further contamination by a fistulous tract and/or allow enteral nutrition during fistula healing, and as such should be familiar to the endoscopist treating chronic fistulae.

Endoscopic Clips

Endoscopic clips are available in two distinct delivery systems, through-the-scope and over-the-scope types. Through-the-scope clips are colloquially referred to as hemoclips, as their intended use was initially hemostasis within the gastrointestinal tract. A myriad of commercially available through-the-scope clips exist, with various degrees of jaw opening, holding power, and maneuverability. There is only one over-the-scope clip system currently commercially available in the United States, OTSC (Ovesco, Tubingen, Germany). The OTSC system is assembled on a standard endoscope and consists of a clear cap holding the clip, a thread and a hand wheel for deployment. To assemble the device, the hand wheel is attached to the working channel. A grasper is then used to grasp the deployment thread and back-feed through the working channel and the thread then wrapped onto the hand wheel. The cap/clip assembly is placed on the scope tip. Suction is then applied and a grasper may be used through the working channel to aid in tissue approximation prior to clip deployment. Clips are typically left in place after deployment. These clips can be removed after placement by application of a bipolar direct current to the hinge portion of the clip, which results in fracture. In addition to three diameters designed to accommodate standard forward viewing endoscopes, OTSC clips are available with three different tooth configurations and two lengths. See Fig. 9.2 for an example of the endoscopic appearance of OTSC application.

Thermal Energy Devices

Thermal energy devices for endoscopy work by either direct thermal contact or by passing electrical current through the target tissue, with either a monopolar or bipolar probe [17]. Argon plasma coagulator (APC) is another type of indirect thermal energy device that utilizes a monopolar alternating current delivered through ionized argon gas [17]. In the treatment of fistulae, these devices are useful for hemostasis when necessary, and for de-epithelialization or ablation of granulation tissue. Ablating the epithelium of a fistulous tract

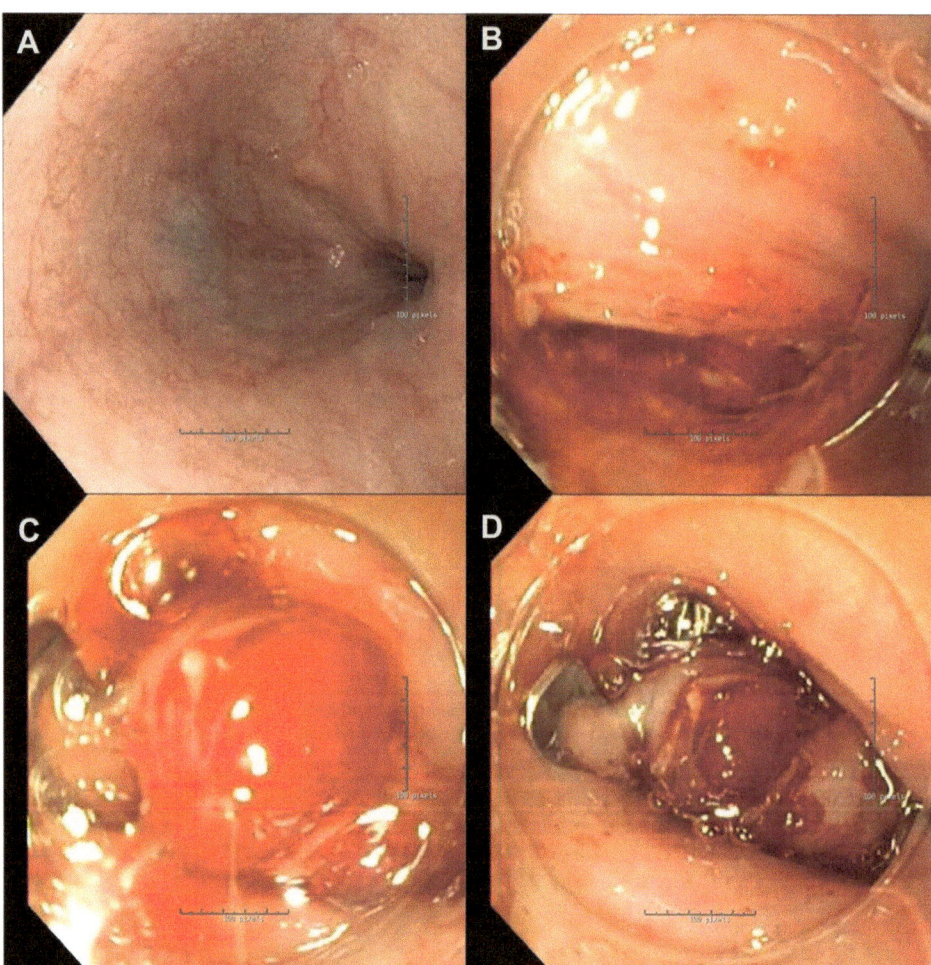

Fig. 9.2 Closure of a gastrointestinal fistula with an OTSC clip (Ovesco, Tubingen, Germany). (**a**) A chronic fistula arising in the esophagus is endoscopically identified. Noted the slightly hyperemic appearance of the mucosal surface. (**b**) Following de-epithelialization of a rim of tissue around the opening with an argon plasma coagulator, the OTSC device is assembled on the endoscope, note the appearance of the endoscopic cap. (**c**) The fistula opening is engaged into the endoscopic cap using suction. The strut of the clip can be seen pre-deployment on the left side of the image. (**d**) Endoscopic appearance of the fistula following OTSC clip deployment

allows apposition of de-epithelialized tissue surfaces, facilitating healing.

Mechanical Debridement

As mentioned above, de-epithelialization aids in healing and closure of fistula tracts [2]. Mechanical debridement may be necessary, especially when debris and/or foreign bodies are additionally present. Various biopsy forceps and brush cytology catheters can be used to accomplish this purpose.

Glue and Sealing Agents

Glue and sealing agents are typically either a cyanoacrylate compound or a fibrin preparation. Cyanoacrylates are solutions that polymerize in the presence of weak bases such as water, and several are commercially available [18]. Cyanoacrylates may be mixed with a lipiodol for use in endoscopy, which has the dual effect of making the glue radiopaque and prolonging the polymerization reaction [18]. Fibrin sealant is a dual component solution containing freeze-dried human fibrinogen and an activator solution that contains human thrombin. The admixture is combined in water, and recreates the terminal process of the natural clotting cascade. Both cyanoacrylates and fibrin glue have been used to successfully manage fistulas [19–24]. Use of sealants in isolation is uncommon in clinical practice when endoscopically managing fistulae, and most are used in conjunction with other devices, such as clips or endoluminal stents [2, 25].

Endoluminal Vacuum-Assisted Closure Therapy

An extension of negative pressure wound therapy has recently been adapted to endoscopic application. Originally described by Wedenmeyer et al., this technique involves endoscopic placement of a polyurethane foam sponge connected to a nasogastric tube, and externally connected to negative pressure suction [26, 27]. In this technique, a nasogastric tube is placed trans-nasally, withdrawn from the mouth, and the sponge attached. A suture loop placed on the distal aspect of the sponge provides a convenient handle for an endoscopic grasper, and allows easier endoscopic manipulation and placement of the device in the GI tract defect [26, 27]. Current published evidence is largely directed to manage acute leaks, but this therapy may also be applicable to chronic fistulas [28]. The combination of gentle mechanical debridement at the time of sponge change, and negative pressure stimulates development of granulation tissue and improved blood flow [27, 29]. Similarly to negative pressure wound therapy devices used externally, endoscopic sponges must be changed regularly. Effectively managing these interval device changes can be a time and resource burden, but for the properly selected patient, this could circumvent a large operation and associated morbidity.

Endoscopic Suturing Devices

Currently, only one endoscopic suturing device is commercially available in the United States, Overstitch (Apollo Endosurgery, Austin TX, USA). Several other devices for endoscopic suture placement have been tested in the past, but are not currently available, including Endocinch (Bard Endoscopic Technologies, Murray Hill NJ, USA) and G Prox (USGI Medical, San Clemente CA, USA). The Overstitch device requires a dual lumen endoscope to operate, and there is technical proficiency to attain; however, the various sutures and anchors that are available make endoscopic closure of some large defects and fistulae possible.

Occlusive Devices and Materials

Off-label use of devices indicated for closure of atrial septal defects has been reported to close gastrointestinal fistulae. Several commercially available devices exist, and are typically either double disk configuration or an umbrella configuration.

In several small cases series, chronic fistulae have been managed with these devices, though none have been following bariatric surgery [30–32]. Prior to use of one of these devices, it is important to measure the defect accurately. One option is to use contrast to fill a balloon passed through the fistula opening [33]. The delivery systems are also not designed to be operated through an endoscope, and are typically passed alongside the endoscope and deployed under endoscopic vision [33].

Endoscopic Dilation and Internal Drainage

In some cases, the best initial treatment of a fistula is internal drainage. Counterintuitively, dilation of the fistula opening may be necessary to allow passage of the endoscope into the tract to accomplish debridement, and/or maintain patency of the fistula to allow for internal drainage (Fig. 9.3) [2, 34, 35]. Bougie or balloon-based systems may be used for dilation. In some cases, short internal plastic stents may be placed as well, similar to a cyst-gastrostomy for pancreatic pseudocysts. These are typically double-pigtail catheters to decrease migrations, as in

pancreatico-biliary stents. As depicted in Fig. 9.3, a large fistula opening may permit the use of an endoscope to reposition a previously placed percutaneous drain.

Principles of Fistula Management

Principles of fistula management can be borrowed from both trauma and the wide body of literature managing enterocutaneous fistulae more generally. Successful management typically follows a relatively predictable pattern: (1) identification of fistula; (2) stabilization of patient; (3) anatomical definition and planning of intervention(s); and (4) intervention [6, 36]. Patient stabilization comprises several elements, including but not limited to control of sepsis, correction of electrolytes abnormalities, diversion of enteric contents away from fistula, and effective nutritional support. Sepsis control is a combination of effective source control, targeted administration of antibiotics, and hemodynamic support when necessary. Addressing nutrition is a key element in the successful management of fistulae, by surgical or endoscopic means [37]. When possible, enteral feeding distal to the fistula is preferred over parenteral nutrition. Enteral

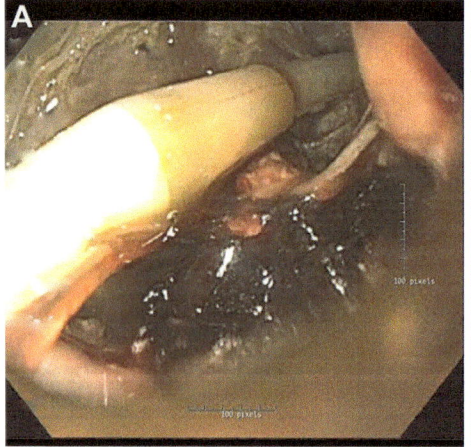
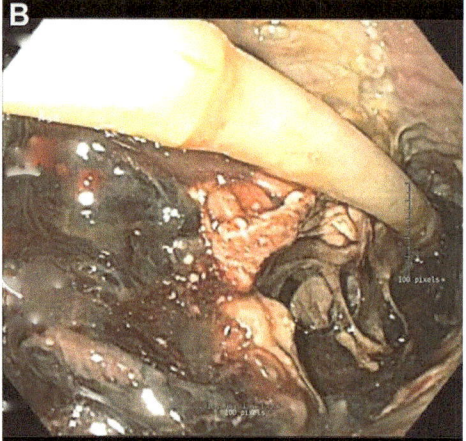
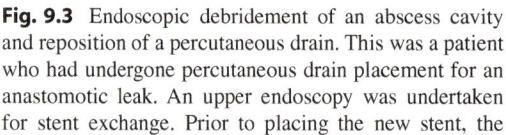

Fig. 9.3 Endoscopic debridement of an abscess cavity and reposition of a percutaneous drain. This was a patient who had undergone percutaneous drain placement for an anastomotic leak. An upper endoscopy was undertaken for stent exchange. Prior to placing the new stent, the large fistulous opening was traversed, as is shown in (**a**). (**b**) Following endoscopic debridement of easily readable necrotic debris within the abscess cavity, the percutaneous drain was slightly repositioned to better allow drainage of the abscess cavity. A stent was then replaced

nutrition preserves intestinal function and integrity of intestinal mucosa [38, 39]. Provision of enteral nutrition may necessitate durable enteral access through feeding tube placement, and planning for this should take place in conjunction with endoscopic intervention of the fistula. Multidisciplinary teams, repeated interventions, and lengthy hospitalizations are common in managing gastrointestinal fistulae.

Owing to their uncommon nature and specialized expertise, only a few centers routinely treat an appreciable number of patients with gastrointestinal fistulae. As such, there is no consensus on management. A number of different types of fistulae have been described following bariatric surgery in case reports, case series, and a few small trials. Nearly all bariatric operations, even revisional bariatric surgery, retain at least a portion of the stomach, and this is commonly the origin of a fistula. We will outline the role of endoscopy in identification and management of gastro-bronchial, gastro-pericardial, gastro-pleural, gastro-gastric, gastro-cutaneous, and gastro-colonic fistulae, and several rare fistulae that exist only in single case reports, as well as fistulae arising from entero-enteric anastomoses associated with several types of bariatric surgery.

Specific Types of Chronic Fistulae Following Bariatric Surgery and Literature Reported Endoscopic Management Techniques

Gastro-pleural Fistulae

Gastro-pleural fistulae are uncommon and generally associated with malignancy or trauma. In the postoperative setting, esophageal reconstruction with a gastric conduit, or fundoplication are other possible antecedent operations [40]. Gastro-pleural fistulae have been reported as a complication following vertical-banded gastroplasty (VBG), Roux-en-Y gastric bypass (RYGB), laparoscopic sleeve gastrectomy (LSG), and laparoscopic adjustable gastric banding (LAGB) [40–43]. Presentation is variable, but may consist of cough, hemoptysis, dyspnea, chest pain, fever, hypoxemia, and may be associated with lung

consolidation, lung abscess, pleural effusion, empyema, and sepsis [40]. Endoscopic identification has been described, but no reports exist of complete endoscopic management [40]. Endoscopic use of APC and application of fibrin sealant was the final step of several operations and drainage procedures that resulted in fistula resolution in one case report [41]. Several surgical interventions are typically necessary on both sides of the diaphragm to completely repair the fistulous tract, and treat the sequelae of the fistula. Some of these interventions may occur prior to the discovery of the underlying etiology.

Gastro-bronchial Fistulae

Different from gastro-pleural fistulae, where the lung parenchyma and large airway remain uninvolved, gastro-bronchial fistulae connect the stomach to the lung tissue and/or bronchi. A systematic review included 36 patients from 11 case series and case reports in which gastro-bronchial fistulae developed after LSG, RYGB, and duodenal switch operations [44]. There are also case reports of gastro-bronchial fistula following LAGB [42, 45]. Presenting symptoms were similar to gastro-pleural fistula and include cough, fever, thoracic pain, vomiting, dyspnea, hypoxemia, recurrent pneumonia, and expectoration of food particles [44]. There were four studies in which upper endoscopy was used for either identification or management of the fistula opening. There were 18 patients who had successful endoscopic management. There are reports with complete resolution of the fistula accomplished by serial stricturotomy and dilation of a stenotic LSG, without attempting mechanical closure of the fistula [46, 47].

Gastro-pericardial Fistulae

Pneumopericardium in the immediate postoperative period following bariatric or foregut surgery would usually be reflective of direct injury during the operation. Pneumopericardium present weeks to years after foregut operation is more enigmatic, but gastro-pericardial fistula should be within the differential (Fig. 9.4). Most of the cases of gastro-pericardial fistula have been described as a complication of peptic ulcer disease, but also present following foregut operations [48]. Presentation is variable, but patients may have pleuritic chest pain, chest pain, or present with pericardial tamponade. Infectious pericarditis is also possible, and enteric debris may be found within the pericardium. Numerous imaging modalities may diagnose pneumopericardium, but discovering the underlying etiology may be more challenging [49]. Endoscopic identification of a gastro-pericardial fistula is possible [50–52]. The few case reports that exist have demonstrated gastro-pericardial fistulae from both the gastric remnant and the gastric pouch/gastro-jejunal anastomosis in patients with RYGB anatomy [50–53]. An additional case report describes erosion of a LAGB through the diaphragm and into the pericardium [54]. Percutaneous or surgical drainage of the pericardium is always necessary, and endoscopic management alone is unlikely to be sufficient for resolution. Experience managing gastro-pleural fistulae at our institution typically involves a combined approach between the bariatric and cardiothoracic surgery teams.

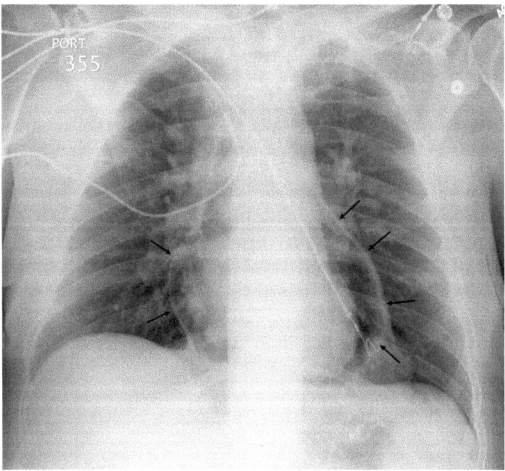

Fig. 9.4 Plain radiograph depicting pneumopericardium (*arrows indicate the edge of the pericardium*). Patient was 8 years post Roux-en-Y gastric bypass, and had a previously known gastrojejunal marginal ulcer, which eventually eroded into the pericardium

Gastro-ventricular Fistula

Gastro-ventricular fistulae are exceptionally rare and associated with a mortality rate of >90% [55]. Gastro-ventricular fistula has been reported as a complication of RYGB surgery, and these authors have treated a case following LAGB [55, 56]. Presentation is profuse gastrointestinal bleeding. While endoscopic identification would likely note brisk bleeding, no reports exist and endoscopic management would be unlikely to be successful. An example of an open repair was reported by Vega-Peralta [55].

Gastro-gastric Fistulae

Gastro-gastric fistulae (GGF) are likely the most familiar to the bariatric surgeon. While GGF are well described following horizontal-banded gastroplasty (HGB) and VBG, they are also common following nondivided open RYGB. In the era of nondivided open RYGB, the rate of GGF formation approached 50% [57]. Routine division of the gastric pouch and remnant has resulted in a GGF rate of 1–6% [58]. Risk factors for development of GGF include failure to completely divide the proximal stomach, foreign body erosions, ischemia usually related to perforations of marginal ulcers, acute or chronic staple line leak, or idiopathic [59]. Foreign body erosions may include sutures, staple material, silastic bands, silicone bands, adjustable gastric bands, or various meshes used historically with VBG [59].

Symptoms of GGF may be absent, or present with an array of nonspecific symptoms that often align with complications following bariatric surgery, including nausea, vomiting, abdominal pain, and gas bloat [59]. Recurrence of diabetes, poor weight loss, and/or weight regain are possible presentations as well, often at further intervals from surgery. Weight recidivism occurs as food bolus travels through the fistula into the bypassed stomach and duodenum [60]. A large GGF allows significant shunting of food into the remnant stomach, and away from the Roux limb [59]. In the case where there is concomitant stenosis of the gastro-jejunal anastomosis and a GGF, complete flow diversion of enteric contents into the gastric remnant and biliopancreatic limb may occur, effectively eliminating the bypass operation. Conversely, patients with asymptomatic GGF may continue to experience adequate weight loss and resolution of comorbid conditions, and thus GGF may not need to be closed [58, 59, 61].

Water-soluble contrast-enhanced upper gastrointestinal series and cross-sectional imaging are often complementary to endoscopic identification of GGF [9]. The order of these studies is debated, with some advocating endoscopy prior to upper gastrointestinal series to avoid contrast interference with endoscopy [59, 62]. Sensitivity of imaging studies is not well reported but is quite high with respect to detection of chronic fistulae [59, 63, 64]. In particular, small fistulae may not be appreciated by endoscopy, and may be revealed by contrast studies. The presence of bile in the pouch after RYGB should alert the endoscopist to the possible presence of a GGF.

Endoscopic evaluation of fistulae is important, giving insight into not only location of the fistula, but also to estimate size and determine suitability for endoscopic therapy (Figs. 9.5, 9.6, and 9.7). Additionally, endoscopy reveals associated sequelae, including gastritis, ulceration, presence of foreign bodies, or necrotic debris [59, 62]. In general, the entirety of the gastric staple line and gastro-jejunal anastomosis should be carefully evaluated. Fistula to the remnant stomach can occur at any point along the staple line, but is more often found at the angle of His. In some cases, use of an endoscopic dissecting cap may be helpful in flattening folds of the gastric mucosa to identify small fistulas. A biopsy forceps or guidewire may also be used as a probe to better elucidate subtle fistulae [59]. Endoscopy with simultaneous fluoroscopy and injection of the tract can be helpful [62]. Prior to detailing specifics of endoscopic management, it is important to note that attempts at endoscopic management of GGF are not usually associated with additional complications if the patients eventually need operative intervention for definitive therapy [65].

Several different endoscopic techniques have been reported to manage GGF following bariatric surgery. The best initial closure rates and most durable results are for GGF <1 cm in diameter [59]. One of the largest series published includes 95 patients with endoscopic management of GGF following RYGB at a single institution using Endocinch (Bard Endoscopic Solutions, Murray Hill, New Jersey) in addition to various other adjuncts, including hemoclip, APC, or cyanoacrylate glue [66]. Technical success rate for initial fistula closure was 95%, but at a median follow-up of 217 days, only 19% remained closed. Fifty-nine patients required at least one additional endoscopic intervention [66]. The endoscopic suturing device used in that series is not commercially available. Another single center study demonstrated endoscopic suture closure of GGF in three patients, which subsequently resulted in additional excess weight loss [67].

The OTSC device has been used in the management of GGF as well. A two-center study of 126 patients undergoing OTSC placement included eight patients with GGF, all post RYBG [68]. The overall conclusion for the study was that immediate technical closure rates were high and long-term durability was low. Within the GGF subgroup immediate technical success was achieved in 75% (6/8) with five needing repeat intervention, and 50% ($n = 4$) showing long-term success of fistula closure with OTSC. In a separate study, OTSC was placed for all types of gastrointestinal fistula, including eight patients after bariatric surgery, with 75% of the patients in this subgroup achieving initial technical closure [69]. Other case reports have similarly demonstrated success with the Overstitch device [70, 71].

Despite promising results of achieving GGF closure with different endoscopic modalities, durability of closure remains challenging [66]. Larger GGF are less likely to close with endoscopic intervention alone, though the size cutoff is not well established. Some series suggest initial fistula size >20 mm was associated with recurrence [66, 72]. Prospective study would be revealing, but the low incidence of GGF may be prohibitive.

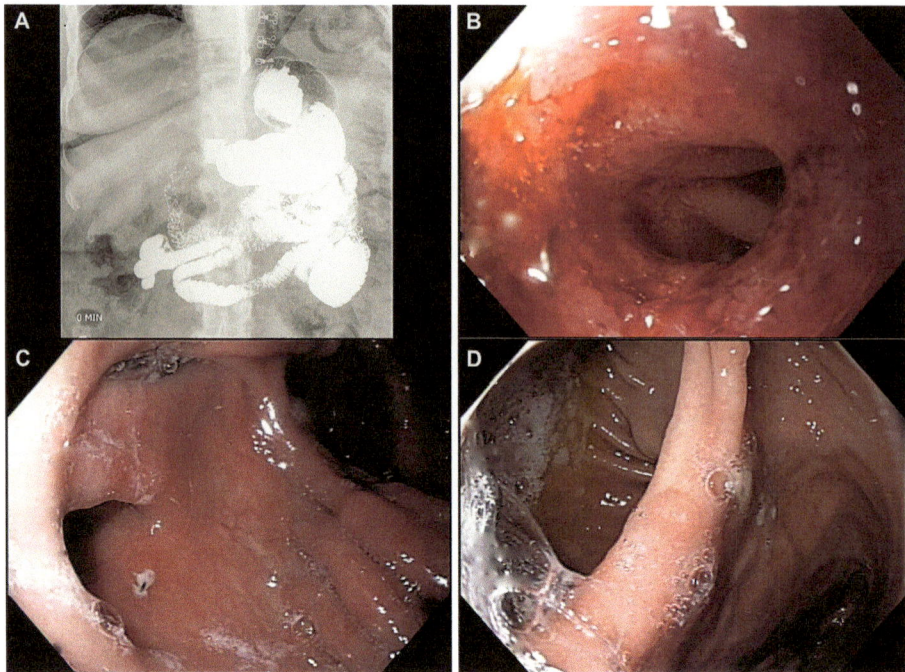

Fig. 9.5 Gastro-gastric fistula following Roux-en-Y gastric bypass (RYGB). Patient is 13 years post RYGB who presented with abdominal pain, weight regain, and de novo diabetes mellitus. (**a**) Barium-enhanced upper gastrointestinal series with opacification of the gastric pouch, excluded remnant, and both the biliopancreatic and Roux limbs. (**b**) Gastro-jejunal anastomosis post dilation. (**c**) Fistula opening in the bottom left, which was easily traversed with the endoscope, and (**d**) the remnant stomach

Gastro-cutaneous Fistula

While gastro-cutaneous fistula (GCF) is less common than GGF, they are likely the second most common fistula type after bariatric surgery. Many endoscopists have familiarity with GCF from treating nonhealing gastrostomy tube sites. GCF closure following bariatric surgery is similar to a PEG site, but may require multimodality therapy. One case report details a patient who had undergone an open conversion from a prior horizontal-banded gastroplasty to a duodenal switch/biliopancreatic diversion. A leak at the gastric cardia failed management with percutaneous drainage, parenteral nutrition, multiple enteral stents and fibrin flue application, eventually developed into a chronic GCF [73]. A Stomaphyx device (EndoGastric Solutions, Redmond, Washington) was used in an off-label manner to plicate the fibrotic tissue around the internal opening of the fistula. This was followed by application of fibrin tissue sealant and multiple through-the-scope clips [73].

In some cases, GCF results from failed attempts at percutaneous management of leaks after surgery. One case report details a patient post-RYGB with a leak from the gastro-jejunal anastomosis that failed to resolve after two surgical interventions. The leak was controlled for 5 months with a percutaneous drain and distal enteral feeding. On referral to a tertiary center, an endoscopy noted intraluminal position of the percutaneous drain, which was withdrawn and revealed a well-epithelialized tract. An APC catheter was used to ablate the tract, and a OTSC clip used to close the internal orifice [74]. Other multimodality strategies have been published as well [75].

A prospective study of 25 patients with GCF following RYGB used a plug made of porcine small intestinal submucosa, typically used to facilitate closure of anal fistulae, to close GCF

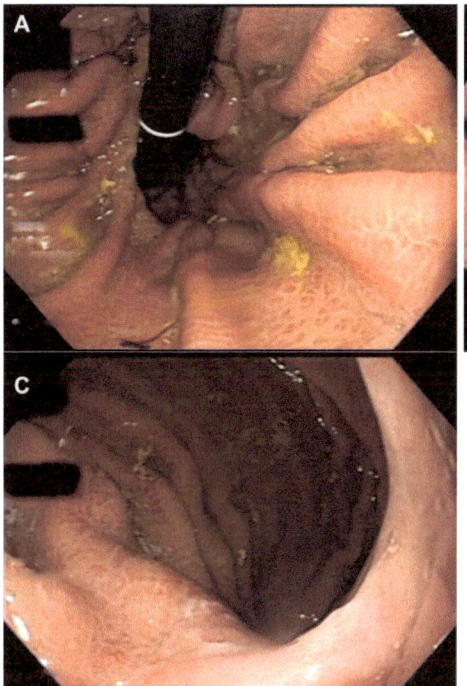
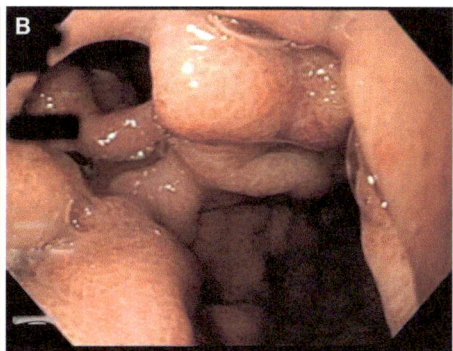
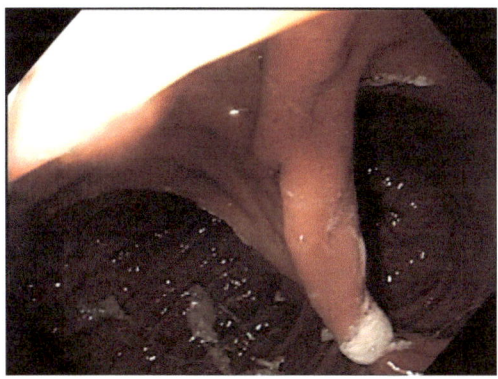

Fig. 9.6 Gastro-gastric fistula after Roux-en-Y gastric bypass (RYGB). Patient was several years post RYGB and presented with weight regain. (**a**) A retroflexed view reveals a dilated gastric pouch and a fistula opening on the upper left of the image alongside the scope. (**b**) More clearly demonstrates a well-matured fistulous opening, which was easily traversed with the endoscope. (**c**) The remnant stomach

Fig. 9.7 Gastro-gastric fistula after vertical-banded gastroplasty (VBG). Patient is 22 years post VBG with a lex ring who developed severe reflux and weight regain. Endoscopy revealed a large gastro-gastric fistula related to patient dehiscence of the staple line. There was no evidence of intraluminal erosion of the lex ring though this is not uncommon

[76]. Porcine small intestinal submucosa is an acellular biologic graft containing collagen and other protein components of the extracellular matrix, which has been shown to facilitate native tissue ingrowth. In this series, a sheet of the biologic graft was rolled into a cone shape and attached to a catheter that was then pulled with an endoscope through the external fistula opening to occlude the tract. 68% of patients experienced fistula closure in this series. While there were no complications noted, most patients required two applications of the plug to achieve complete closure [76, 77]. This approach not only necessitates an external opening, but it was never commercially developed for this specific application.

Gastro-peritoneal Fistulae: A Persistent Fistula to a Chronic Abscess Cavity

The final type of fistulae to discuss is not a true fistula per se, in that it does not connect two tubular organs, but rather connects the gastrointestinal tract to a chronic fistula cavity (Fig. 9.8 and see Fig. 9.1). Generally these arise from an acute leak after surgery that was contained either in the lesser sac or by the omentum. Typically these have small internal openings that have likely undergone a repeat process of partial healing and subsequent chronic inflammation. Treatment of these fistulae was described by Baretta et al., in a case series of 27 patients, which included 14 patients after RYGB, nine patients after LSG, and four patients after duodenal switch [78]. The authors describe the typical appearance of a septum between the gastric pouch and the abscess cavity, in conjunction with a stenosed gastric outlet. Their endoscopic technique was to fully evacuate the abscess cavity by aspiration and saline irrigation followed by a septotomy with an electrocautery knife or APC catheter. Patients with a sleeve anatomy (both duodenal switch and LSG) underwent dilation of the angularis incisura to 30 mm with a pneumatic balloon, while patients with RYGB anatomy underwent balloon dilation of the gastro-jejunal anastomosis to 20 mm. This combined approach allowed internal drainage of the persistent abscess cavity and relieved any concomitant outflow obstruction. Without mechanically closing the fistula tract, the mean time to fistula closure was 18 days. Moreover, most the patients were able to tolerate a liquid diet by mouth on the first day following the procedure [78].

Gastro-colonic Fistulae

Gastro-colonic fistulae most commonly develop as a complication of malignancy, gastrostomy tube misplacement, or peptic ulcer disease. However, gastro-colonic fistula can occur from staple lines, marginal ulcers, or foreign body erosion following bariatric operations. Presentation may range from no symptoms, to emesis of feculent content, to diarrhea and passage of recently ingested food per rectum; typically neither of the latter conditions is well tolerated by patients. A case report details simultaneous erosion of an adjustable gastric band into both the colon and stomach, resulting in gastro-colonic fistula [79]. This case demonstrates that endoscopic evaluation of fistulae following bariatric surgery may also be noted on lower endoscopy. Another case report of a gastro-colonic fistula developed after revision of LSG [80]. In this case the fistula, identified both endoscopically and radiographically, was temporarily managed with an internal stent, allowing sufficient time for the patient to gain better nutritive indices from a combination of peroral and

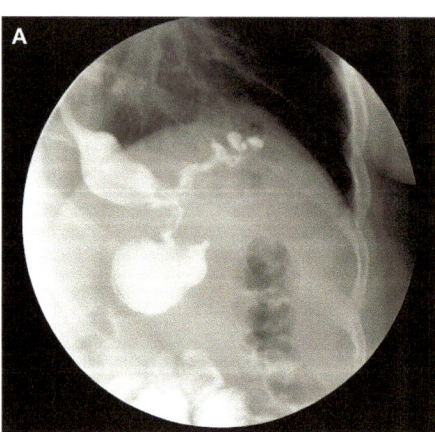
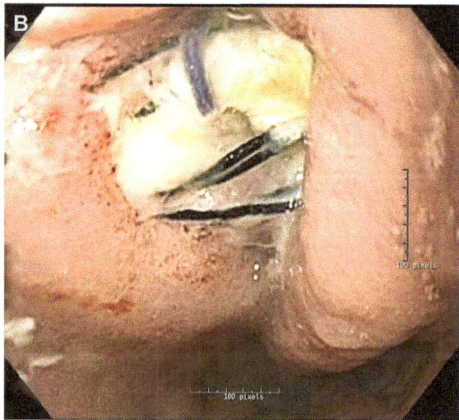
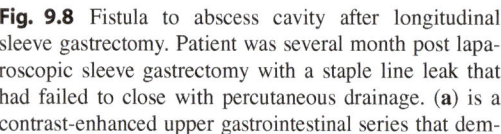

Fig. 9.8 Fistula to abscess cavity after longitudinal sleeve gastrectomy. Patient was several month post laparoscopic sleeve gastrectomy with a staple line leak that had failed to close with percutaneous drainage. (**a**) is a contrast-enhanced upper gastrointestinal series that demonstrates extraluminal contrast extravasation from the upper portion of the stomach. (**b**) Endoscopically the presence of multiple pieces of staple and suture material, as well as other debris likely prohibited effective neo-epithelialization

parenteral nutrition, prior to surgical repair [80]. Endoscopic management of gastro-colonic fistulae arising from diverticula have been described after diagnosis by combined upper and lower endoscopy [81].

Rare Gastro-enteric Fistulae

Other less common types of fistulae have been reported. These include gastro-colic-aortic [82], gastro-splenic [83], and jejuno-colic [84]. The authors of this chapter have also treated patients with a fistulous connection between the gastric pouch and the blind limb of the gastrojejunostomy. While isolated case reports are insufficient to determine efficacy of endoscopic management, diagnosis by endoscopy is typically part of the evaluation.

Conclusion

Bariatric surgery has proven to be durable and effective with a low complication rate. Post-bariatric surgery fistulae are rare, and challenging clinical scenarios. Endoscopy plays an important role in diagnosis and treatment of these conditions. In the appropriate setting, endoscopic management of fistulae can be definitive. In cases when further surgical intervention is necessary, endoscopy can provide a valuable intervention, to lessen or ameliorate sepsis, improve nutritional status, and maximize performance status of a patient prior to a definitive surgical procedure.

References

1. Yimcharoen P, Heneghan HM, Tariq N, Brethauer SA, Kroh M, Chand B. Endoscopic stent management of leaks and anastomotic strictures after foregut surgery. Surg Obes Relat Dis. 2011;7(5):628–36.
2. Bhayani NH, Swanström LL. Endoscopic therapies for leaks and fistulas after bariatric surgery. Surg Innov. 2014;21(1):90–7.
3. Rebibo L, Dhahri A, Berna P, Yzet T, Verhaeghe P, Regimbeau J-M. Management of gastrobronchial fistula after laparoscopic sleeve gastrectomy. Surg Obes Relat Dis. 2014;10(3):460–7.
4. Nedelcu AM, Skalli M, Deneve E, Fabre JM, Nocca D. Surgical management of chronic fistula after sleeve gastrectomy. Surg Obes Relat Dis. 2013;9(6):879–84.
5. Rosenthal RJ, International Sleeve Gastrectomy Expert Panel, Diaz AA, Arvidsson D, Baker RS, Basso N, et al. International sleeve Gastrectomy expert panel consensus statement: best practice guidelines based on experience of >12,000 cases. Surg Obes Relat Dis. 2012;8(1):8–19.
6. Schecter WP, Hirshberg A, Chang DS, Harris HW, Napolitano LM, Wexner SD, et al. Enteric fistulas: principles of management. J Am Coll Surg. 2009;209(4):484–91.
7. Edmunds LH, Williams GM, Welch CE. External fistulas arising from the gastro-intestinal tract. Ann Surg. 1960;152:445–71.
8. Bège T, Emungania O, Vitton V, Ah-Soune P, Nocca D, Noël P, et al. An endoscopic strategy for management of anastomotic complications from bariatric surgery: a prospective study. Gastrointest Endosc. 2011;73(2):238–44.
9. ASGE Standards of Practice Committee, Fukami N, Anderson MA, Khan K, Harrison ME, Appalaneni V, et al. The role of endoscopy in gastroduodenal obstruction and gastroparesis. Gastrointest Endosc. 2011;74(1):13–21.
10. Feitoza AB, Baron TH. Endoscopy and ERCP in the setting of previous upper GI tract surgery. Part I: reconstruction without alteration of pancreaticobiliary anatomy. Gastrointest Endosc. 2001;54(6):743–9.
11. Malli CP, Sioulas AD, Emmanouil T, Dimitriadis GD, Triantafyllou K. Endoscopy after bariatric surgery. Ann Gastroenterol. 2016;29(3):249–57.
12. Lee JK, Van Dam J, Morton JM, Curet M, Banerjee S. Endoscopy is accurate, safe, and effective in the assessment and management of complications following gastric bypass surgery. Am J Gastroenterol. 2009;104(3):575–82; quiz 583.
13. Eisendrath P, Cremer M, Himpens J, Cadière G-B, Le Moine O, Devière J. Endotherapy including temporary stenting of fistulas of the upper gastrointestinal tract after laparoscopic bariatric surgery. Endoscopy. 2007;39(7):625–30.
14. ASGE Technology Committee, Varadarajulu S, Banerjee S, Barth B, Desilets D, Kaul V, et al. Enteral stents. Gastrointest Endosc. 2011;74(3):455–64.
15. Chang J, Sharma G, Boules M, Brethauer S, Rodriguez J, Kroh MD. Endoscopic stents in the management of anastomotic complications after foregut surgery: new applications and techniques. Surg Obes Relat Dis. 2016;12(7):1373–81.
16. Puig CA, Waked TM, Baron TH, Wong Kee Song LM, Gutierrez J, Sarr MG. The role of endoscopic stents in the management of chronic anastomotic and staple line leaks and chronic strictures after bariatric surgery. Surg Obes Relat Dis. 2014;10(4):613–7.
17. Committee AT, Conway JD, Adler DG, Diehl DL, Farraye FA, Kantsevoy SV, et al. Endoscopic hemostatic devices. Gastrointest Endosc. 2009;69(6):987–96.

18. Technology Committee ASGE, Bhat YM, Banerjee S, Barth BA, Chauhan SS, Gottlieb KT, et al. Tissue adhesives: cyanoacrylate glue and fibrin sealant. Gastrointest Endosc. 2013;78(2):209–15.

19. Kowalski C, Kastuar S, Mehta V, Brolin RE. Endoscopic injection of fibrin sealant in repair of gastrojejunostomy leak after laparoscopic Roux-en-Y gastric bypass. Surg Obes Relat Dis. 2007;3(4):438–42.

20. Papavramidis ST, Eleftheriadis EE, Apostolidis DN, Kotzampassi KE. Endoscopic fibrin sealing of high-output non-healing gastrocutaneous fistulas after vertical gastroplasty in morbidly obese patients. Obes Surg. 2001;11(6):766–9.

21. Papavramidis ST, Eleftheriadis EE, Papavramidis TS, Kotzampassi KE, Gamvros OG. Endoscopic management of gastrocutaneous fistula after bariatric surgery by using a fibrin sealant. Gastrointest Endosc. 2004;59(2):296–300.

22. Papavramidis TS, Kotzampassi K, Kotidis E, Eleftheriadis EE, Papavramidis ST. Endoscopic fibrin sealing of gastrocutaneous fistulas after sleeve gastrectomy and biliopancreatic diversion with duodenal switch. J Gastroenterol Hepatol. 2008;23(12):1802–5.

23. Cameron R, Binmoeller KF. Cyanoacrylate applications in the GI tract. Gastrointest Endosc. 2013;77(6):846–57.

24. Vilallonga R, Himpens J, Bosch B, van de Vrande S, Bafort J. Role of percutaneous glue treatment after persisting leak after laparoscopic sleeve gastrectomy. Obes Surg. 2016;26(7):1378–83.

25. Walsh C, Karmali S. Endoscopic management of bariatric complications: a review and update. World J Gastrointest Endosc. 2015;7(5):518–23.

26. Wedemeyer J, Schneider A, Manns MP, Jackobs S. Endoscopic vacuum-assisted closure of upper intestinal anastomotic leaks. Gastrointest Endosc. 2008;67(4):708–11.

27. Mennigen R. Novel treatment options for perforations of the upper gastrointestinal tract: endoscopic vacuum therapy and over-the-scope clips. World J Gastroenterol. 2014;20(24):7767.

28. Bludau M, Hölscher AH, Herbold T, Leers JM, Gutschow C, Fuchs H, et al. Management of upper intestinal leaks using an endoscopic vacuum-assisted closure system (E-VAC). Surg Endosc. 2014;28(3):896–901.

29. Ku A. Assessment of year 2 FCM seminars 2011. Cleveland Clinic Lerner College of Medicine Portal. http://cclcm.ccf.org/eportfolio/s_assess.aspx?instanceid=57748. Accessed 20 Apr 2017.

30. Technology Committee ASGE, Banerjee S, Barth BA, Bhat YM, Desilets DJ, Gottlieb KT, et al. Endoscopic closure devices. Gastrointest Endosc. 2012;76(2):244–51.

31. Kumta NA, Boumitri C, Kahaleh M. New devices and techniques for handling adverse events: claw, suture, or cover? Gastrointest Endosc Clin N Am. 2015;25(1):159–68.

32. Melmed GY, Kar S, Geft I, Lo SK. A new method for endoscopic closure of gastrocolonic fistula: novel application of a cardiac septal defect closure device (with video). Gastrointest Endosc. 2009;70(3):542–5.

33. Rogalski P, Daniluk J, Baniukiewicz A, Wroblewski E, Dabrowski A. Endoscopic management of gastrointestinal perforations, leaks and fistulas. World J Gastroenterol. 2015;21(37):10542–52.

34. Kumbhari V, Abu Dayyeh BK. Keeping the fistula open: paradigm shift in the management of leaks after bariatric surgery? Endoscopy. 2016;48(9):789–91.

35. Bouchard S, Eisendrath P, Toussaint E, Le Moine O, Lemmers A, Arvanitakis M, et al. Trans-fistulary endoscopic drainage for post-bariatric abdominal collections communicating with the upper gastrointestinal tract. Endoscopy. 2016;48(9):809–16.

36. Turégano F, García-Marín A. Anatomy-based surgical strategy of gastrointestinal fistula treatment. Eur J Trauma Emerg Surg. 2011;37(3):233–9.

37. Willingham FF, Buscaglia JM. Endoscopic management of gastrointestinal leaks and fistulae. Clin Gastroenterol Hepatol. 2015;13(10):1714–21.

38. Segaran E. Provision of nutritional support to those experiencing complications following bariatric surgery. Proc Nutr Soc. 2010;69(4):536–42.

39. Kaafarani HMA, Shikora SA. Nutritional support of the obese and critically Ill obese patient. Surg Clin North Am. 2011;91(4):837–55.

40. Garcia-Quintero P, Hernandez-Murcia C, Romero R, Derosimo J, Gonzalez A. Gastropleural fistula after bariatric surgery: a report of two cases. J Robot Surg. 2015;9(2):163–6.

41. Doumit M, Doumit G, Shamji FM, Gregoire S, Seppala RE. Gastropulmonary fistula after bariatric surgery. Can J Gastroenterol. 2009;23(3):215–6.

42. Garrett KA, Rosati C. Gastro-broncho-pleural fistula after laparoscopic gastric band placement. Obes Surg. 2009;19(7):941–3.

43. Sakran N, Assalia A, Keidar A, Goitein D. Gastrobronchial fistula as a complication of bariatric surgery: a series of 6 cases. Obes Facts. 2012;5(4):538–45.

44. Silva LB, Moon RC, Teixeira AF, Jawad MA, Ferraz ÁAB, Neto MG, et al. Gastrobronchial fistula in sleeve gastrectomy and Roux-en-Y gastric bypass—a systematic review. Obes Surg. 2015;25(10):1959–65.

45. Chin PL. Gastrobronchial fistula as a complication of laparoscopic adjustable gastric banding. Surg Obes Relat Dis. 2008;4(5):671–3.

46. Campos JM, Siqueira LT, Ferraz AAB, Ferraz EM. Gastrobronchial fistula after obesity surgery. J Am Coll Surg. 2007;204(4):711.

47. Campos JM, Siqueira LT, Meira MRL, Ferraz AA, Ferraz EM, Guimarães MJ. Gastrobronchial fistula as a rare complication of gastroplasty for obesity: a report of two cases. J Bras Pneumol. 2007;33(4):475–9.

48. Murthy S, Looney J, Jaklitsch MT. Gastropericardial fistula after laparoscopic surgery for reflux disease. N Engl J Med. 2002;346(5):328–32.

49. Davidson JP, Connelly TM, Libove E, Tappouni R. Gastropericardial fistula: radiologic findings and literature review. J Surg Res. 2016;203(1):174–82.

50. Rodriguez D, Heller MT. Pneumopericardium due to gastropericardial fistula: a delayed, rare complication of gastric bypass surgery. Emerg Radiol. 2013;20(4):333–5.

51. Launey Y, Nesseler N, Larralde A. Pyopneumopericardium after total gastrectomy. Arch Cardiovasc Dis. 2010;103(10):561–2.

52. Huyskens J, Macken E, Schurmans J, Parizel PPM, Salgado R. A case of pneumopericardium as a late complication of gastric bypass surgery. Circulation. 2014;130(18):1633–5.

53. Gagné DJ, Papasavas PK, Birdas T, Lamb J, Caushaj PF. Gastropericardial fistula after Roux-en-Y gastric bypass: a case report. Surg Obes Relat Dis. 2006;2(5):533–5.

54. Rudd AA, Lall C, Deodhar A, Chang KJ, Smith BR. Gastropericardial fistula as a late complication of laparoscopic gastric banding. J Clin Imaging Sci. 2017;7:3.

55. Vega-Peralta J, Van Camp J, Freeman M. Gastroventricular fistula in a patient with Roux-en-Y gastric bypass (with video). Gastrointest Endosc. 2008;68(2):392–3.

56. Rutkoski JD, Schrope BA, Lee BE. Survival following gastro-left ventricular fistula in a patient post Roux-en-Y gastric bypass. Ann Thorac Surg. 2017;103(1):e51–3.

57. Capella JF, Capella RF. Gastro-gastric fistulas and marginal ulcers in gastric bypass procedures for weight reduction. Obes Surg. 1999;9(1):22–7; discussion 28.

58. Carrodeguas L, Szomstein S, Soto F, Whipple O, Simpfendorfer C, Gonzalvo JP, et al. Management of gastrogastric fistulas after divided Roux-en-Y gastric bypass surgery for morbid obesity: analysis of 1,292 consecutive patients and review of literature. Surg Obes Relat Dis. 2005;1(5):467–74.

59. Pauli EM, Beshir H, Mathew A. Gastrogastric fistulae following gastric bypass surgery-clinical recognition and treatment. Curr Gastroenterol Rep. 2014;16(9):405.

60. O'Brien CS, Wang G, McGinty J, Agénor KK, Dutia R, Colarusso A, et al. Effects of gastrogastric fistula repair on weight loss and gut hormone levels. Obes Surg. 2013;23(8):1294–301.

61. Stanczyk M, Deveney CW, Traxler SA, McConnell DB, Jobe BA, O'Rourke RW. Gastro-gastric fistula in the era of divided Roux-en-Y gastric bypass: strategies for prevention, diagnosis, and management. Obes Surg. 2006;16(3):359–64.

62. Valli PV, Gubler C. Review article including treatment algorithm: endoscopic treatment of luminal complications after bariatric surgery. Clin Obes. 2017;7(2):115–22.

63. Chandler RC, Srinivas G, Chintapalli KN, Schwesinger WH, Prasad SR. Imaging in bariatric surgery: a guide to postsurgical anatomy and common complications. AJR Am J Roentgenol. 2008;190(1):122–35.

64. Carucci LR, Turner MA. Imaging following bariatric procedures: Roux-en-Y gastric bypass, gastric sleeve, and biliopancreatic diversion. Abdom Imaging. 2012;37(5):697–711.

65. Flicker MS, Lautz DB, Thompson CC. Endoscopic management of gastrogastric fistulae does not increase complications at bariatric revision surgery. J Gastrointest Surg. 2011;15(10):1736–42.

66. Fernandez-Esparrach G, Lautz DB, Thompson CC. Endoscopic repair of gastrogastric fistula after Roux-en-Y gastric bypass: a less-invasive approach. Surg Obes Relat Dis. 2010;6(3):282–8.

67. Raman SR, Holover S, Garber S. Endolumenal revision obesity surgery results in weight loss and closure of gastric-gastric fistula. Surg Obes Relat Dis. 2011;7(3):304–8.

68. Law R, Wong Kee Song LM, Irani S, Baron TH. Immediate technical and delayed clinical outcome of fistula closure using an over-the-scope clip device. Surg Endosc. 2015;29(7):1781–6.

69. Winder JS, Kulaylat AN, Schubart JR, Hal HM, Pauli EM. Management of non-acute gastrointestinal defects using the over-the-scope clips (OTSCs): a retrospective single-institution experience. Surg Endosc. 2016;30(6):2251–8.

70. Wu E, Garberoglio R, Scharf K. Endoluminal closure of gastrogastric fistula. Surg Obes Relat Dis. 2016;12(3):705–6.

71. Gómez V, Lukens FJ, Woodward TA. Closure of an iatrogenic bariatric gastric fistula with an over-the-scope clip. Surg Obes Relat Dis. 2013;9(2):e31–3.

72. Storm AC, Thompson CC. Endoscopic treatments following bariatric surgery. Gastrointest Endosc Clin N Am. 2017;27(2):233–44.

73. Schweitzer M, Steele K, Mitchell M, Okolo P. Transoral endoscopic closure of gastric fistula. Surg Obes Relat Dis. 2009;5(2):283–4.

74. Shehab HM, Elas HM. Combined endoscopic techniques for closure of a chronic post-surgical gastrocutaneous fistula: case report and review of the literature (with video). Surg Endosc. 2013;27(8):2967–70.

75. Mejía AF, Bolaños E, Chaux CF, Unigarro I. Endoscopic treatment of gastrocutaneous fistula following gastric bypass for obesity. Obes Surg. 2007;17(4):544–6.

76. Maluf-Filho F, Hondo F, Halwan B, de Lima MS, Giordano-Nappi JH, Sakai P. Endoscopic treatment of Roux-en-Y gastric bypass-related gastrocutaneous fistulas using a novel biomaterial. Surg Endosc. 2009;23(7):1541–5.

77. Ku N, Thompson CC. Endoscopic therapy for postoperative leaks and fistulae. Gastrointest Endosc Clin N Am. 2013;23(1):123–36.

78. Baretta G, Campos J, Correia S, Alhinho H, Marchesini JB, Lima JH, et al. Bariatric postoperative fistula: a life-saving endoscopic procedure. Surg Endosc. 2015;29(7):1714–20.

79. Póvoa AA, Soares C, Esteves J, Gandra A, Maciel R, Cardoso JM, et al. Simultaneous gastric and colic laparoscopic adjustable gastric band migration. Complication of bariatric surgery. Obes Surg. 2010;20(6):796–800.

80. Trelles N, Gagner M, Palermo M, Pomp A, Dakin G, Parikh M. Gastrocolic fistula after re-sleeve gastrectomy: outcomes after esophageal stent implantation. Surg Obes Relat Dis. 2010;6(3):308–12.

81. Nici A, Hussain S, Rubin M, Kim S. Repair of a gastrocolic fistula using a wire-guided, simultaneous dual scope approach. Endoscopy. 2013;45(Suppl 2 UCTN):E307–8.

82. Villalba MR, Villalba MR. Development of a gastric pouch-aorto-colic fistula as a complication of a revisionary open Roux-en-Y gastric bypass. Obes Surg. 2009;19(2):265–8.

83. Nguyen D, Dip F, Hendricks L, Lo Menzo E, Szomstein S, Rosenthal R. The surgical management of complex fistulas after sleeve gastrectomy. Obes Surg. 2016;26(2):245–50.

84. Fronza JS, Martin JA, Nagle AP. Jejunocolic fistula after Roux-en-Y gastric bypass. Surg Obes Relat Dis. 2012;8(5):e60–2.

Role of Endoscopy in Managing Foreign Body Erosions After Bariatric Surgery

10

Sofiane El Djouzi

Introduction

Since its inception, the field of bariatric surgery has witnessed extensive dedicated research leading to ongoing innovation [1]. The journey started several decades ago with the need to overcome the obesity epidemic that only recently has become recognized as a disease [2]. The pioneers of this arena mastered successive surgical weight loss procedures through endless laboratory experimentations and clinical investigations [3]. As various operations were conducted through the years, surgeons and bench researchers gained more in-depth knowledge and better understanding of the pathophysiology of obesity. Consequently, prior surgeries lost their popularity and fell out of favor due to the emergence of conceptually newer and more efficient procedures. The current weight loss procedural armamentarium has narrowed down to very few operations that have proven safe and effective. Furthermore, the future of bariatrics appears to be favoring endoluminal procedures whether with short-term goals [4–6] or with durable effects [7].

Throughout the years, surgeons have implemented different techniques to enhance the performance of bariatric surgeries at any given time. It was not uncommon, although it has become less practiced, to apply synthetic materials as a boosting adjunct to the index weight loss surgery. Foreign body materials were heavily used at some point in time with surgeons liberally wrapping or encircling targeted parts of the upper stomach to optimize weight loss. Such procedures led to the genesis of the adjustable gastric band, and hundreds of thousands of bands were subsequently inserted worldwide. Embracing its so many attributes (same day surgery, minimal operative risks, and reversibility), the adjustable band became the ideal procedure for so many. Similarly, the nonadjustable bands have been and yet still are being used in some parts of the world. Among all the potential adverse events, these devices and others have introduced a new complication entity called "foreign body erosion." It represents one of the most dreadful complications of such devices and procedures. The erosion could be asymptomatic [8] or might lead to a large spectrum of manifestations including multiorgan erosions, bleeding [9–11], gastric emphysema [12], and gastropericardial fistula [13]. One of those situations that could be deemed unreachable for endoscopic retrieval is when the band migrates distally into the jejunum [14–17]. Equivalently, but seen less often, are other prosthetic material erosions (i.e., prosthetic mesh).

10

10

S. El Djouzi, M.D., M.Sc. (✉)
Division of GI/Minimally Invasive Surgery, Strich School of Medicine, Loyola University Medical Center, 2160 S 1st Ave., Maywood, Chicago, IL 60153, USA
e-mail: sofiane.eldjouzi@lumc.edu

© Springer International Publishing AG 2018
B. Chand (ed.), *Endoscopy in Obesity Management*, DOI 10.1007/978-3-319-63528-6_10

Biomaterials in the Bariatric Patient

Intuitively, any prosthetic (synthetic or biologic) material is regarded as foreign to self and could trigger a cascade of responses [18]. Nonetheless, experimental biologic material from pigs (i.e., porcine and bovine collagen) has resulted in no tissue reaction [19] or histologic rejection [20] on postoperative microscopic analyses. The human immunological system has a varied reaction extending from local periprosthetic wall fibrosclerosis [21] to formal rejection. Some of those fibrotic responses are favorable, like when a metallic rod or similar material is used for bone fracture consolidation. However, the response can become troublesome and certainly unwanted when eroding into the gastrointestinal tract. Foreign body erosions is one of the most feared imperfections and drawbacks to the use of biomedical devices as either adjunct to or as a proper weight loss surgery. Erosion speaks of the process of migration of the foreign body through the gastrointestinal wall.

The rate of such foreign body erosions depends on several factors, with the nature of the biomaterial being the most important. There are many garment materials that have been used with adequate human biocompatibility [22], namely, Gore-Tex, silicone, polypropylene, etc. Considering the large number of adjustable gastric bands inserted (300,000+ worldwide) [23] over the past couple of decades, it is common sense to expect some long-term complications from those devices. Although less popular, nonadjustable bands and wrapping meshes have also been associated with gastric erosions. Permanent sutures and staple line reinforcement materials eroding into the gastrointestinal lumen have also been reported in the literature, yet with less of a major clinical significance. Considering that bands and rings are the main source of gastric erosions in the bariatric population (Fig. 10.1), this chapter will mainly focus on their review. Asymptomatic erosions are not that uncommon [8, 24] but the most common presentation of an eroded adjustable gastric band is that of loss of satiety with weight regain followed by abdominal pain [25]. Port-site sepsis may reveal an erosion of the adjustable band. Interestingly,

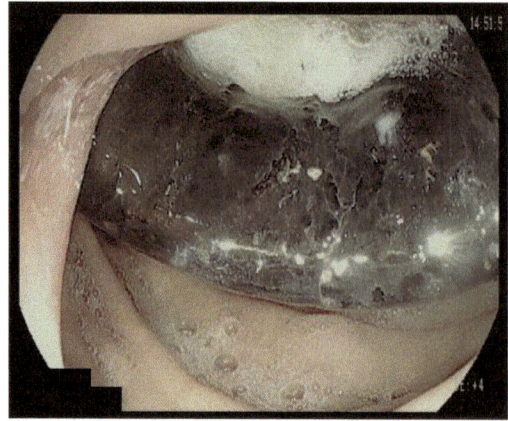

Fig. 10.1 Retroflexed endoscopic view of full thickness gastric erosion of an adjustable band

even the band tubing could lead to visceral erosion especially targeting the colon [26, 27]. In expert's hands, laparoscopic omental plugging and band removal through a separate anterior gastrotomy proved to be an effective method for managing those complications [28]. Furthermore, other laparoscopic methods [29, 30] and even laparotomy have been successfully attempted in such circumstances. This should prompt the bariatric surgeon to learn about the different available modalities of managing such complications.

Foreign Body (FB) Erosion of the Gastrointestinal Tract

The current trend of weight loss surgery has shown that close to 30% of bariatric patients will require revision surgery after their index surgery [31]. Such surgeries could be categorized as corrective for complications from the index surgery or conversional when facing weight recidivism and failures [32]. When a foreign body erosion is detected, one must consider several factors in the decision-making process, namely, severity of presentation and preservation of gastric anatomy for potential future procedures.

Transabdominal corrective gastrointestinal surgery, whether through laparoscopy or laparotomy, is undoubtedly complex and could be disruptive with potential increased morbidity. In contrary and due to its rightly perceived lesser invasiveness, endoscopic therapy of complications following bariatric surgery has gained steady popularity and acceptance [33]. Furthermore, endoscopic management, when feasible, could positively impact outcomes of gastric erosions by allowing faster healing and minimal morbidity [34]. It has been well accepted that endoscopy has evolved from a diagnostic test to viable treatment modality [35]. That being said, it is not until more recently that the "Standards of Practice Committee of the American Society for Gastrointestinal Endoscopy" changed its position statement on [36] endoscopy being a diagnostic tool to now having a therapeutic role in the management of foreign body erosions. [37].

Endoluminal Therapy for Eroded Nonadjustable Gastric Bands

The application of a gastric segmentation procedure using a banding apparatus was initially described by Wilkinson and Peloso [38] in 1978. The authors used a Marlex mesh placed around the proximal stomach. Molina and Oria modified the technique by using a Dacron graft around the proximal stomach resulting in a smaller proximal pouch than the former authors' experience. Although the long-term weight loss from the later was reported to be significantly better, the patient food intolerance was problematic. The gastric partition concept triggered the emergence of subsequent weight loss procedures incorporating banding with foreign bodies (i.e., vertical band gastroplasty [VBG]). The resulted weight loss might have been satisfactory but at the expense of numerous banding-related complications, erosions being the most problematic [39]. In fact, up to 50% of the VBGs require reintervention due to one or more of those complications [40].

Bands consisting of silastic material are technically easier to remove given a lack of incorporation of surrounding tissue or structures. In contrary, bands made of marlex [41] or nonsilastic materials can be more difficult to remove

because of integration into surrounding tissue (Fig. 10.2). The resulting scar tissue that encompasses bands and makes laparoscopic retrieval difficult may very well be protecting the patient after gastric wall erosion.

Fobi [42] reported one of the first endoscopic experiences in removing eroded silastic rings after transected banded vertical gastric bypass (TBVGB) surgeries. Out of a total of 2949 TBVGB, 48 cases of erosions were encountered. Only 40 patients were managed by the author and his team. Eighteen patients were treated conservatively and allowed for spontaneous extrusion of the band into the lumen. Fourteen patients had their band removed endoscopically. The paper does not discuss the management algorithm but does report that the remaining cases were managed through different surgical modalities. Interestingly, three patients underwent revisional surgery (distal Roux-en-Y gastric bypass) with a new ring placed that subsequently leaked and healed. Out of these three leak cases, two developed band erosion that were endoscopically removed. Although endoscopic retrieval of band erosions was successful in 14 patients and failed in 5, the author reports no technical details. This could well be because those endoscopies were

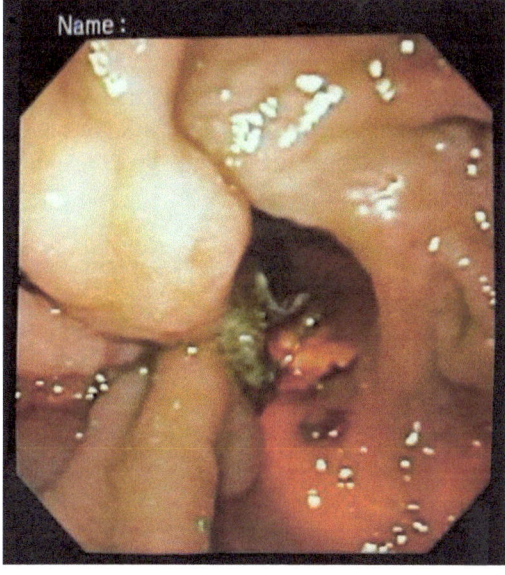

Fig. 10.2 Endoscopic forward view of eroded nonadjustable silastic band

performed by GI endoscopists, and failed attempts were secondary to initial limited experience or technical issues. However, subsequent endoscopic retrieval in the last four patients was done as an outpatient procedure with patients discharged on diet after no leaks were shown on contrast studies. It clearly reflects the team's developing expertise and confidence in managing such complications.

Another challenge in endoscopic retrieval of foreign body erosion is the thickness and amount of material eroded into the lumen. The less the material and more the degree of luminal erosion, inherently easier is endoscopic removal. Removal is also contingent on two other parameters: the architecture of the FB (i.e., suture removal is intuitively easier than debulking a partially embedded Marlex mesh) and the site of erosion. Method of removal may be as simple as using biopsy forceps to extract the material, to a much more complex technique with refined instruments. Argon beam coagulation has been used in dividing the remaining gastric bridge of tissue holding a portion of a gastric band [43]. This allowed subsequent endoscopic retrieval of the band after the port was surgically disconnected from the tubing. In the first report, a penetrated Dacron band was vaporized with a Nd:YAG laser; removal was incomplete, and portions of the Dacron band were left behind. Similarly, favorable experience was reported with the application of Nd:YAG laser at the time of upper endoscopy to vaporize a Dacron band in a bariatric patient. Only part of the band could be explanted with some of the FB left imbedded in the gastric wall.

One of the most challenging complications of the VBG, reported to occur in 1–3% of the cases, is the partial or total Gore-Tex (W. L. Gore Inc., Elkton, Md) band erosion through the vertical staple line or through the lesser curvature of the gastric pouch. Unless a band has freely eroded from the gastric wall, allowing spontaneous elimination or simple endoscopic retrieval, surgical removal may be required. The first endoscopic use of flexible scissors was reported in a European experience [44] when authors removed an eroded vascular prosthesis placed at the time of gastric

surgery. Similarly, Evans et al. [45] replicated analogous experience in the USA when the authors explanted eroded Gore-Tex bands from two sisters that had VBG 4 years prior. The authors describe the use of an Olympus double-channel endoscope and flexible scissors with flexible alligator grasper. Both procedures were completed as outpatient surgery and patients subsequently underwent Roux-en-Y gastric bypass.

Karmali et al. [48] shared their favorable experience with using endoscopic removal of eroded silastic bands in VBG patients. Under conscious sedation, in the endoscopy suite, endoscopic scissors were used through Pentax double-channel endoscope (EG-3870 TK) to retrieve the eroded bands in nine patients. The authors used rat-toothed grasping forceps (GF-49L-1; Olympus) to grab the band and with straight endoscopic scissors (FS-3 1-1; Olympus) cut it. The band was pulled out through the mouth after an average procedure time of 30 min (28.0 ± 8.8 min). All nine patients went home the same day without any reported immediate or long-term complications.

The Molina nonadjustable gastric band was used to create an hourglass effect on the stomach, thereby restricting the size of the proximal gastric pouch and causing early satiety [46]. This weight loss procedure was very popular for a decade (1970s–1980s) but led to a number of significant complications [47]. The morbidity of the operation led to its abandonment. One of the most common indications for surgical exploration was band erosion. The Dacron nature of the band created an extensive inflammatory response around the proximal stomach and in most instances the left lobe of the liver. This led to a hostile environment and made any corrective surgery a challenge.

Blero et al. [49] reported their innovative algorithm (Fig. 10.3) in managing 13 cases of symptomatic band or ring dysfunction at a tertiary-care university center. A total of 10 silastic rings and 3 laparoscopic adjustable gastric bands (AGBs) were reported on. Using a therapeutic gastroscope (GIF-1T 160 or GIF-2T 160, Olympus, Tokyo, Japan), initial upper endoscopy under general anesthesia was diagnostic and therapeutic in all

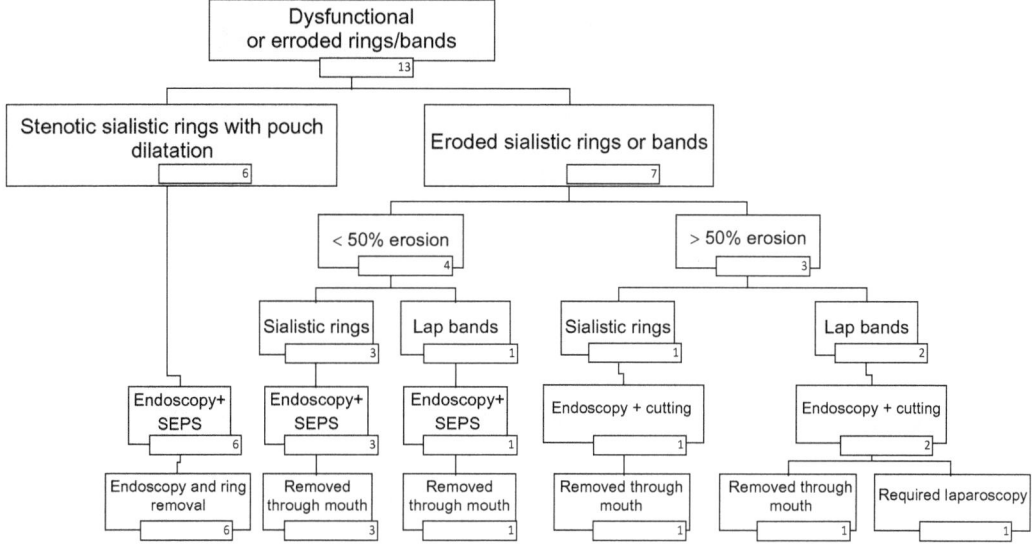

Fig. 10.3 Algorithm of the endoscopic management of 13 cases of symptomatic band/ring dysfunction

cases. Two AGBs and one silastic ring were found to be more than 50% eroded into the lumen and were cut under fluoroscopic guidance using an Atkinson extractor (Olympus Keymed, Southend-on-Sea, UK). One of the two AGBs could not be removed endoscopically as the associated tubing was, at the time of laparoscopy, found to be densely adherent to the gastric lesser curve and liver. Interestingly, the authors deployed SEPS (Polyflex, Boston Scientific, Natick, MA, USA) stents in patients with stenotic silastic rings or partially eroded (<50%) bands. Such approach was meant to trigger some targeted necrosis of the gastric wall between the stent and the ring or AGB. With an average time of 6 weeks (range 3–14 weeks) for the second endoscopy, and like Hookey's [50] prior experience, complete intra-gastric migration was achieved in 6 rings (6 of 9) and 1 AGB (1 of 1). This allowed for both SEPS and foreign body erosion at the same time using a rat tooth forceps. All the patients were discharged on regular diet, within 24 h from their successful endoscopic procedures.

Wilson et al. [51] published their results on 15 patients presenting with erosions of nonadjust-able bands requiring explantation also using plastic stents. Similarly, Campos et al. [52] reported their favorable prospective study deploying self-expandable plastic stent (SEPS) in 41 patients with non-eroded banded (rings) Roux-en-Y gastric bypass suffering from food intolerance. The authors managed to retrieve all bands endoscopically. Most bands were removed (with full erosion) at the time of SEPS removal and the remaining (only partial erosion) a month later. No complications were noted initially; however, nine patients needed endoscopic dilation after stent removal to treat fibrotic strictures. The patient satisfaction was recorded as good in 78% of patients with food tolerance.

Shehab and Gawdat [53] shared their experience with endoscopic management of 16 eroded nonadjustable bands following 2030 banded gastric bypass surgeries. The authors acknowledged a change in their practice favoring an endoscopic approach after eight band erosions treated surgically. All erosions were visualized at the level of the gastrojejunal anastomosis with only two bands presenting with partial thickness gastric erosion. These were deemed not amenable to endoscopic removal. Interestingly, the authors stated that the amount of intraluminal circumference of band erosion was not considered a factor affecting removability. Under moderate sedation, without endotracheal intubation, endoscopic explantation of the remaining 14 full thickness eroded bands (9 Prolene and 5 Gore-Tex bands) was attempted. With an average of 37.5 min (22–55 min) procedural time, all 14 bands were split with endoscopic scissors (13254 MS, Karl Storz, Tuttlingen, Germany) with three cases requiring the additional use of argon plasma coagulation (APC) at a setting of 90 W and 1.5 L/min flow to complete the process. Two of these three were Prolene meshes and could only be partially removed as they were found to be well embedded in the gastric wall. The band fragments were retrieved through either standard (in eight patients) or double-channel (in six patients) adult gastroscopes. These patients were started on clear liquid diet and were discharged home the same day of their procedures. The authors reported high patient satisfaction without any associated complications at 6-month follow-up.

Karmali et al. [54] investigated a novel approach in removing eroded bands which they named TGER standing for "transgastric endoscopic rendezvous technique." Such approach consists of a combo laparoscopic and endoscopic procedure allowing for the retrieval of eroded Molina bands. The retroflexed gastroscope provides intragastric direct view of the eroded segment of the Molina band, which was divided with laparoscopic scissors through a transgastric laparoscopic port. The band was then pulled out through the mouth and the small gastrostomy was sutured closed. The two patients reported in the authors' series had uneventful post-procedural course.

Endoluminal Therapy for Eroded Adjustable Gastric Bands

Adjustable band erosion through the gastric wall is an uncommon phenomenon, yet a serious complication [55] reported in both adults and adolescents [56]. Large series [57, 58] have reported an incidence of 1–2%, but, in small series, it has ranged from 7.5 to 12% [59]. Such variability is likely multifactorial with surgical removal being the most commonly reported technique. The corresponding pathophysiology is also multifactorial [60, 61] with partial stomach damage or microperforation when found early after place-

ment and chronic ischemia for the later presentations. The timing of erosion can be weeks (early erosions) to years after placement (delayed erosions) with up to 75% presenting as silent erosion. Asymptomatic erosions often present with unexpected weight gain [62]. Nonetheless, case reports of unusual acute presentations such as catastrophic hemorrhage [63–65], complete erosion with associated bowel obstruction [17, 66], and septic complications [67, 68] have also been described.

Even though the prevalence of AGB erosions is low, management is still a challenge. A myriad of surgical approaches exists for band explantation and many pioneers have described novel techniques including laparoscopic transabdominal division of the AGB with transgastric retrieval [69]. Laparotomy is a valid approach yet remains the most invasive. The laparoscopic approach for band replacement [25] or explanation [28, 70] has been embraced by many but could prove difficult for several reasons. Adhesions from previous surgery would make it difficult to safely identify the anatomy. A posterior rotation of the band buckle makes it exceedingly difficult to free. Traditionally, the human body walls off such inflammatory process into a contained capsule. Ideally, such FB erosions would benefit from an endoscopic management. This approach preserves the outer gastric wall from any disruption. Additionally, the endoscopic approach is intuitively safer and least invasive of all.

Despite several authors reporting their supportive experience with the endoscopic approach and advocated for its widespread adoption, a 2011 systematic review (1998–2010) of 25 authors' experience on 231 eroded AGBs omitted the endoluminal approach [71]. Similarly, Cherian et al. [57, 72] reviewed the outcome of 865 adjustable gastric bands and found 18 events relating to band erosions. The endoscopic approach was not attempted in any of those patients. Hamdan et al. [73] wrote a paper reviewing the management of complications of different weight loss surgeries. Laparoscopy was thought of as the first line in managing eroded bands without any reference to the role of endoscopy. Furthermore, a recent large 15-year review paper

[25] speculated on higher costs of endoscopic treatments in managing migrated bands. Interestingly, the cost analysis conducted by Chisholm et al. [74] unveiled a lower cost by over $1000 in favor of endoscopic therapy. Brown et al. [25] supported an editorial comment [75] discussing technical burdens of such advanced endoscopy and procedural time. They also disliked delayed endoscopic band explantation when the buckle was not seen within the gastric lumen. They felt repeated endoscopy and separate anesthesia for port and tubing removal was less favorable when compared to surgical one-time intervention. Obviously, all of those concerns are real but can be mitigated with increased experience and an endoscopic combined surgical approach in the operating room.

In a case report by El-Hayek et al. [76] a combined endoscopic and transgastric approach using a standard 8 mm laparoscopic trocar was positioned similar to a percutaneous gastrostomy tube. The endoscope functioned as the "eyes" while the trocar allowed for the use of ultrasonic shears to divide the eroded gastric band. The cut band and tubing were removed transorally using a polypectomy snare. The port of the gastric band was removed through a small skin incision. The entire procedure was done at one setting, under general anesthesia, and did not require full erosion of the band or buckle. Baldinger et al. [77] reported a 1% rate of eroded bands out of the 714 implanted Swedish Adjustable Gastric Bands (SAGB) (Obtech, Zug, Switzerland) over a 3 and half year period. The four patients were asymptomatic with the erosion and initial diagnostic endoscopy revealed a 50–75% erosion of the AGB. In order to promote further erosion and complete intraluminal migration, the authors advocated deliberate overfilling of the bands. At the time of a subsequent visit, under local anesthesia the tubing was cut allowing for port removal concomitantly with the endoscopic retrieval of now a fully migrated band using a polypectomy snare. All four patients experienced no immediate complications.

Similar to Karmali et al. [54] approach but more recently, Prathanvanich [78] presented a video showing successful combination of endoscopic and percutaneous technique. Using the same concept of gastric access as in percutaneous gastrostomy tube placement, a small laparoscopic trocar was inserted into the inflated stomach and under endoscopic guidance. The trocar allowed for the eroded (more than 50%) band to be cut with an ultrasonic shear and retrieved through the mouth. Intelligently, the laparoscopic port was used for a percutaneous gastrostomy tube placement at the end of the procedure.

Specially designed instruments have been manufactured to allow endoscopically cutting eroded bands. Mozzi et al. [79] described the use of therapeutic endoscopy in 20 patients presenting with erosions of adjustable bands from four different manufacturers of AGBs. The authors required that the erosion involves more than 50% thickness and the use of a gastric band cutter (Agency for Medical Innovation GmbH, Gotzis, Austria). Sixteen bands were explanted through the described technique while three patients were found to have perigastric adhesions preventing transoral retrieval. One patient faced technical issues with the cutting wire leading to twisting and blockage of the band at the level of the gastric cardia. All four cases required laparoscopic intervention. Herreros de Tejada et al. [80] illustrated their stepwise technique using the same band cutter (A.M.I. Gastric Band Cutter; CJ Medical, Haddenham, UK). The solo patient treated by the authors had no immediate post-procedure complication and she was discharged home after a 24-h observation. Regusci et al. [81] reported comparable positive experience adopting the same device and technique. Using general anesthesia in five patients and local anesthesia in one, ports were first removed before bands were explanted in the same setting. All patients were sent home the same day without any subsequent complications. The technique is well described but the amount of band erosion or procedural time is not reported. Although no clear explanations were provided, another patient was subjected to laparoscopic removal. Similarly, Lattuda et al. [82] report on seven patients subjected to this technique with the band cutter. Five had their band uneventfully removed endoscopically. One band could not be cut due to twisting of the cutter and required laparoscopy and the other had the band cut but required laparotomy secondary to dense adhesions preventing retrieval. The authors of this review stressed the importance of conducting such procedures in an operating room setting as it allows easy conversion to surgery when needed. Both authors had satisfactory outcomes with the band cutter. However the device is not readily available in all centers secondary to cost and regulatory standards. The device is not available in the USA. Alternatively, and creatively speaking, Flor et al. [83] replicated the same technique but with the use of a 0.035-in. guidewire (Jagwire; Boston Scientific, El Coyol, Costa Rica) passed endoscopically around the eroded band. The wire was then allowed to cut through the band with the aid of a mechanical lithotriptor (Soehendra Lithotriptor, Cook Medical, Bloomington IN, USA). The end result was a cut band that was subsequently removed through the patient's mouth.

Chisholm et al. [74] reviewed similar data with 50 eroded SAGB (Ethicon Endosurgery®, Cincinnati, OH) gastric bands approached in the OR under general anesthesia using the gastric band cutter (AMI® Gastric Band Cutter, Agency for Medical Innovation GmbH, Götzis, Austria). Interestingly, the endoscopic removal was only attempted when the buckle of the band was seen inside the stomach. The authors had to convert earlier in their experience three patients to surgery for incomplete erosions (buckle not visible within the stomach). With the median duration of the procedure approximating 46 min (range 17–118 min), the reported success rate was close to 92% (46 patients). This favorable outcome was at a cost, five patients (10%) presented with complications of which three required interventions: laparoscopy for two patients with symptomatic pneumoperitoneum and surgical debridement for one patient with port infection. Conversely, Weiss et al. [84] conducted their cases in the endoscopic suite under sedation. They describe their procedure as being of two concomitant steps. Initially a SLT-

LASER®, Neodym-YAG 100 is introduced through a two-channel gastroscope (Olympus GIF-2T100, Vienna) to deliver 25 watts cutting energy to the eroded band. Subsequently, the port is removed through a skin incision. The authors found the N-YAG to be more time efficient than traditional endoscopic scissors. This technique was employed on five patients who were discharged home after normal gastrografin upper GI study on Day 2.

Neto et al. [85] shared their experience with the largest series of endoscopic management of eroded bands. The authors treated a total of 82 band erosions over the span of 5 years. Different band types were reported with predominance of the Swedish type (SAGB). Similar to Lattuda et al. [82] recommendations, the authors conducted all their cases in the OR and under general anesthesia. The endoscopic technique is well illustrated and explained in their paper. They were conservative with erosions involving less than 50% of the band thickness with the reasoning that such bands would not be explanted easily or without significant complications. They hastened the erosion speed by inflating the band to full capacity with subsequent endoscopy in 2–3 months' interval at which point the band was cut with a band cutter and removed by biopsy forceps. Only 4 out of the 82 bands could not be removed after they were split. A total of 19 patients required 2 endoscopic sessions for retrieval but the authors did not provide the explanations to why. The cases took anywhere from 25 to 150 min with an average duration of 55 min. The immediate complication from this series included five patients (6.4%) who presented with painful pneumoperitoneum. Three of these patients only required conservative measures while one patient needed a veress needle decompression of severely distended abdomen and another patient was taken for laparotomy for a nondisclosed indication. The use of carbon dioxide during endoscopy should be performed in all these cases to mitigate the amount of distention both in the bowel and if distention occurs in the abdominal cavity.

Contrary to the established conservative practice of bands with less than 50% erosion [86–88], Campos and his group [89] used an endoscopic needle knife to cut the residual gastric bridge over the wall of an eroded LAGB (Ethicon Endosurgery, Cincinnati, OH, USA). One week later, a follow-up endoscopy showed hastened band erosion which allowed cutting of the band before its removal through the mouth with uneventful patient recovery. The authors concluded that minimal gastric band erosion does not always warrant watchful course as such shallow band penetration could be deepened by endoscopic means (i.e., needle knife). This approach is thought to be safe leading to an earlier endoscopic retrieval of the gastric band.

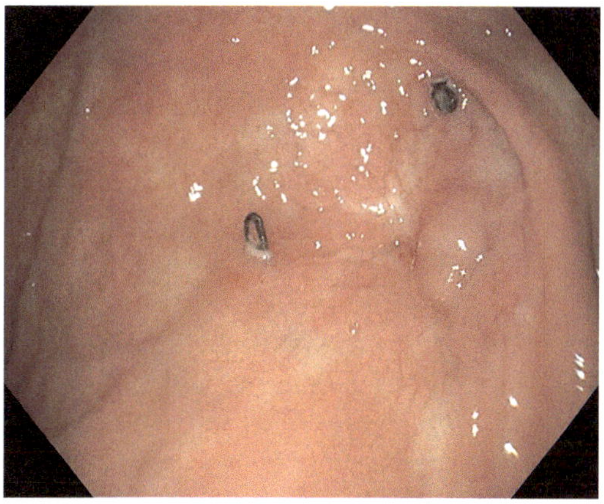

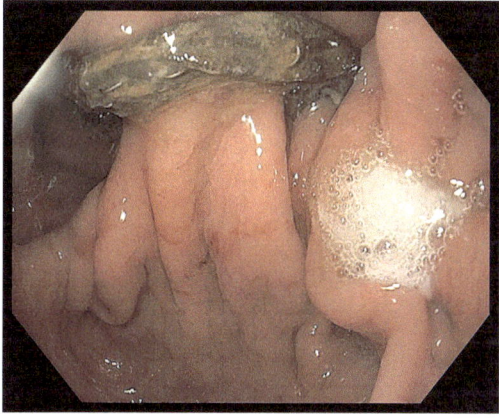

Fig. 10.5 Erosion of permanent suture material through the gastric wall of a former vertical banded gastroplasty patient

Endoluminal Therapy of the Miscellaneous Erosions

Permanent suture erosion (Figs. 10.4 and 10.5) and staple line reinforcement erosion (Fig. 10.6) are relatively uncommon nowadays but the associated symptoms could be sometimes overwhelming [90]. I have personally treated few of both erosions endoscopically. Kaimal and colleagues [91] reported the endoscopic excision and removal of an eroded Prolene suture at the gastrojejunal anastomosis in a patient 4 years out of Roux-en-Y gastric bypass. Yu et al. [92]

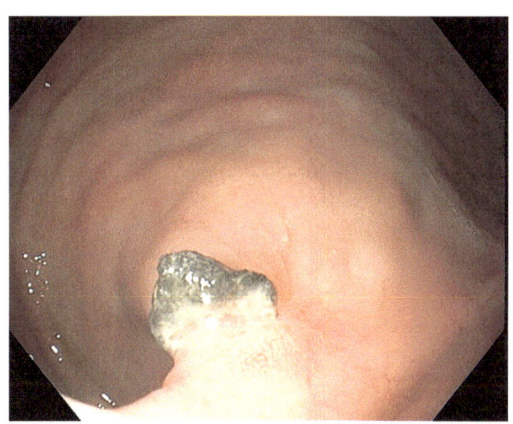

Fig. 10.4 Erosion of permanent suture material through the wall of a gastric pouch

Fig. 10.6 Full thickness erosion of permanent staple line reinforcement material through the gastric wall of a Roux-en-Y gastric bypass patient

reported their institutional experience in the endoluminal management of the Roux-en-Y gastric bypass patient with eroding non-dissolvable material, such as Peri-Strips (Synovis Life Technologies Inc., St Paul, MN, USA) (six patients) and silk sutures (21 patients). The authors report the use of endo-shears and biopsy forceps on all 23 patients they encountered. There were no resulting complications and either a resolution or improvement of the pre-procedural complaints in 83% of the patients. Other possibly eroding materials are exceedingly rare and mostly not reported in the medical literature.

Conclusion

Foreign body erosions following bariatric surgery are luckily of an overall low prevalence. Hence most of the endoscopic experience in their management is either from small case series or case reports. As evidenced by the innovative practice at several centers across the globe, the endoscopic approach in treating this atrocious complication has become a safe and efficient option. Nonetheless, formal training and expert coaching are paramount to the successful implementation of therapeutic endoscopy in the management of this often-challenging complication.

References

1. Ahuja NK, Nimgaonkar A. Precision Bariatrics: toward a new paradigm of personalized devices in obesity therapeutics. Obes Surg. 2016;26(7):1642–5.
2. Funk LM, Jolles SA, Voils CI. Obesity as a disease: has the AMA resolution had an impact on how physicians view obesity? Surg Obes Relat Dis. 2016;12(7):1431–5.
3. Moshiri M, Osman S, Robinson TJ, Khandelwal S, Bhargava P, Rohrmann CA. Evolution of bariatric surgery: a historical perspective. AJR Am J Roentgenol. 2013;201(1):W40–8.
4. Kumar N, Bazerbachi F, Rustagi T, McCarty TR, Thompson CC, Galvao Neto MP, et al. The influence of the Orbera Intragastric balloon filling volumes on weight loss, tolerability, and adverse events: a systematic review and meta-analysis. Obes Surg. 2017.
5. Buzga M, Kupka T, Siroky M, Narwan H, Machytka E, Holeczy P, et al. Short-term outcomes of the new intragastric balloon end-ball(R) for treatment of obesity. Wideochir Inne Tech Maloinwazyjne. 2016;11(4):229–35.
6. Yorke E, Switzer NJ, Reso A, Shi X, de Gara C, Birch D, et al. Intragastric balloon for Management of Severe Obesity: a systematic review. Obes Surg. 2016;26(9):2248–54.
7. Sullivan S, Edmundowicz SA, Thompson CC. Endoscopic bariatric and metabolic therapies: new and emerging technologies. Gastroenterology. 2017;152(7):1791–801.
8. Yun GY, Kim WS, Kim HJ, Kang SH, Moon HS, Sung JK, et al. Asymptomatic gastric band erosion detected during routine gastroduodenoscopy. Clin Endosc. 2016;49(3):294–7.
9. Al-Bahri S, Gonzalvo JP, Murr M. Simultaneous gastric and colonic band erosion presenting as lower gastrointestinal bleeding. Surg Obes Relat Dis. 2017;13(3):538–9.
10. Manatakis DK, Terzis I, Kyriazanos ID, Dontas ID, Stoidis CN, Stamos N, et al. Simultaneous gastric and duodenal erosions due to adjustable gastric banding for morbid obesity. Case Rep Surg. 2014;2014:146980.
11. Povoa AA, Soares C, Esteves J, Gandra A, Maciel R, Cardoso JM, et al. Simultaneous gastric and colic laparoscopic adjustable gastric band migration. Complication of bariatric surgery. Obes Surg. 2010;20(6):796–800.
12. Su MZ, Munro WS. Gastric emphysema secondary to laparoscopic gastric band erosion. Int J Surg Case Rep. 2014;5(10):727–30.
13. Rudd AA, Lall C, Deodhar A, Chang KJ, Smith BR. Gastropericardial fistula as a late complication of laparoscopic gastric banding. J Clin Imaging Sci. 2017;7:3.
14. Creedon L, Leeder P, Awan A. Laparoscopic adjustable gastric band erosion and migration into the proximal jejunum. Surg Obes Relat Dis. 2014;10(2):e19–21.
15. Parmar C, Mamtora S, Balupuri S. Endoscopic removal of intrajejunal migrated gastric band. Surg Obes Relat Dis. 2016;12(9):e75–e6.
16. Salar O, Waraich N, Singh R, Awan A. Gastric band erosion, infection and migration causing jejunal obstruction. BMJ Case Rep. 2013;2013.
17. Egbeare DM, Myers AF, Lawrance RJ. Small bowel obstruction secondary to intragastric erosion and migration of a gastric band. J Gastrointest Surg. 2008;12(5):983–4.
18. Anderson JM, Rodriguez A, Chang DT. Foreign body reaction to biomaterials. Semin Immunol. 2008;20(2):86–100.
19. Nocca D, Gagner M, Aggarwal R, Deneve E, Millat B, Pourquier D, et al. Is collagen a good banding material for outlet control of vertical gastroplasty? Preliminary study in pigs. Obes Surg. 2006;16(1):39–44.
20. Nocca D, Aggarwal R, Deneve E, Picot MC, Sanders G, Pourquier D, et al. Use of collagen wrap from bovine origin for the management of colic perforation. Preliminary study in a pig model. J Laparoendosc Adv Surg Tech A. 2009;19(1):79–83.
21. Lattuada E, Zappa MA, Mozzi E, Gazzano G, Francese M, Antonini I, et al. Histologic study of tissue reaction to the gastric band: does it contribute to the problem of band erosion? Obes Surg. 2006;16(9):1155–9.
22. Williams DF. On the mechanisms of biocompatibility. Biomaterials. 2008;29(20):2941–53.
23. York DA, Rossner S, Caterson I, Chen CM, James WP, Kumanyika S, et al. Prevention conference VII: obesity, a worldwide epidemic related to heart disease and stroke: group I: worldwide demographics of obesity. Circulation. 2004;110(18):e463–70.
24. Spinosa SR, Valezi AC. Endoscopic findings of asymptomatic patients one year after Roux-en-Y gastric bypass for treatment of obesity. Obes Surg. 2013;23(9):1431–5.
25. Brown WA, Egberts KJ, Franke-Richard D, Thodiyil P, Anderson ML, O'Brien PE. Erosions after laparoscopic adjustable gastric banding: diagnosis and management. Ann Surg. 2013;257(6):1047–52.

26. Strahan A, Aseervatham R. Laparoscopic adjustable gastric band tubing erosion into large bowel. ANZ J Surg. 2015.
27. Blouhos K, Boulas KA, Katsaouni SP, Salpigktidis II, Mauroeidi B, Ioannidis K, et al. Connecting tube colonic erosion and gastrocolic fistula formation following late gastric band erosion. Clin Obes. 2013;3(5):158–61.
28. Kohn GP, Hansen CA, Gilhome RW, McHenry RC, Spilias DC, Hensman C. Laparoscopic management of gastric band erosions: a 10-year series of 49 cases. Surg Endosc. 2012;26(2):541–5.
29. Quadri P, Gonzalez-Heredia R, Masrur M, Sanchez-Johnsen L, Elli EF. Management of laparoscopic adjustable gastric band erosion. Surg Endosc. 2017;31(4):1505–12.
30. Spitali C, De Vogelaere K, Delvaux G. Removal of eroded gastric bands using a Transgastric SILS device. Case Rep Surg. 2013;2013:852747.
31. Brethauer SA, Kothari S, Sudan R, Williams B, English WJ, Brengman M, et al. Systematic review on reoperative bariatric surgery: American Society for Metabolic and Bariatric Surgery Revision Task Force. Surg Obes Relat Dis. 2014;10(5):952–72.
32. Fournier P, Gero D, Dayer-Jankechova A, Allemann P, Demartines N, Marmuse JP, et al. Laparoscopic Roux-en-Y gastric bypass for failed gastric banding: outcomes in 642 patients. Surg Obes Relat Dis. 2016;12(2):231–9.
33. Cai JX, Schweitzer MA, Kumbhari V. Endoscopic Management of Bariatric Surgery Complications. Surg Laparosc Endosc Percutan Tech. 2016;26(2):93–101.
34. Zorron R, Galvao-Neto MP, Campos J, Branco AJ, Sampaio J, Junghans T, et al. From complex evolving to simple: current revisional and endoscopic procedures following bariatric surgery. Arq Bras Cir Dig. 2016;29(Suppl 1):128–33.
35. Patel N, Darzi A, Teare J. The endoscopy evolution: 'the superscope era'. Frontline Gastroenterol. 2015;6(2):101–7.
36. Asge Standards of Practice C, Evans JA, Muthusamy VR, Acosta RD, Bruining DH, Chandrasekhara V, et al. The role of endoscopy in the bariatric surgery patient. Surg Obes Relat Dis. 2015;11(3):507–17.
37. Asge Standards of Practice C, Anderson MA, Gan SI, Fanelli RD, Baron TH, Banerjee S, et al. Role of endoscopy in the bariatric surgery patient. Gastrointest Endosc. 2008;68(1):1–10.
38. Wilkinson LH, Peloso OA. Gastric (reservoir) reduction for morbid obesity. Arch Surg. 1981;116(5):602–5.
39. Moreno P, Alastrue A, Rull M, Formiguera X, Casas D, Boix J, et al. Band erosion in patients who have undergone vertical banded gastroplasty: incidence and technical solutions. Arch Surg. 1998;133(2):189–93.
40. Miller K, Pump A, Hell E. Vertical banded gastroplasty versus adjustable gastric banding: prospective long-term follow-up study. Surg Obes Relat Dis. 2007;3(1):84–90.
41. Subramanyam K, Robbins HT. Erosion of Marlex band and silastic ring into the stomach after gastroplasty: endoscopic recognition and management. Am J Gastroenterol. 1989;84(10):1319–21.
42. Fobi M, Lee H, Igwe D, Felahy B, James E, Stanczyk M, et al. Band erosion: incidence, etiology, management and outcome after banded vertical gastric bypass. Obes Surg. 2001;11(6):699–707.
43. Meyenberger C, Gubler C, Hengstler PM. Endoscopic management of a penetrated gastric band. Gastrointest Endosc. 2004;60(3):480–1.
44. Fonnest GF, Jess P. [Gastroscopic removal of penetrating gastric band]. Ugeskr Laeger 1999;161(43):5930–1.
45. Evans JA, Williams NN, Chan EP, Kochman ML. Endoscopic removal of eroded bands in vertical banded gastroplasty: a novel use of endoscopic scissors (with video). Gastrointest Endosc. 2006;64(5):801–4.
46. Oria HE. Gastric banding for morbid obesity. Eur J Gastroenterol Hepatol. 1999;11(2):105–14.
47. Vassallo C, Andreoli M, La Manna A, Turpini C. 60 reoperations on 890 patients after gastric restrictive surgery. Obes Surg. 2001;11(6):752–6.
48. Karmali S, Snyder B, Wilson EB, Timberlake MD, Sherman V. Endoscopic management of eroded prosthesis in vertical banded gastroplasty patients. Surg Endosc. 2010;24(1):98–102.
49. Blero D, Eisendrath P, Vandermeeren A, Closset J, Mehdi A, Le Moine O, et al. Endoscopic removal of dysfunctioning bands or rings after restrictive bariatric procedures. Gastrointest Endosc. 2010;71(3):468–74.
50. Hookey LC, Mehdi A, Le Moine O, Deviere J. Removal of a gastroplasty ring. Gastrointest Endosc. 2005;61(4):594.
51. Wilson TD, Miller N, Brown N, Snyder BE, Wilson EB. Stent induced gastric wall erosion and endoscopic retrieval of nonadjustable gastric band: a new technique. Surg Endosc. 2013;27(5):1617–21.
52. Marins Campos J, Moon RC, Magalhaes Neto GE, Teixeira AF, Jawad MA, Bezerra Silva L, et al. Endoscopic treatment of food intolerance after a banded gastric bypass: inducing band erosion for removal using a plastic stent. Endoscopy. 2016;48(6):516–20.
53. Shehab H, Gawdat K. Endoscopic management of eroded bands following banded-gastric bypass (with video). Obes Surg. 2017.
54. Karmali S, Sweeney JF, Yee K, Brunicardi FC, Sherman V. Transgastric endoscopic rendezvous technique for removal of eroded Molina gastric band. Surg Obes Relat Dis. 2008;4(4):559–62.
55. Owers C, Ackroyd R. A study examining the complications associated with gastric banding. Obes Surg. 2013;23(1):56–9.
56. Treadwell JR, Sun F, Schoelles K. Systematic review and meta-analysis of bariatric surgery for pediatric obesity. Ann Surg. 2008;248(5):763–76.
57. Cherian PT, Goussous G, Ashori F, Sigurdsson A. Band erosion after laparoscopic gastric banding: a retrospective analysis of 865 patients over 5 years. Surg Endosc. 2010;24(8):2031–8.

58. Nocca D, Frering V, Gallix B, de Seguin des Hons C, Noel P, Foulonge MA, et al. Migration of adjustable gastric banding from a cohort study of 4236 patients. Surg Endosc. 2005;19(7):947–50.

59. Silecchia G, Restuccia A, Elmore U, Polito D, Perrotta N, Genco A, et al. Laparoscopic adjustable silicone gastric banding: prospective evaluation of intragastric migration of the lap-band. Surg Laparosc Endosc Percutan Tech. 2001;11(4):229–34.

60. Abu-Abeid S, Keidar A, Gavert N, Blanc A, Szold A. The clinical spectrum of band erosion following laparoscopic adjustable silicone gastric banding for morbid obesity. Surg Endosc. 2003;17(6):861–3.

61. Kurian M, Sultan S, Garg K, Youn H, Fielding G, Ren-Fielding C. Evaluating gastric erosion in band management: an algorithm for stratification of risk. Surg Obes Relat Dis. 2010;6(4):386–9.

62. Forsell P, Hallerback B, Glise H, Hellers G. Complications following Swedish adjustable gastric banding: a long-term follow-up. Obes Surg. 1999;9(1):11–6.

63. Rao AD, Ramalingam G. Exsanguinating hemorrhage following gastric erosion after laparoscopic adjustable gastric banding. Obes Surg. 2006;16(12):1675–8.

64. Campos J, Ramos A, Galvao Neto M, Siqueira L, Evangelista LF, Ferraz A, et al. Hypovolemic shock due to intragastric migration of an adjustable gastric band. Obes Surg. 2007;17(4):562–4.

65. Iqbal M, Manjunath S, Seenath M, Khan A. Massive upper gastrointestinal hemorrhage: an unusual presentation after laparoscopic adjustable gastric banding due to erosion into the celiac axis. Obes Surg. 2008;18(6):759–60.

66. Bueter M, Thalheimer A, Meyer D, Fein M. Band erosion and passage, causing small bowel obstruction. Obes Surg. 2006;16(12):1679–82.

67. Wylezol M, Sitkiewicz T, Gluck M, Zubik R, Pardela M. Intra-abdominal abscess in the course of intragastric migration of an adjustable gastric band: a potentially life-threatening complication. Obes Surg. 2006;16(1):102–4.

68. De Roover A, Detry O, Coimbra C, Hamoir E, Honore P, Meurisse M. Pylephlebitis of the portal vein complicating intragastric migration of an adjustable gastric band. Obes Surg. 2006;16(3):369–71.

69. Basa NR, Dutson E, Lewis C, Derezin M, Han S, Mehran A. Laparoscopic transgastric removal of eroded adjustable band: a novel approach. Surg Obes Relat Dis. 2008;4(2):194–7.

70. Yoon CI, Pak KH, Kim SM. Early experience with diagnosis and management of eroded gastric bands. J Korean Surg Soc. 2012;82(1):18–27.

71. Egberts K, Brown WA, O'Brien PE. Systematic review of erosion after laparoscopic adjustable gastric banding. Obes Surg. 2011;21(8):1272–9.

72. Cherian PT, Goussous G, Sigurdsson A. Management of band erosion with omental plugging: case series from a 5-year laparoscopic gastric banding experience. Obes Surg. 2009;19(10):1409–13.

73. Hamdan K, Somers S, Chand M. Management of late postoperative complications of bariatric surgery. Br J Surg. 2011;98(10):1345–55.

74. Chisholm J, Kitan N, Toouli J, Kow L. Gastric band erosion in 63 cases: endoscopic removal and rebanding evaluated. Obes Surg. 2011;21(11):1676–81.

75. O'Brien P. Comment on: endoscopic removal of eroded adjustable gastric band: lessons learned after 5 years and 78 cases. Surg Obes Relat Dis. 2010;6(4):427–8.

76. El-Hayek K, Timratana P, Brethauer SA, Chand B. Complete endoscopic/transgastric retrieval of eroded gastric band: description of a novel technique and review of the literature. Surg Endosc. 2013;27(8):2974–9.

77. Baldinger R, Mluench R, Steffen R, Ricklin TP, Riedtmann HJ, Horber FF. Conservative management of intragastric migration of Swedish adjustable gastric band by endoscopic retrieval. Gastrointest Endosc. 2001;53(1):98–101.

78. Prathanvanich P, Chand B. Complete endoscopic/transgastric retrieval of eroded gastric band: a novel technique. Gastrointest Endosc. 2013;78(6):816.

79. Mozzi E, Lattuada E, Zappa MA, Granelli P, De Ruberto F, Armocida A, et al. Treatment of band erosion: feasibility and safety of endoscopic band removal. Surg Endosc. 2011;25(12):3918–22.

80. Herreros de Tejada A, Calleja JL, Jimenez M, Rojo V, Santander C, Rial JC, et al. Gastric band cutter to remove a migrated gastric band. Endoscopy. 2012;44(Suppl 2 UCTN):E40–1.

81. Regusci L, Groebli Y, Meyer JL, Walder J, Margalith D, Schneider R. Gastroscopic removal of an adjustable gastric band after partial intragastric migration. Obes Surg. 2003;13(2):281–4.

82. Lattuada E, Zappa MA, Mozzi E, Fichera G, Granelli P, De Ruberto F, et al. Band erosion following gastric banding: how to treat it. Obes Surg. 2007;17(3):329–33.

83. Flor L, Gornals JB, Ruiz-de-Gordejuela AG. Endoscopic removal of eroded gastric band using strangulation technique with a mechanical lithotriptor as a minimally invasive procedure. Dig Endosc. 2014;26(2):296–7.

84. Weiss H, Nehoda H, Labeck B, Peer R, Aigner F. Gastroscopic band removal after intragastric migration of adjustable gastric band: a new minimal invasive technique. Obes Surg. 2000;10(2):167–70.

85. Neto MP, Ramos AC, Campos JM, Murakami AH, Falcao M, Moura EH, et al. Endoscopic removal of eroded adjustable gastric band: lessons learned after 5 years and 78 cases. Surg Obes Relat Dis. 2010;6(4):423–7.

86. Di Lorenzo N, Lorenzo M, Furbetta F, Favretti F, Giardiello C, Boschi S, et al. Intragastric gastric band migration: erosion: an analysis of multicenter experience on 177 patients. Surg Endosc. 2013;27(4):1151–7.

87. Angrisani L, Alkilani M, Basso N, Belvederesi N, Campanile F, Capizzi FD, et al. Laparoscopic Italian experience with the lap-band. Obes Surg. 2001;11(3):307–10.

88. Ventienen B, Vaneerdeweg W, D'Hoore A, Hubens G, Chapelle T, Eyskens E. Intragastric erosion of lapa-

roscopic adjustable silicone gastric band. Obes Surg. 2000;10(5):474–6.

89. Campos JM, Evangelista LF, Galvao Neto MP, Ramos AC, Martins JP, dos Santos MA Jr, et al. Small erosion of adjustable gastric band: endoscopic removal through incision in gastric wall. Surg Laparosc Endosc Percutan Tech. 2010;20(6):e215–7.

90. Consten EC, Dakin GF, Gagner M. Intraluminal migration of bovine pericardial strips used to rein-

force the gastric staple-line in laparoscopic bariatric surgery. Obes Surg. 2004;14(4):549–54.

91. Kaimal N, Al-Rashedy M, Ammori BJ, Syed AA. Suture erosion after gastric bypass surgery. QJM. 2013;106(5):483–4.

92. Yu S, Jastrow K, Clapp B, Kao L, Klein C, Scarborough T, et al. Foreign material erosion after laparoscopic Roux-en-Y gastric bypass: findings and treatment. Surg Endosc. 2007;21(7):1216–20.

Eric Marcotte

Introduction

Laparoscopic Roux-en-Y gastric bypass (RYGB) is a procedure that has proven to have long-term benefits of weight loss as well as of improvement/resolution of comorbidities in the morbidly obese patient [1–3]. These benefits from surgery are counterbalanced by some risks of complications, both medical and surgical, most often presenting in the early perioperative period [4, 5]. Long-term complications are more often related to nutritional deficiencies. Marginal ulceration is a complication that arises long term and has been reported to occur at a time varying from 1 month to 6 years after surgery [6]. Marginal ulcers are defined as ulceration at the site of the gastrojejunal (GJ) anastomosis, classically on the jejunal side [7]. A systematic review of 41 studies (16,987 patients) reported a marginal ulcer incidence of 4.6% (787 patients) but individual cohorts report an incidence ranging from 0.6 to 16% [5–16]. The majority of these studies are retrospective in which endoscopies were performed when patients presented with gastrointestinal-type symptoms. Csendes et al. performed prospective routine endoscopy on 441 consecutive patients after RYGB, independent of symptoms, at 4 weeks and at 1–2 years post-op [8]. They reported an incidence of marginal ulcer of 6% "early" and 0.6% "late" [8, 9]. Seven of the 25 patients (28%) that presented as an "early" marginal ulcer were asymptomatic.

The most common presentation consists of epigastric pain/burning and/or nausea (over half of patients), but it can also lead to a stricture with associated dysphagia and, less frequently, bleeding (with melena and/or hematemesis and subsequent anemia) [6, 7, 16, 17]. Normal postoperative anatomy was the most common finding (43% of the cases) [18]. Therefore the positive predictive value of any individual upper gastrointestinal symptom was low in this series (40%). Wilson et al. reported similar results in a study of 226 patients that underwent upper endoscopy for symptoms post-RYGB and found "normal anatomy" in 44% of cases [19].

Perforation with peritonitis and sepsis is rare (less than 1% of patients after RYGB) but it is a potentially fatal presentation of a marginal ulcer [6, 20, 21]. Efforts should therefore be made to control risk factors for ulceration formation. Once diagnosed, it is imperative to initiate effective therapy in order to prevent a potentially fatal complication.

Risk Factors for Marginal Ulceration

The exact etiology of marginal ulcers is widely unknown due to a paucity of small retrospective studies. However, the leading pathophysiology is

E. Marcotte, M.D., M.Sc. (✉)
Department of Surgery, Stritch School of Medicine,
Loyola University Medical Center,
2160 S. First Avenue, Maywood, IL 60153, USA
e-mail: eric.marcotte@lumc.edu

thought to be from inflammation, acid, and ischemia secondary to faulty microcirculation or tension on the gastrojejunal anastomosis [7, 22].

Smoking

El Hayek et al. reviewed the experience from Cleveland Clinic in a retrospective study of 328 consecutive symptomatic patients with epigastric pain after RYGB and found 34% incidence of marginal ulcer [7]. When studying different variables, tobacco smoking was the only factor that led to an increased risk of marginal ulcer development. Smoking was also found to be a cause for nonhealing (recalcitrant) and recurrent ulceration. Wilson et al. similarly identified smoking as the single most predictive independent factor for the development of anastomotic ulcer with an adjusted odds ratio (AOR) of 30.6 (95% CI [6.4–146], $P < 0.001$) [19]. Azagury et al. also found an association between smoking and marginal ulcer development with an odds ratio (OR) of 2.5 ($P = 0.02$) [23]. Patel et al. noted 3 "heavy smokers" presenting with recurrent ulcer after revisional surgery for refractory marginal ulcers [24]. It is hypothesized that tobacco creates inflammation and also alters microperfusion of the anastomosis. It is therefore recommended that patients quit smoking at a minimum of 4 weeks prior to a RYGB. Abstinence can be confirmed with a negative urine nicotine test prior to surgery. If a marginal ulcer develops, confirming a patient is tobacco free by confirmatory laboratory testing is essential to allow for healing.

Nonsteroidal Anti-inflammatory Drugs (NSAIDs) and Antiplatelet Use

In line with the theory of inflammation/local damage, NSAID usage has been identified as an independent risk factor for developing marginal ulceration in multiple studies [19]. They are found to cause mucosal disruption due to inhibition of cyclooxygenase, causing decreased prostaglandin E_2 levels and subsequent disruption of the gastric barrier [17, 25]. In a systematic review,

out of 365 patients with marginal ulcers, 98 (27%) were on NSAIDs [6]. Higa et al. attributed "the majority" of the marginal ulcers in their cohort (1.4% of 1040 patients) to the use of NSAIDs "despite written and verbal precautions" [5]. In the Wilson study, NSAIDs use was found to be an independent risk factor for the development of marginal ulcer with an AOR of 11.5 (95% CI [4.8–28], $P < 0.001$) [19]. NSAID usage not only leads to marginal ulcers but delays their healing [26]. A population-based cohort study of the Swedish Patient Registry on 20,294 subjects that underwent gastric bypass over a 5-year period was performed by Sverden et al. to identify risk factors for marginal ulcer [22]. Mean follow-up was 2 years and the incidence of marginal ulcer was 3.3% (694 patients). They report that "higher doses" of aspirin are associated with marginal ulcer development. The study did not find a significant correlation between NSAID use and marginal ulceration formation. However, this registry does not contain data on over-the-counter use of NSAIDs and might therefore explain this observation. Kang et al. reported on their cohort taking low-dose (81 mg daily) aspirin. Marginal ulcer rates were 8.3 and 10.3% in patients taking and not taking low-dose aspirin, respectively. They therefore deemed low-dose aspirin to be safe after RYGB [15]. Another study reported outcomes with clopidogrel for coronary artery disease in the context of RYGB [27]. Of 11 patients on Plavix, 4 (36%) presented with upper GI bleeding 25–234 days after surgery, two were found to have a marginal ulcer and the other two were bleeding at the anastomosis without ulcers. Bleeding resolved after stopping clopidogrel and administering intravenous protein pump inhibitors (PPIs); no adverse effects were observed after stopping Plavix. Based on these findings, the authors recommended the administration of PPIs while a patient is on clopidogrel, based on studies demonstrating that PPIs prevent recurrent gastrointestinal bleeding in patients with a history of peptic ulcer disease [28].

Although no specific studies for the purpose of screening for NSAIDs use in the post-RYGB population has been published yet, human whole blood assays have been described to test for

NSAIDs and are based on cyclooxygenase-2 activity [29]. Platelet aggregation studies can be done to screen for antiplatelet products [7].

Helicobacter pylori

Helicobacter pylori is a well-recognized cause of peptic ulcer disease but its causative effect in marginal ulcerations remains inconclusive with many contradictory findings in the literature. A systematic review revealed the incidence of pre-operative *H. pylori* infection in patients who were screened varied widely between studies, between 22 and 67%, although only 10.5% of patients that developed a marginal ulcer had a positive test demonstrating infection [6].

A report of 260 patients that were routinely tested for *H. pylori* antibodies before RYGB showed that 44 (17%) tested positive and were treated preoperatively with a standard eradication packet [16]. Nineteen patients (7%) developed a marginal ulcer and *H.pylori* seropositivity was identified as an independent risk factor (32% vs. 12%, $P = 0.02$). Half of patients who were sero-positive for *H. pylori* preoperatively and presented with an ulcer were retested by upper GI endoscopy (biopsy) and were all negative, leading the authors to postulate that the ulcer formation may be potentiated by preoperative injury to the gastric mucosa since they were able to confirm lack of active infection post-op. However, the accuracy of *H. pylori* in the gastric pouch is questionable and may be tested best with stool antigen. Loewen et al. reported on 448 patients that underwent screening endoscopy before bariatric surgery, which revealed positive (minor) findings in 32% of the patients including 61 cases of gastritis, 9 (2%) associated to *H. pylori* [30]. Thirty-seven (17%) out of the 223 subjects that underwent RYGB developed a marginal ulcer but *H. pylori* was not found to be a risk factor. The presence of gastritis on preoperative EGD was however found to be a significant factor, supporting the theory of preoperative injury leading to postoperative ulceration. D'Hondt et al. screened 449 consecutive patients pre-RYGB with endoscopic biopsies for *H. pylori* [12]. Eighty-two (19%) patients were found to be positive and were given standard eradication treatment. Sixty-five were retested with an endoscopic biopsy to confirm eradication and two patients were found to have persistent infection and were treated with a second line of eradication therapy with 100% success. Forty-eight (10.7%) patients developed a marginal ulcer after RYGB and *H. pylori* status was not found to be a predictive factor. About half of the overall patients received 1 month of prophylactic daily PPI. Although there was no difference in the proportion of marginal ulcers in the *H. pylori* negative group (10.7% vs. 11.86%, $P = 0.74$), there was a significant reduction in the *H. pylori* positive group (0% vs. 15.6%, $P = 0.01$). Moreover, the *H. pylori* positive patients were found to have gastritis on preoperative endoscopy more often than their counterparts (93% vs. 38%, $P < 0.0001$), leading the authors to believe the preoperative gastritis led to a higher rate of ulceration. PPIs may have prevented an injury to the weakened gastric lining by optimizing its protective function, reinforcing their utility. There are however numerous smaller retrospective studies that have reported no association between H. pylori status and the development of marginal ulcers [31–34]. Kelly et al. reported the influence of *H. pylori* status diagnosed histologically on intraoperative full-thickness biopsies of the stomach at the time of RYGB in 694 patients [31]. Sixty-six (9.5%) were found to be *H. pylori* positive and did not get eradication therapy. Nonetheless, the development of a marginal ulcer was more frequent in the *H. pylori* negative group than for patients who tested *H. pylori* positive (17.1% vs. 7.6%, $p = 0.05$). Lastly, Schulman et al. surveyed the 2012 Nationwide Inpatient Sample (NIS) database, one of the largest in the United States with a sample size of 253,765 patients that underwent bariatric surgery (not RYGB specifically) [35]. Only 340 patients (0.001%) were found to have an *H. pylori* infection but 31% of those patients developed a marginal ulcer, as opposed to 4% in *H. pylori* negative patients, making *H. pylori* positive status the strongest predictor of the development of a marginal ulcer with an AOR of 10.88 (95% CI [6.46–18.30], $P < 0.01$). Tobacco use was also found to be a risk factor for the development of ulceration with an AOR of 1.28 (95% CI [1.16–1.43], $P < 0.01$).

Diabetes

In the study of 20,294 patients after RYGB in the Swedish Patient Registry, Sverden et al. identified diabetes as an independent risk factor in the development of marginal ulcers with a hazard ratio (HR) of 1.26 (95% CI [1.03–1.55], $P < 0.05$) [22]. The reports of the Harvard group experience also showed a correlation of marginal ulcer with diabetes with an OR of 2.5 ($P = 0.03$) [23]. However, numerous other studies did not find such association [12, 16, 36].

Acid

It is well recognized that extra acid leads to gastric lining injury and subsequent ulceration, hence the recommendation for PPIs to treat peptic ulcer disease. In the setting of a GJ anastomosis, the jejunum (proximal Roux limb) may be exposed to acid (if still produced in the pouch) and is extra vulnerable, since it usually faces a milder pH environment [7, 37]. Whereas the main location for acid-producing gastric parietal cells is the antrum, they were found in all parts of the stomach when patients were randomly biopsied [7, 38]. El-Hayek et al. found no association between the presence of parietal cells on random biopsies and the presence of a marginal ulcer [7]. Nevertheless, it was reported by Mason et al. that making the gastric pouch smaller (more proximal) to a volume from about 200 mL to under 50 mL reduced the marginal ulcer rate from 4.2 to 0.9% in a series of 653 patients [10, 39]. In a 2005 study of 23 patients in Sweden that underwent a RYGB, the authors performed their "standard pouch" measuring 4 × 3 cm for 13 cases and on 10 patients they performed a "smaller pouch" measuring 2 × 3 cm to reduce the parietal cell mass [38]. Two patients (15%) with a "standard pouch" were believed to have developed a marginal ulcer (one confirmed by endoscopy, the other with epigastric pain that resolved with PPIs) and no patient developed an ulcer in the "smaller pouch" group. The same authors confirmed this finding by surveying the Scandinavian Obesity Registry and studying 14,168 patients that underwent a "highly standardized" laparoscopic RYGB in Sweden with a stapled GJ technique, especially looking at the length of the total firings to create the pouch [37]. Although marginal ulcers were a rare complication (0.9% at 1 year), they report a relative risk of marginal ulcer increase of 14% for every additional centimeter of stapler used to create the pouch. The authors believe this is due to a more acidic environment in the larger pouch. Other studies support the theory that a larger pouch is associated with an increased risk of developing marginal ulcers [23, 40, 41]. Additionally, Hedberg et al. reported their experiment of wireless pH testing with the Bravo reflux testing system (Medtronic, Minneapolis MN, USA) for 24 h at the GJ anastomosis on patients 2–8 years after RYGB [42]. Sixteen asymptomatic patients were studied and demonstrated an acid environment with pH < 4 a median of 10.5% of the time and no correlation was found between the number of cartridges used to create the pouch and the measured levels of acidity. Four patients had epigastric symptoms and were placed on PPIs (presuming this was from a marginal ulceration) and 2 of them were unable to stop their PPIs before testing. On PPIs, the percentage of time with pH < 4 was 0% therefore supporting the efficacy of PPIs to normalize pH in the pouch. Two symptomatic patients were able to stop PPIs 2 weeks prior to testing and the measurements confirmed an acidic environment in the pouch with a marginal ulcer confirmed on endoscopy for one patient.

Gastro-gastric fistulas lead to an increased risk of ulceration because of the acid from the gastric remnant refluxing into the gastric pouch due to a communication between the two. Fistulas were more common with open gastric bypass, especially with the nondivided technique. The current technique using cutting linear staplers has decreased the risk of gastro-gastric fistulas from 49% to 3–6% [43, 44]. Carrodeguas et al. reported that of 1292 patients that underwent a divided

RYGB, 15 (1.2%) presented with a gastro-gastric fistula after surgery, of which 8 (53%) developed a marginal ulcer, compared to a 4% rate for the entire series [45]. When diagnosed, gastro-gastric fistulas can be managed either endoscopically or through revisional surgery [43].

Surgical Technique

It is believed that early ulcers (within the first months) are usually due to ischemia, either because of a vascular injury at the time of surgery or because of tension on the mesentery of the Roux limb [7].

The technique to create the gastrojejunal anastomosis has been shown to be an important risk factor for the development of marginal ulcer. A study by Sacks et al. reported a significant reduction in the marginal ulceration rate by switching the suture to close the inner layer of the common enterotomy of a linear stapled GJ from nonabsorbable to absorbable [36]. Ulceration rates dropped from 2.6% (28/1095) to 1.3% (29/2190), respectively [36, 44]. They also noted a significant reduction in the frequency of visible sutures at the site of the marginal ulcer, 64.3% (18/28) to 3.4% (1/29), respectively [36].

A study of the 32,284 RYGB patients in the Scandinavian Obesity Registry reported that a circular stapled GJ anastomosis leads to more marginal ulcer development than a linear stapled GJ with 2.9% and 1% rates, respectively [46]. However, the circular stapled group represented less than 2% of the study population and those procedures were performed specifically at only three smaller hospitals, therefore presenting a bias. The same authors presented their experience; they started with a circular stapled GJ and then changed their technique for a linear stapler GJ due to the increased frequency of surgical site infection and pain [40]. The rate of marginal ulceration was found to be 2.4% (7/288) for the circular stapler and 0.4% (1/272) for the linear stapler. The authors however believe that the reason is that the pouch they created for the circular stapler technique was made larger in order to fit a 25-mm anvil, and not the stapler itself, which is highly probable, as previously discussed [37, 40].

All and all, no specific RYGB technique seems to constitute an increased risk for development of marginal ulcer. However, it is believed to be beneficial to avoid nonabsorbable sutures and other foreign bodies near the GJ anastomosis. It is also important to respect the usual principles of an adequately perfused, healthy and tension-free anastomosis to promote healing and prevent early ulceration.

Prevention

The key to management of a complication is ultimately preventing it from happening. A systematic review and meta-analysis of cohort studies (7) on benefits of PPIs demonstrated an OR of 0.50 (95% CI [0.28–0.90], $P = 0.02$), meaning postoperative PPI administration was found to reduce the risk of marginal ulcer by half [13, 47]. Wilson et al. reported that PPI prophylaxis is of higher value for patients that are NSAIDs users [19]. As previously mentioned, D'Hondt et al. stated that PPI prophylaxis led to reduction of marginal ulcers only in the patients with a history of a *H. pylori* infection [12]. The duration of prophylactic treatment and dosage is not standardized with different studies reporting a daily dose of PPI (sometimes with H2 blocker or cytoprotective agent such as sucralfate) for 1–6 months postoperatively [14, 48]. Some groups will only administer PPI prophylaxis for patients that endorse a recognized factor that would put patients at a higher risk of developing marginal ulcers, such as being *H. pylori* positive, using NSAIDs or antiplatelets and smoking [27, 48]. An international survey from 2014 of 189 bariatric surgeons that was conducted by Steinemann et al. revealed that 88% prescribe prophylactic therapy for their patients after RYGB, 91% of which prefer PPIs [48].

Another element of prophylaxis is that if a patient post-RYGB undergoes an upper GI endoscopy and a foreign body is seen coming through inside the lumen (a clip, a suture, or staples), it is recommended to remove it due to the increased risk of marginal ulceration because of the inflammatory reaction it creates [36, 49]. The preferred approach is with a dual-channel therapeutic gastroscope in order to be able to grasp the foreign body and put it on tension with one instrument and cut the suture with endoscopic shears through the other channel [49].

Treatment

Once a marginal ulcer is endoscopically confirmed, it is important to treat it promptly in order to avoid complications such as bleeding and perforation. We recommend starting empirical medical treatment even prior to confirming the marginal ulcer through an upper GI endoscopy. The first step after the diagnosis (and even at the time of clinical suspicion) is to assess the patient's risk factors for a marginal ulcer and modify them, as previously discussed. This includes smoking cessation (and possibly urine nicotine testing to confirm use or lack thereof), avoidance of NSAIDs and stopping antiplatelets if clinically possible, as well as testing for *H. pylori* using stool antigen with subsequent eradication if positive. Diabetes management should also be optimized to achieve better control of the disease.

Medication

The mainstay of treatment of marginal ulcers is high-dose PPI [12, 48]. Inhibition of gastric acid secretion is successful in treating 68–100% of ulcers and those refractory usually have anatomic abnormalities, such as a stricture, a gastro-gastric fistula, a foreign body, or a large pouch [6, 7, 16, 17, 24]. In the international survey conducted by Steinemann et al., participants revealed that 32% of respondents add sucralfate to the "therapeutic dose" of PPIs and a minority (6%) also add an H2 blocker to the regimen [48]. Forty-nine percent of surgeons continue treatment until resolution of marginal ulcer is proven by endoscopy and others continue for a fixed period of 3 months (31%) while 20% of participants choose to continue therapy for up to 2 years. Once the ulcer has healed, more than half of surgeons continue the therapeutic medical regimen for a median of 6 months to prevent recurrence. A recent study by Schulman et al. noted the superiority of opening PPI capsules for the healing of marginal ulcer [50]. It is postulated that the small gastric pouch and rapid small bowel transit limits the opportunity for capsular breakdown and absorption of the medication. For 164 patients that developed a marginal ulcer after RYGB in a 15-year period, patients were prescribed PPIs twice daily for treatment, the regimen and method of administration being dependent on (and consistent for) each provider. Each patient underwent an upper GI endoscopy every 3 months until the ulcer was healed and the median time to ulcer healing was 91 days for opened PPI capsules compared to 342 days for intact PPI capsules. This was the only significant factor related to the time to ulcer healing with a calculated OR of 6.04 (95% CI [3.74–9.76], $P < 0.001$). Although the concomitant administration of sucralfate was more common in the "opened PPI capsule" group, this factor alone was not found to lead to a significant reduction of the time to heal.

Revisional Surgery

El-Hayek et al. described that about 15% of patients underwent repeat endoscopy because of persistence of symptoms; half had documented healing of the ulcer, 38% had persistence and 12% had recurrence after initial healing [7]. Some authors expect marginal ulcers to heal with conservative management within 3 months and therefore their persistence after 3 months warrants revisional surgery [24, 48]. One hundred and five (56%) respondents in the international survey would consider continuing the conservative approach and consider surgery only if complications occur, but 41% (77 surgeons) would choose to resect and redo the GJ anastomosis [48]. That decision seemed to be related to a more extensive surgical experience with higher volumes of cases (over 200 RYGB performed in their career) [48, 51].

Patel et al. reported the experience of a single surgeon over 22 years, performing 2282 RYGB operations (1621 open, 661 laparoscopic) between

1982 and 2006 [24]. The overall marginal ulcer rate was 5.3% (5.4% for open and 5.1% in laparoscopic) and 68% of those were successfully treated with conservative management (PPIs and smoking cessation). Thirty-nine patients (32% of the patients that presented with an ulcer) required revision and were more common in the open group (2.2% vs. 0.6% for the laparoscopic group, $P \leq 0.003$), most probably related to the increased number of gastro-gastric fistulas. The operations consisted of open resection of the ulcer and revision of the GJ anastomosis, except for one "particularly noncompliant" patient who underwent a reversal of the RYGB. Postoperative complications were rare with 2 (5%) anastomotic leaks and 2 (5%) wound infections. Eighty-seven percent of the patients remained asymptomatic after the revision. Three patients (7.7%), all "heavy smokers" developed recurrent ulcers after the revision and underwent another surgery (subtotal gastrectomy of the remnant +/− revision of the GJ) with favorable outcomes in 2 of the 3 patients.

In the experience of the Cleveland Clinic, twelve patients (4% of the initial cohort) went on to undergo revisional surgery (resection and revision of the GJ anastomosis) for intractability, most often associated with an "anatomic abnormality" as previously described [7]. Unfortunately, 5 of these patients were found to have a recurrence of a marginal ulcer, with half associated with tobacco use. Steinemann et al. report a case of a 50-year-old male that presented a recurrence of marginal ulcer after resection of the ulcer and revision of the GJ anastomosis [52]. Once the patient stopped smoking, he underwent a laparoscopic resection of the pouch and gastric remnant and a reconstruction with esophagojejunostomy (EJ). The patient did not present a recurrence with 6 months of follow-up. However, it is hard to confirm that success was because of the revision or the fact the patient stopped smoking, thereby proving the importance of smoking cessation. Jirapinyo et al. reported their experience of endoscopic suturing of 3 patients with a recalcitrant ulcer that failed medical management, 2 for recurrent bleeding, and the other one for severe abdominal pain [53]. Two were deemed poor surgical candidates due to medical comorbidities.

One to three interrupted stitches of 2–0 polypropylene sutures were necessary to cover the ulcer and they applied fibrin glue to the sutured area at the end of the procedure. Two patients had complete resolution of the symptoms and the healing of the ulcer was confirmed on endoscopy 6 weeks after the procedure. The third patient reported significant improvement but developed an unrelated complication (intussusception) that required two surgical revisions and ultimately presented with a new marginal ulcer, 11 weeks after the suturing.

Bleeding

The systematic review by Coblijn et al. reported that 15.1% of patients with a marginal ulcer presented with bleeding [6]. This is usually managed endoscopically by injecting epinephrine (diluted 1:10,000), bipolar cautery, and hemostatic clips, combination therapy being recommended [53–55]. Barola et al. described successful management of a refractory ulcer that was massively bleeding by endoscopically suturing it closed [54]. Moon et al. reported two patients and Patel et al. reported five patients who required urgent surgical revision (resection of the ulcer and revision of the GJ anastomosis) for actively bleeding ulcer [14, 24].

Perforation

Felix et al. reported their experience over an 8-year period of 3430 patients that underwent RYGB and found an incidence of perforation due to marginal ulcer of 1% (35 patients), presenting 3–70 months post-RYGB [56]. Eighty percent of the patients possessed a risk factor such as smoking tobacco, using NSAIDs or steroids. They maintained all perforated patients on PPIs and four patients had a second episode of perforation; these four were all smokers. Kalaiselvan et al. also presented their experience and noted a marginal ulcer perforation in about 1% of their 1213 patients who underwent RYGB over an 8-year period [20]. All ten patients underwent a surgery with closure and omental patch, half of them laparoscopically (if they were treated by a bariatric surgeon) and the other half open (by nonbariatric surgeon at different local hospitals). The majority presented with high-risk factors such as smoking, NSAID use, and not taking their prophylactic PPIs. Morbidity and mortality rates were lower amongst the patients treated laparoscopically and the length of stay was also shorter (6 vs. 24 days). Wendling et al. compared the outcomes of omental patch repair (in 16 patients) to resection and revision of the GJ anastomosis (in 2 patients) and found that operative time is shorter, estimated blood loss are less, and the length of stay is also shorter [21]. They therefore recommended omental patch repair in an acute setting of perforation and resection with revision of the GJ anastomosis in a more controlled elective setting such as for a refractory ulcer, as discussed earlier.

Summary

In summary, marginal ulcers are not uncommon complications of RYGB and can present in various ways, from mild nausea to perforation and sepsis. We believe risk factors such as smoking, NSAIDs use, *H. pylori* infection, and diabetes should be controlled as much as possible in order to reduce the incidence of development of ulceration. We also think that prophylactic PPIs should be ordered for at least 3 months post-RYGB and the duration should be prolonged in the setting of NSAIDs or antiplatelets use, with possibly adding a cytoprotective agent such as sucralfate for the latter group. If a marginal ulcer is found, all risk factors should be controlled as much as possible and the ulcer should be treated with optimal medical management with a therapeutic dose of PPIs (ideally open capsules) and sucralfate. Any foreign body present in the ulcer bed or near the anastomosis should be removed endoscopically and any other associated abnormality such as a gastro-gastric fistula should be addressed in order to optimize the chance of healing. In case of refractory ulceration or recalcitrant ulceration, a laparoscopic resection and revision of the GJ

anastomosis should be performed. Bleeding should be managed endoscopically or surgically in case of hemodynamic instability or failure of endoscopic control. Cases of perforation from a marginal ulcer should undergo omental patch repair in a timely manner. The surgery should be performed laparoscopically if the patient's hemodynamics are favorable and depending on the surgeon's comfort level with minimally invasive techniques.

Acknowledgment The author has nothing to disclose.

References

1. Buchwald H, Avidor Y, Braunwald E, Jensen MD, Pories W, Fahrbach K, Schoelles K. Bariatric surgery: a systematic review and meta-analysis. JAMA. 2004;292(14):1724–37.
2. Buchwald H, Estok R, Fahrbach K, Banel D, Jensen MD, Pories WJ, et al. Weight and type 2 diabetes after bariatric surgery: systematic review and meta-analysis. Am J Med. 2009;122(3):248–56.e5.
3. Hanipah ZN, Schauer PR. Surgical treatment of obesity and diabetes. Gastrointest Endosc Clin N Am. 2017;27(2):191–211.
4. Marcotte E, Chand B. Management and prevention of surgical and nutritional complications after bariatric surgery. Surg Clin North Am. 2016;96(4):843–56.
5. Higa KD, Boone KB, Ho T. Complications of the laparoscopic Roux-en-Y gastric bypass: 1,040 patients—what have we learned? Obes Surg. 2000;10(6):509–13.
6. Coblijn UK, Goucham AB, Lagarde SM, Kuiken SD, van Wagensveld BA. Development of ulcer disease after Roux-en-Y gastric bypass, incidence, risk factors, and patient presentation: a systematic review. Obes Surg. 2014;24(2):299–309.
7. El-Hayek K, Timratana P, Shimizu H, Chand B. Marginal ulcer after Roux-en-Y gastric bypass: what have we really learned? Surg Endosc. 2012;26(10):2789–96.
8. Csendes A, Burgos AM, Altuve J, Bonacic S. Incidence of marginal ulcer 1 month and 1 to 2 years after gastric bypass: a prospective consecutive endoscopic evaluation of 442 patients with morbid obesity. Obes Surg. 2009;19(2):135–8.
9. Csendes A, Torres J, Burgos AM. Late marginal ulcers after gastric bypass for morbid obesity. Clinical and endoscopic findings and response to treatment. Obes Surg. 2011;21(9):1319–22.
10. Printen KJ, Scott D, Mason EE. Stomal ulcers after gastric bypass. Arch Surg. 1980;115(4):525–7.
11. Garrido AB Jr, Rossi M, Lima SE Jr, Brenner AS, Gomes CA Jr. Early marginal ulcer following Roux-en-Y gastric bypass under proton pump inhibitor

treatment: prospective multicentric study. Arq Gastroenterol. 2010;47(2):130–4.

12. D'Hondt MA, Pottel H, Devriendt D, Van Rooy F, Vansteenkiste F. Can a short course of prophylactic low-dose proton pump inhibitor therapy prevent stomal ulceration after laparoscopic Roux-en-Y gastric bypass? Obes Surg. 2010;20(5):595–9.

13. Coblijn UK, Lagarde SM, de Castro SM, Kuiken SD, van Tets WF, van Wagensveld BA. The influence of prophylactic proton pump inhibitor treatment on the development of symptomatic marginal ulceration in Roux-en-Y gastric bypass patients: a historic cohort study. Surg Obes Relat Dis. 2016;12(2):246–52.

14. Moon RC, Teixeira AF, Goldbach M, Jawad MA. Management and treatment outcomes of marginal ulcers after Roux-en-Y gastric bypass at a single high volume bariatric center. Surg Obes Relat Dis. 2014;10(2):229–34.

15. Kang X, Hong D, Anvari M, Tiboni M, Amin N, Gmora S. Is daily low-dose aspirin safe to take following laparoscopic Roux-en-Y gastric bypass for obesity surgery? Obes Surg. 2017;27(5):1261–5.

16. Rasmussen JJ, Fuller W, Ali MR. Marginal ulceration after laparoscopic gastric bypass: an analysis of predisposing factors in 260 patients. Surg Endosc. 2007;21(7):1090–4.

17. Carr WR, Mahawar KK, Balupuri S, Small PK. An evidence-based algorithm for the management of marginal ulcers following Roux-en-Y gastric bypass. Obes Surg. 2014;24(9):1520–7.

18. Huang CS, Forse RA, Jacobson BC, Farraye FA. Endoscopic findings and their clinical correlations in patients with symptoms after gastric bypass surgery. Gastrointest Endosc. 2003;58(6):859–66.

19. Wilson JA, Romagnuolo J, Byrne TK, Morgan K, Wilson FA. Predictors of endoscopic findings after Roux-en-Y gastric bypass. Am J Gastroenterol. 2006;101(10):2194–9.

20. Kalaiselvan R, Exarchos G, Hamza N, Ammori BJ. Incidence of perforated gastrojejunal anastomotic ulcers after laparoscopic gastric bypass for morbid obesity and role of laparoscopy in their management. Surg Obes Relat Dis. 2012;8(4):423–8.

21. Wendling MR, Linn JG, Keplinger KM, Mikami DJ, Perry KA, Melvin WS, Needleman BJ. Omental patch repair effectively treats perforated marginal ulcer following Roux-en-Y gastric bypass. Surg Endosc. 2013;27(2):384–9.

22. Sverdén E, Mattsson F, Sondén A, Leinsköld T, Tao W, Lu Y, Lagergren J. Risk factors for marginal ulcer after gastric bypass surgery for obesity: a population-based cohort study. Ann Surg. 2016;263(4):733–7.

23. Azagury DE, Abu Dayyeh BK, Greenwalt IT, Thompson CC. Marginal ulceration after Roux-en-Y gastric bypass surgery: characteristics, risk factors, treatment, and outcomes. Endoscopy. 2011;43(11):950–4.

24. Patel RA, Brolin RE, Gandhi A. Revisional operations for marginal ulcer after Roux-en-Y gastric bypass. Surg Obes Relat Dis. 2009;5(3):317–22.

25. Soll AH, Weinstein WM, Kurata J, McCarthy D. Nonsteroidal anti-inflammatory drugs and peptic ulcer disease. Ann Intern Med. 1991;114(4):307–19.

26. Konturek SJ, Konturek PC, Brzozowski T. Prostaglandins and ulcer healing. J Physiol Pharmacol. 2005;56(Suppl 5):5–31.

27. Caruana JA, McCabe MN, Smith AD, Panemanglore VP, Sette CD. Risk of massive upper gastrointestinal bleeding in gastric bypass patients taking clopidogrel. Surg Obes Relat Dis. 2007;3(4):443–5.

28. Liberopoulos EN, Elisaf MS, Tselepis AD, Archimandritis A, Kiskinis D, Cokkinos D, Mikhailidis DP. Upper gastrointestinal haemorrhage complicating antiplatelet treatment with aspirin and/or clopidogrel: where we are now? Platelets. 2006;17(1):1–6.

29. Laufer S, Greim C, Luik S, Ayoub SS, Dehner F. Human whole blood assay for rapid and routine testing of non-steroidal anti-inflammatory drugs (NSAIDs) on cyclo-oxygenase-2 activity. Inflammopharmacology. 2008;16(4):155–61.

30. Loewen M, Giovanni J, Barba C. Screening endoscopy before bariatric surgery: a series of 448 patients. Surg Obes Relat Dis. 2008;4(6):709–12.

31. Kelly JJ, Perugini RA, Wang QL, Czerniach DR, Flahive J, Cohen PA. The presence of Helicobacter pylori is not associated with long-term anastomotic complications in gastric bypass patients. Surg Endosc. 2015;29(10):2885–90.

32. Rawlins L, Rawlins MP, Brown CC, Schumacher DL. Effect of Helicobacter pylori on marginal ulcer and stomal stenosis after Roux-en-Y gastric bypass. Surg Obes Relat Dis. 2013;9(5):760–4.

33. Hartin CW Jr, ReMine DS, Lucktong TA. Preoperative bariatric screening and treatment of Helicobacter pylori. Surg Endosc. 2009;23(11):2531–4.

34. Papasavas PK, Gagné DJ, Donnelly PE, Salgado J, Urbandt JE, Burton KK, Caushaj PF. Prevalence of Helicobacter pylori infection and value of preoperative testing and treatment in patients undergoing laparoscopic Roux-en-Y gastric bypass. Surg Obes Relat Dis. 2008;4(3):383–8.

35. Schulman AR, Abougergi MS, Thompson CC. H. Pylori as a predictor of marginal ulceration: a nationwide analysis. Obesity (Silver Spring). 2017;25(3):522–6.

36. Sacks BC, Mattar SG, Qureshi FG, Eid GM, Collins JL, Barinas-Mitchell EJ, et al. Incidence of marginal ulcers and the use of absorbable anastomotic sutures in laparoscopic Roux-en-Y gastric bypass. Surg Obes Relat Dis. 2006;2(1):11–6.

37. Edholm D, Ottosson J, Sundbom M. Importance of pouch size in laparoscopic Roux-en-Y gastric bypass: a cohort study of 14,168 patients. Surg Endosc. 2016;30(5):2011–5.

38. Siilin H, Wanders A, Gustavsson S, Sundbom M. The proximal gastric pouch invariably contains acid-producing parietal cells in Roux-en-Y gastric bypass. Obes Surg. 2005;15(6):771–7.

39. Mason EE, Ito C. Gastric bypass in obesity. Surg Clin North Am. 1967;47(6):1345–51.

40. Sima E, Hedberg J, Ehrenborg A, Sundbom M. Differences in early complications between circular and linear stapled gastrojejunostomy in laparoscopic gastric bypass. Obes Surg. 2014;24(4):599–603.

41. Sapala JA, Wood MH, Sapala MA, Flake TM Jr. Marginal ulcer after gastric bypass: a prospective 3-year study of 173 patients. Obes Surg. 1998;8(5):505–16.

42. Hedberg J, Hedenstrom H, Sundbom M. Wireless pH-metry at the gastrojejunostomy after Roux-en-Y gastric bypass: a novel use of the BRAVO system. Surg Endosc. 2011;25(7):2302–7.

43. Corcelles R, Jamal MH, Daigle CR, Rogula T, Brethauer SA, Schauer PR. Surgical management of gastrogastric fistula. Surg Obes Relat Dis. 2015;11(6):1227–32.

44. Capella JF, Capella RF. Gastro-gastric fistulas and marginal ulcers in gastric bypass procedures for weight reduction. Obes Surg. 1999;9(1):22–7; discussion 28.

45. Carrodeguas L, Szomstein S, Soto F, Whipple O, Simpfendorfer C, Gonzalvo JP, et al. Management of gastrogastric fistulas after divided Roux-en-Y gastric bypass surgery for morbid obesity: analysis of 1,292 consecutive patients and review of literature. Surg Obes Relat Dis. 2005;1(5):467–74.

46. Edholm D, Sundbom M. Comparison between circular- and linear-stapled gastrojejunostomy in laparoscopic Roux-en-Y gastric bypass—a cohort from the Scandinavian Obesity Registry. Surg Obes Relat Dis. 2015;11(6):1233–6.

47. Ying VW, Kim SH, Khan KJ, Farrokhyar F, D'Souza J, Gmora S, Anvari M, Hong D. Prophylactic PPI help reduce marginal ulcers after gastric bypass surgery: a systematic review and meta-analysis of cohort studies. Surg Endosc. 2015;29(5):1018–23.

48. Steinemann DC, Bueter M, Schiesser M, Amygdalos I, Clavien PA, Nocito A. Management of anastomotic ulcers after Roux-en-Y gastric bypass: results of an international survey. Obes Surg. 2014;24(5):741–6.

49. Frezza EE, Herbert H, Ford R, Wachtel MS. Endoscopic suture removal at gastrojejunal anastomosis after Roux-en-Y gastric bypass to prevent marginal ulceration. Surg Obes Relat Dis. 2007;3(6):619–22.

50. Schulman AR, Chan WW, Devery A, Ryan MB, Thompson CC. Opened proton pump inhibitor capsules reduce time to healing compared with intact capsules for marginal ulceration following roux-en-y gastric bypass. Clin Gastroenterol Hepatol. 2017;15(4):494–500.e1.

51. Racu C, Dutson EP, Mehran A. Laparoscopic gastrojejunostomy revision: a novel approach to intractable marginal ulcer management. Surg Obes Relat Dis. 2010;6(5):557–8.

52. Steinemann DC, Schiesser M, Clavien PA, Nocito A. Laparoscopic gastric pouch and remnant resection: a novel approach to refractory anastomotic ulcers after Roux-en-Y gastric bypass: case report. BMC Surg. 2011;11:33.

53. Jirapinyo P, Watson RR, Thompson CC. Use of a novel endoscopic suturing device to treat recalcitrant marginal ulceration (with video). Gastrointest Endosc. 2012;76(2):435–9.

54. Barola S, Magnuson T, Schweitzer M, Chen YI, Ngamruengphong S, Khashab MA, Kumbhari V. Endoscopic suturing for massively bleeding marginal ulcer 10 days post roux-en-y gastric bypass. Obes Surg. 2017;27(5):1934–6.

55. Liu JJ, Saltzman JR. Endoscopic hemostasis treatment: how should you perform it? Can J Gastroenterol. 2009;23(7):481–3.

56. Felix EL, Kettelle J, Mobley E, Swartz D. Perforated marginal ulcers after laparoscopic gastric bypass. Surg Endosc. 2008;22(10):2128–32.

Melissa Felinski, Maamoun A. Harmouch,
Erik B. Wilson, and Shinil K. Shah

Introduction

Morbid obesity is a chronic relapsing disease that
has become one of the most important public
health problems. While bariatric surgery is the
most effective therapy for sustained weight loss
with resolution or improvement of obesity-
related comorbidities and increased life expectancy, there are a subset of patients who fail to
attain or maintain treatment goals. The reasons
that drive this failure are multifactorial.
Nonetheless, the timing and choice of intervention as well as the need to repeat therapy plays a
significant role when one considers that the treatment of obesity should parallel the lifelong nature
of the disease.

M. Felinski, D.O. • M.A. Harmouch, M.D.
E.B. Wilson, M.D.
Department of Surgery, McGovern Medical School,
University of Texas Health, 6431 Fannin Street,
MSB 4.156, Houston, TX 77030, USA
e-mail: melissa.felinski@uth.tmc.edu;
maamoun.a.harmouch@uth.tmc.edu;
erikbwilson@yahoo.com

S.K. Shah, D.O. (✉)
Department of Surgery, McGovern Medical School,
University of Texas Health, 6431 Fannin Street,
MSB 4.156, Houston, TX 77030, USA

Michael E. DeBakey Institute for Comparative
Cardiovascular Science and Biomedical Devices,
Texas A&M University, College Station, TX, USA
e-mail: shinil.k.shah@uth.tmc.edu

Weight recidivism is a challenging problem
for patients and bariatric surgeons alike. Besides
the emotional and psychosocial toll on the
patient, the significant improvements in overall
health seen after surgery will diminish with subsequent weight regain. This may lead to the
recurrence of prior comorbid conditions [1, 2]
and their array of consequences. To prevent this,
bariatric surgeons must be able to evaluate the
causes for failure and then determine the best
options for managing the patient's future treatment. There exists no standardized approach for
revisional intervention for weigh regain. Any
combination of surgical or nonsurgical therapy
may be used, but the management plan must be
tailored to each individual.

Weight Failure: Defining Weight Regain Versus Insufficient Weight Loss

Roux-en-Y gastric bypass (RYGB) is a well-
established bariatric procedure that results in
65–80% excess weight loss (EWL) over an average of 12–24 months after surgery [3, 4]. Studies
have shown, though, that %EWL lessens over
time from 66% at 1–2 years to 50% at 10 years
[5]. It is estimated that 25–35% of patients will
experience weight regain from the nadir weight
2–5 years after surgery [6–8]. Yet the true
incidence of weight recidivism after RYGB
remains unknown. This may be largely due to
the way we characterize weight failure and the

B. Chand (ed.), *Endoscopy in Obesity Management*, DOI 10.1007/978-3-319-63528-6_12

not insignificant percentage of patients who are lost to follow-up. Additionally, studies often report weight failure outcomes by grouping together patients with insufficient weight loss and weight regain after bariatric surgery; however, it is important to differentiate between the two. Primary insufficient weight loss is generally regarded as a weight loss <50% of excess body weight [9] or total body weight loss (TBWL) <15% [10] at 18 months after gastric bypass. On the contrary, weight regain is a progressive increase in weight after initial successful weight loss [9].

Currently, there is no consensus on how we should define weight loss or regain. A number of different metrics are used when assessing these weight loss outcomes, including the absolute number of pounds or body mass index (BMI) units lost, BMI achieved after weight loss nadir, the % EWL, or %TBWL [11–13]. Percentage TBWL is a more frequently used metric to evaluate the response with pharmacological and behavioral therapy whereas %EWL, defined as the number of pounds lost above the patient's ideal body weight, is the historical precedent among surgical literature. Because %EWL is based on a somewhat arbitrary target of "ideal" weight, it is heavily influenced by preoperative BMI and will disproportionally favor those starting at a lower BMI. To further clarify, a super-obese patient (i.e., BMI > 50) will lose more absolute body weight, but a smaller percentage of excess body weight when compared to a patient with a lower starting BMI. Such a significant variation in %EWL resulting from BMI is eliminated by using %TBWL. Percentage TBWL has the benefit of characterizing absolute weight loss that is independent of the preoperative BMI. It has been proposed that such a standardized measure be used to facilitate communication among the surgical and nonsurgical communities. Perhaps then can the growing number of obesity therapies and their outcomes can be better directly compared and provide guidance on which patient would benefit from additional treatment and what type of procedure to choose.

Predictors of Weight Regain (Preoperative BMI, Time Since Surgery, Age, Comorbidities, Etc.)

Obesity is a multifactorial and overlapping disease with genetics/epigenetics, neurobehavioral, environmental, cultural, immune, endocrine, medical causes, etc. all contributing to the complex disease [14]. There is a limited understanding of how to predict which patients are more likely to be successful or unsuccessful after bariatric surgery. Identifying predictors of post-RYGB weight regain could provide further insight into the underlying pathogenesis of this disease and the therapies used to manage it, but more importantly, may help lead to better preoperative patient education and selection.

High preoperative BMI [15], younger age, iron deficiency, longer duration after surgery [16], and certain psychological disorders, such as binge eating [17], have been associated with weight regain in long-term follow-up. Additional studies failed to demonstrate the influence of higher preoperative BMI on post-RYGB weight maintenance, but further support the role of age and time since surgery [18]. Additional research into the influence of these and many other factors on the outcomes of bariatric surgery is paramount.

Etiological Factors

The underlying causes leading to weight recidivism tend to be complex and multifactorial. Both patient-specific (lifestyle choices, mental health issues, hormonal/metabolic conditions) and surgical-specific etiologies contribute to this increasing problem. The extent and magnitude of these factors is currently uncertain and likely differs between each patient [19, 20].

Lifestyle Choices

Prior to surgery, the patient should have realistic goals regarding their weight loss, knowledge about nutrition, and willingness to adhere to a diet and exercise plan. It is imperative that they understand that bariatric surgery is not a quick fix for their obesity, as obesity is a chronic disease. Noncompliance and inadequate follow-up is a cause for failure in all weight loss operations. Poor habits such as regular intake of high-fat, high-sugar foods and beverages, grazing, large portioned meals, and sedentary lifestyle will lead to suboptimal results regardless of the procedure performed. The evolution of this noncompliance is facilitated by poor follow-up. A bariatric patient may revert to their old habits if not adequately monitored. A dietary and physical activity interview should be performed routinely to identify any unhealthy choices or behaviors, followed by ongoing counseling. Often, such interventions may be enough to get these patients back on track while also promoting greater adherence to long-lasting lifestyle changes. Early identification of the symptoms and behaviors that may contribute to failure is key. It is imperative that patients are compliant with follow-up, as it is at these appointments that weight loss plateaus and small regains can be addressed early with intervention. Expectations of routine follow-up, especially after 2 years postoperatively, should be emphasized with patients even prior to surgery.

Mental Health Issues

Patients who suffer from obesity may be especially prone to a number of mental health issues. Depression, mood and anxiety disorders, negative coping mechanisms, maladaptive eating disorders, and substance use are just a few of the challenges that this population faces [21, 22]. These issues may interfere with durable weight loss by undermining motivation and adherence to diet, exercise, and overall general health recommendations. Maladaptive eating patterns such as binge eating, night eating, and mindless or emotional eating lead to weight regain [20]. To add to the dilemma, several of the antidepressants and antipsychotics commonly used in the management of mental health conditions are associated with weight gain [23]. Patients should be encour-

aged to seek support via support groups, family, friends, or professional counseling. It is important that the patient continues postoperative psychological/psychiatric follow-up, especially if experiencing distress or having difficulty adjusting to the many changes that occur after surgery.

Hormonal/Metabolic Imbalance

RYGB-induced restriction of food intake is only a part of the underlying mechanism behind the weight reducing effects of the procedure. Perhaps even more important is the alteration in gastrointestinal hormones, which have a considerable impact on glucose hemostasis, appetite regulation, and weight loss. Changes in secretion of glucagon-like peptide (GLP-1), glucose-dependent insulinotropic polypeptide (GIP), ghrelin, and other gastrointestinal hormones have been well studied [20, 24]. However, it appears that these hormonal changes vary between patients with durable weight loss when compared to those who experience weight regain [24]. Further investigation of gastrointestinal hormone secretion profiles and their effect on hunger and satiety perception is ongoing.

Several studies describe the role of reactive hypoglycemia on weight regain. It is believed that the augmented secretion of GLP-1 and GIP after RYGB may induce B cell proliferation and insulin hypersecretion, resulting in hypoglycemia [20, 25]. Hypoglycemia is an appetite stimulant, thus driving snacking or grazing tendencies and subsequent weight gain. In order to avoid the insulin surge and subsequent hypoglycemia, post-RYGB patients should eat 3 meals plus 2–3 snacks, and minimize their consumption of simple carbohydrates while increasing fiber and protein [20].

Surgical Factors

With time, the construction of the RYGB may undergo unwanted anatomic changes and are potential causes behind weight recidivism. The gastric pouch may enlarge, the gastrojejunal stoma outlet can dilate, or in some cases, a gastrogastric fistula (GGF) may develop.

Pouch and/or stoma outlet dilation may lead to loss of perceived and actual restriction. Though somewhat anecdotal, the gastric pouch is considered enlarged if dimensions measure >5 cm wide and >6 cm long and the stoma outlet is considered dilated if >2 cm [26, 27].

Staple line failure can result in a leak with abscess formation, which then drains into the nearby remnant stomach forming a GGF. A chronic GGF allows food to pass from the pouch to the remnant stomach, hence reducing the restrictive, malabsorptive, and potential hormonal effects of the RYGB. Although the prevalence of GGF has dramatically decreased since completely dividing the pouch from the remnant stomach, its presence can contribute to weight gain and identification of a possible fistula should be part of the workup for patients who experience weight regain or insufficient weight loss [28].

Evaluation

The presence of an insufficient response, regardless of whether is it inadequate weight loss or weight recidivism after bariatric surgery, deserves further evaluation and management. As previously stated, weight failure tends to be multifactorial. Determining which of these factors is contributing to weight failure requires a systematic and multidisciplinary approach. A comprehensive review of medical, psychological, educational, and surgical issues must be performed in order to identify and correct the reasons for suboptimal success. The preoperative evaluation should involve a full history and physical exam, review of the technical details of the primary operation, thorough examination of the anatomical and functional aspects of the relevant gastrointestinal tract, and nutritional and behavioral assessment. Once a patient is considered a candidate for revisional intervention, they should attend dedicated revisional seminars with surgeons, obesity medicine specialists, dieticians, and psychologists.

The history should focus on salient features such as whether they initially achieved postsurgical weight loss and/or improvement of comorbidities. Reviewing the operative report will help elicit understanding of the patient's RYGB construction, including pouch size and type (divided, nondivided), limb lengths (biliopancreatic (BP) limb, roux limb, and common channel), limb configuration (Roux-en-Y, loop) and route (antecolic, retrocolic). The most useful radiological study to evaluate the functional features of the gastrointestinal tract is an upper gastrointestinal (UGI) series. The UGI study may detect esophageal or RYGB abnormalities such as dilatations, strictures, and fistulas that frequently require additional evaluation. As stated previously, the post-RYGB anatomy may alter with time. Thus, upper endoscopy is a mandatory step to assess current pouch and stoma outlet sizes. Care should be taken to accurately measure the dimensions of the pouch and diameter of the gastrojejunal stoma outlet using a measurement tool (snare, etc.). Upper endoscopy also provides more useful intraluminal information regarding the presence of mucosal inflammation, foreign body erosions, marginal ulcers, and staple line integrity. Staple line failure leading to a GGF may often be clinically silent but is typically discovered with the combination of UGI, upper endoscopy, +/− computed tomography (CT) imaging [26, 28]. The presence of air or contrast within the remnant stomach on CT is highly suggestive of a GGF. The presence of bile in the gastric pouch can alert the endoscopist to GGF or a short roux limb. CT is also a helpful adjunct to evaluate for internal hernia, small bowel intussusception, or other intra-abdominal anomalies.

Although laboratory testing is unlikely to reveal why weight recidivism occurs, the patient's underlying nutritional state must be evaluated. This is especially true when considering revisional interventions. Albumin, prealbumin, vitamin, and mineral levels should be assessed and corrected. Vitamin deficiency may be a sign of noncompliance, which may require targeted intervention prior to recommendation of a revisional surgical or endoscopic procedure. Baseline physiologic and other metabolic set points may also influence weight failure and deserve further study. Consideration should be given in measuring resting metabolic rate and body composition in order to optimize successful weight loss maintenance.

While the anatomical and functional causes of weight recidivism may be easily identified and subsequently treated, addressing the underlying psychological or behavioral issues may prove to be a formidable challenge. Early recognition of behaviors that are resilient to intervention and being prepared to manage them is essential. In fact, the initial step in evaluation of a patient with weight failure is to review food records. These may help highlight poor choices or habits and will allow for the reinforcement of appropriate behaviors.

It is important to recognize that weight recidivism may even occur despite finding any anatomical or functional abnormalities in a patient that is adherent to nutritional and behavioral measures. This further supports the complex relapsing nature of the disease and deserves further study.

Treatment Options

There are a number of treatment options to consider for the treatment of weight regain or inadequate weight loss and includes pharmacotherapy, surgical and endoscopic therapies.

Pharmacotherapy

Anti-obesity drugs (AODs) have been shown to be an effective component of the multimodal treatment approach to obesity. Currently, there are five different US Food and Drug Administration (FDA) approved medications for long-term use in obese patients with BMI > 30 or BMI > 27 with at least 1 weight-associated comorbidity (type 2 diabetes, hypertension, hyperlipidemia, etc.). These medications include orlistat, lorcaserin, naltrexone-bupropion, phentermine-topiramate, and liraglutide. With the exception of orlistat, which induces weight loss by lipid malabsorption, the rest of these agents work in part by inducing a state of appetite suppression. Liraglutide is given via injection and its mechanism is related to GLP-1. They all have some effect on lipid profiles and

average weight loss is generally between 5.8 and 10.2 kg [29]. In a recent systemic review, all five medications were associated with higher odds of achieving weight loss compared to placebo with at least 1 year of therapy. Among these agents, phentermine-topiramate followed by liraglutide was found to be associated with higher odds of achieving total body weight loss (TBWL) of at least 5 and 10% from baseline weight [30].

There is paucity of literature looking at the role of AOD in patients with weight regain after bariatric surgery. In a recent study, liraglutide has been shown to be effective in patients who have poor weight loss or weight regain after surgery (gastric band, RYGB, sleeve gastrectomy, and duodenal switch) when no technical problem has been identified [31]. A recent study evaluating patients with weight regain or inadequate weight loss after sleeve gastrectomy or RYGB demonstrated that AODs resulted in additional weight loss. This was true in patients who received AODs at the time of plateau of weight loss or at time of weight regain. Topiramate was noted to be the most effective, and patients who had undergone RYGB were more likely to achieve >5% total weight loss [23]. There are a number of other studies that demonstrate efficacy of AODs when prescribed after weight loss surgery, including combination of phenteramine and fenfluramine in patients with RYGB or biliopancreatic diversion [32] and phenteramine and combination phentermine-topiramate in patients with RYGB or gastric band [33]. Overall, studies are small and mostly retrospective, and certainly this area is ripe for future research.

Surgical Options

When considering surgical options to address failure after RYGB, it is important to remember that surgical approaches generally deal with anatomical changes that result in loss of the restrictive and/or malabsorptive mechanisms. It is critical to establish anatomic failure prior to considering revisional surgery [34]. Loss of restriction secondary to pouch enlargement, stoma dilation (increased diameter of the gastrojejunostomy

(GJ)), and GGF may all contribute to weight regain or poor weight loss. To date, there is paucity of research regarding revisional surgery. Revisional surgery has been associated with high perioperative morbidity, inconsistent long-term results, and a high risk to benefit ratio when compared to the primary procedure [34]. Furthermore, there are no standardized protocols to aid in selecting the best revisional option for the individual patient. Various endoscopic and surgical revisional options have been suggested. In patients without documented GGFs, the surgical options are numerous and focus on two main mechanisms. These include reestablishing restriction and increasing malabsorption.

Reduction of pouch size/stoma diameter. Reestablishing restriction is often accomplished by reducing the gastric pouch size as well as the diameter of the stoma. As discussed previously, preoperative UGI series and upper endoscopy are crucial to the evaluation of degree of dilation of the pouch and stoma. Revisions are often done with minimally invasive techniques. The gastric pouch, stoma, and roux limb must be freed from all surrounding structures. This also aids in confirmation of no occult GGF, which may contribute to weight regain/inadequate weight loss. An intraluminal tube/bougie is passed orally to help identify the gastroesophageal (GE) junction and the GJ anastomosis [19, 20]. Once the anatomy has been established, several surgical options can be implemented to address a dilated pouch and or GJ diameter. If the stoma diameter was found to be satisfactory on preoperative evaluation, one can spare it and focus and resize the pouch with or without transecting the blind end of the alimentary limb. This can be accomplished by firing serial staple loads longitudinally along the gastric pouch to further narrow it (sleeving the pouch). If the stoma was found to be dilated on preoperative assessment, one should start the new staple line at the dilated roux limb across the GJ and gastric pouch up to the GE junction. Alternatively, the GJ anastomosis can be resected, the pouch recreated, and a new GJ anastomosis fashioned [34–37].

Several retrospective series have shown safety and modest efficacy of gastric pouch and stoma revision. Similar to what is seen with primary surgery, efficacy decreases over time; overall, the mean percent excess BMI loss was 43.3% at 1 year but dropped to 14% at up to 3 years. This highlights the need for comprehensive management of these patients. In a recent systematic review, as compared to other options for RYGB revision, surgical pouch/stoma revision had the lowest complication rates at approximately 3.5% [34, 38].

Banding after Roux-en-Y gastric bypass. Gastric banding has been performed as a primary bariatric procedure, as an adjunct to RYGB in the super-obese patients, and as a revisional procedure in patients with weight regain after RYGB. Salvage banding using an adjustable gastric band (AGB) was suggested as a safe and easily performed procedure. Early reports showed low incidence of early major complications with no mortalities reported [39, 40]. The procedure entails placing an AGB either around the gastric pouch distal to the GE junction, or at the GJ anastomosis, or around the proximal dilated roux limb [39–41]. This provides further restriction and decrease in pouch compliance, which may help prevent overeating behaviors. It also allows the clinician easy access to alter the degree of restriction if more weight loss is desired. In a recent systemic review, revisional gastric banding had % excess BMI loss of 47.6 and 47.3% at 1 and 3 years of follow-up, respectively [34]. Although the early perioperative morbidity and mortality is low following salvage gastric banding, the rates of long-term complication and reoperation are not insignificant (approximately 17–18%). Reported complications include gastric volvulus, small bowel obstruction, band erosions, and band slippage [34].

Distalization of Roux-en-Y gastric bypass. Distal gastric bypass (D-RYGB) can be done as a primary procedure in the super-obese patients or as a revisional procedure in patients with failed RYGB. Unlike other strategies that focused on increasing the restriction, D-RYGB increases the degree of malabsorption in patients with failed RYGB. The first technique was described in the mid-1980s by Sugerman et al. and later underwent slight variation in technique by other investigators. It generally involves taking down the jejunojejunostomy (JJ) at the alimentary side and re-anastomosis to the distal ileum approximately 150 cm proximal to the ileocecal valve. This generally results in a 150 cm common channel, an unchanged alimentary limb length, and a very long unmeasured BP limb. Another technique later reported entails taking down the JJ at the BP limb and re-anastomosis to the distal ileum at a point 75 cm proximal to ileocecal valve. This resulted in a shorter 75 cm common channel and a longer unmeasured BP limb [42].

Investigators that performed the former technique in which the common channel is 100–150 cm reported %EWL of 61–90%, 68–85%, and 77% at 1, 5, and 10 years, respectively [34, 43, 44]. These excellent results were however accompanied by significant major metabolic complications, mainly protein calorie malnutrition (PCM) that required total parenteral nutrition (TPN) in 14–21% of patients and reoperation to lengthen the common channel in 5–14% of patients [34, 42–44]. Brolin et al. studied the second technique and reported 48% EWL at 1 year with PCM seen in 7% of patients, with some requiring either temporary TPN or reversal [45]. In general, D-RYGB is a very effective revisional procedure with % excess BMI loss of 54% at 1 year and 52.2% at 3 years [34]. As would be expected with increasing the malabsorptive nature of this operation, D-RYGB has a high complication rate, the majority being related to PCM.

Conversion to biliopancreatic diversion/duodenal switch. Conversion to biliopancreatic diversion/duodenal switch (BPD/DS) as a revisional option for a failed RYGB is considered the most effective option and has been shown to have the best long-term weight loss. Despite that, it has not gained wide acceptance due to the complexity of the procedure and the concern for long-term severe malnutrition [34]. Initially, this complex procedure was performed via laparotomy and soon afterwards was shown to be feasible via laparoscopy. The procedure can be done as a one- or two-stage operation. It entails disconnecting the gastrojejunal anastomosis. Gastric continuity is then reestablished followed by a sleeve gastrectomy. The construction of the gastrogastric anastomosis can be accomplished with hand sewn or stapled (generally circular stapler) techniques. A standard technique for BPD/DS is then followed [46–48]. This new orientation results in an approximately 150 cm alimentary limb, 100 cm common channel, and long unmeasured BP limb. According to current reports, this revisional procedure generally results in %EWL reported at 62.7% at 1 year and 71% EWL at up to 3 years, corresponding to % excess BMI loss of 63.7% and 76%, respectively [34].

Endoscopic Therapy

Endoluminal surgery is an emerging technology and may be an attractive solution to address some of the complications seen after RYGB, including weight regain. These interventions focus on reducing the gastric pouch size and the GJ anastomotic diameter. Historically and currently, this has been accomplished by either injection of a sclerosing agent, over the scope clips, argon plasma coagulation, or utilization of an endoscopic suturing platform. Endoscopic suturing is rapidly gaining traction as the endoscopic technique of choice. It appears to be more effective in reducing stoma size, improving eating behaviors, and inducing post-procedure weight loss [49].

Sclerotherapy. Endoscopic sclerotherapy was first introduced in 2003. This technique entails injecting a sclerosing agent circumferentially around the gastrojejunostomy [50]. The most commonly used agent is sodium morrhuate. The amount to be injected has not been standardized, and can be anywhere between 6 and 20 cm^3. According to published literature, patients that underwent this procedure had a mild to moderate response at best. Spaulding et al. reported that 75% of patients had 9% EWL at 6 months (2). The same author published another study with 1 year follow-up showing that 90% of subjects that received the intervention had lost weight or stopped regaining weight [51]. Catalano et al. studied 28 patients over a 3-year period. Patients underwent a mean of 2.3 sessions, and 18/28 patients (64%) had what was considered successful therapy (postinjection stoma size of <12 mm and >75% loss of regained weight). Mean weight loss at 18 months in patients who underwent successful sclerotherapy was 22.3 kg (+/− 9.2 kg). Commonly reported side effects including pain (75% of patients) requiring prescription pain medications, superficial ulcers (10/28 patients) that responded to PPI therapy, and GJ stenosis requiring balloon dilation (one patient) [52]. Abu Dayyeh et al. reported a series of 231 patients with weight regain after RYGB. Increased weight regain from nadir after RYGB (similar to other smaller studies [53]) and increased number of sclerotherapy sessions predicted response. Adverse reported outcomes included bleeding, dysphagia/chest discomfort, transient elevations in diastolic blood pressure, pain, and ulcers [54, 55]. Other smaller series have reported similar outcomes [53, 55].

Overall, endoscopic sclerotherapy is an easily performed procedure, with a low complication profile, and can be repeated over multiple treatment sessions [54]. Data to support this procedure is limited to small, retrospective case series with limited short-term follow-up [6]. In one of the only series to report longer term follow-up (up to 60 months, mean of 22 months), only 58% of patients had weight loss or stabilization, but average weight loss when compared pre and post sclerotherapy was not statistically significant. This was a small study of only 48 patients [56].

There is a single study reporting the combination of sclerotherapy and endoscopic suturing. Sclerotherapy with hypertonic saline combined with endoscopic suturing in 11 patients trended towards greater weight loss at 22 months as compared to suturing only [57].

Over the scope clip. A single study has described the use of an over the scope clip (OTSC-clip, Ovesco AG, Tubingen, Germany) in 94 patients who have undergone a gastric bypass with silastic ring band (Fobi pouch RYGB) who experienced 10% or more weight regain. GJ anastomotic diameter was reduced from an average of 35 mm to 8 mm. Reported adverse events included sore throat and dysphagia (2/5 required anastomotic dilation). BMI reduced from 45.8 to 27.4 at a mean of 1 year of follow-up [58].

A small series has reported use of an over the scope clip to close GGFs. Although there was initial technical success in 12/14 patients, long-term success was only 33%, similar to other endoscopic interventions for GGFs [59].

Argon plasma coagulation. The use of argon plasma coagulation has been utilized in small series to decrease GJ stoma size as way to induce weight loss in patients who have had weight regain after RYGB [60]. Baretta et al. reported a series of 30 patients in which patients with a GJ diameter of 15 mm or more underwent argon plasma coagulation of the entire circumference of the anastomosis. Patients underwent two additional treatments at 8 week intervals. Mean weight loss was 15.48 kg with average reduction of GJ diameter by 66.89%. All patients had a diameter of 12 mm or less after the three endoscopic treatments, and increased weight loss was observed with smaller GJ diameters. Follow-up was limited, which was 8 weeks after the third treatment session [61]. The largest series reported 53 patients with a mean stoma diameter of 16 mm. At 6 months, %EWL was 16% (5.3 kg). Patients underwent an average of 1.3 endoscopic treatments [62]. While argon plasma coagulation is not widely utilized as a sole intervention for weight regain in post-RYGB patients, it is used as part of the GJ outlet reduction procedure using the OverStitch endoluminal suturing platform (described below).

Endoscopic suturing. Endoscopic suturing devices used for the treatment of weight regain after RYGB focus on reducing gastric pouch and gastrojejunal stoma diameter. Early platforms for endoscopic suturing utilized suction as opposed to tissue retraction devices to assist with suturing, which had the disadvantage of usually only allowing for partial thickness bites. As this technology evolved, helical and other tissue retraction adjuncts have allowed for full thickness suturing which has expanded the potential indications for endoscopic suturing devices and appear to result in improved weight loss outcomes [63].

EndoCinch. Swain et al. contributed to the development of one of the first commercially available endoscopic suturing platforms (EndoCinch device

[CR Bard, Murray Hill, NJ]) [6]. This device utilized suction to capture tissue to allow for suturing. Sutures were secured by a cinch device. This device allowed for partial thickness suturing and has been used in multiple applications in post-RYGB patients.

An initial series of four patients utilized this device to narrow GJ anastomotic diameter from >20 mm to <15 mm with or without plication of the gastric pouch. The authors reported weight loss and increased restriction; however, no absolute numbers were provided [64]. Thompson et al. reported a series of 8 patients, in which the EndoCinch was used to reduce GJ anastomotic diameter from an average of 25 mm to 10 mm. Average weight loss in 6/8 patients who lost weight was 10 kg. One of the patients in the initial series and 3 of the patients in the series reported by Thompson et al. underwent repeat procedures [65]. Follow-up in both series was extremely limited.

A multicenter randomized prospective sham controlled trial evaluating EndoCinch versus sham (RESTORe trial) for weight regain or inadequate weight loss after RYGB was also conducted. At 6 months of follow-up, patients who underwent GJ stoma plication as opposed to sham procedure had 3.5% as compared to 0.4% absolute weight loss ($p = 0.021$). The majority of patients in the EndoCinch group achieved weight stabilization/loss (96%) as compared to 78% in the sham procedure group ($p = 0.019$) [66, 67].

The EndoCinch device has also been used to close GGFs. Fernandez-Esparrach et al. reported a series of 95 patients in which the device and/or hemoclips (with or without combinations of glue and/or argon plasma coagulation) was utilized to close the fistula. Long-term success was reported in only 19% of patients, with all patients with fistula size >20 mm recurring in follow-up. Thirty-two percent of patients with GGFs <10 mm in diameter had success during the follow-up period [68].

With the advent of commercially available endoscopic suturing platforms that allow for full thickness suturing, this device is not generally used in current endoscopic revisional weight loss procedures.

Stomaphy-X. The Stomaphy-X device (Endogastric Solutions, Redmond, WA) was one of the first devices to allow for full thickness tissue plication utilizing tissue fasteners. Later generations of this device have been used for transoral incisionless fundoplication for reflux. This device was utilized in multiple studies for post-RYGB weight regain to address pouch dilation. Individual series of 39 patients [69] and 64 patients [70] were published, reporting 10 kg (19.5% EWL loss, 1 year) and 7.6 kg (mean follow-up 5.8 months) of weight loss, respectively. Adverse reported events included pharyngeal irritation, epigastric pain, nausea and vomiting, and bleeding [69, 70]. In both series, improvement in dumping syndrome as well as reflux was reported, and in the larger series, four patients were noted to have closure of GGFs [69, 70]. It is unclear as to the durability of the GGF closure, as only a mean of 5.8 months of follow-up was reported. Another series of 59 patients reported that at 41 months of mean follow-up, average weight loss was 1.7 kg (%EWL of 4.3). In 12 patients who underwent repeat endoscopy, there was no sustained reduction in stoma or pouch size (average time to repeat endoscopy was 18 months). This series raised serious questions about the durability of this procedure [71].

A randomized trial compared Stomaphy-X versus sham procedure in patients who had undergone RYGB with at least 60% excess BMI initial loss and a resultant BMI of 35 or less. Patients included had a BMI of 35–40 and the primary endpoint was excess BMI loss of 15% or more and a BMI of <35 at 1 year. Less than 50% of patients who underwent the procedure met the endpoint and the study was terminated early. 10/45 patients who underwent the Stomaphy-X procedure achieved the primary endpoint as compared to 1/29 sham patients [72].

Restorative obesity surgery endoscopic. The Incisionless Operating Platform (USGI Medical, San Clemente, CA) is one of the devices that have been used for endoscopic revision of RYGB. The current generation of the device (Transport® Endoscopic Access Device—Retroflex) has four working channels to accommodate a flexible pediatric endoscope, tissue approximation devices and graspers, and tissue anchors. This device has been utilized for the restorative obesity surgery endoscopic (ROSE) procedure. It allows for full thickness plication of gastric pouch as well as reduction in stoma diameter.

Initial experience with this device was reported in small series. An initial five patient experience noted a mean weight loss of 7.8 kg (3 months of follow-up). Stoma diameter was reduced on average by 21 mm and pouch length reduced by 4.4 cm [73]. A larger series of 20 patients was later published by the same group. The procedure was completed in 17 patients with a mean weight loss of 8.8 kg at 3 months, reduction of stoma diameter from an average of 25 mm to 16 mm, and reduction of pouch length by 2.5 cm. Adverse events reported included bloating, sore throat, nausea and vomiting, and bleeding not requiring transfusion or repeat endoscopy [74]. Borao et al. published a single center series of 21 patients. Twenty of twenty-one patients successfully underwent the procedure, with reductions of GJ stoma diameter of 53% and pouch length of 41%. Follow-up endoscopy at 12 months confirmed the presence of anchors with %EWL reported to be 18% (6 months follow-up) [75]. Raman et al. reported a series of 37 patients with similar results; with a mean follow-up of 4.69 months, there was 23.5% EWL. Two patients underwent endoscopic dilation after the procedure for PO intolerance. In this series, three patients with GGF were noted to have closure of the fistula on follow-up imaging and endoscopy [76].

A multicenter registry of 116 patients reported a technical success rate of 97%, with reductions of stoma size and pouch length of 50 and 44%, respectively. Percent EWL was approximately 18% at 6 months, and in 13 patients who underwent follow-up endoscopy at 12 months, anchors were noted to be in place with intact plications [77]. Further follow-up of 73 patients at 12 months after the procedure reported %EWL of 14.5% with anchors confirmed to be present endoscopically in 92% of patients (61/66 patients). Factors noted to predict increased %EWL included a pre-procedure stoma diameter > 12 mm and a post-procedure stoma diameter < 10 mm [75].

OverStitch. Currently, the most widely utilized platform for endoscopic revision of RYGB is the OverStitchTM Endoscopic Suturing System (Apollo Endosurgery, Austin, TX). This platform has been utilized for reduction of GJ stoma diameter as well as pouch plication. This device allows for both interrupted and running placement of permanent or absorbable sutures. The device fits over therapeutic upper endoscope. Full thickness suturing is facilitated by a helical tissue retractor [6].

There are a number of small studies evaluating the use of the OverStitch platform for reduction in GJ stomal diameter in patients with weight regain after RYGB. One of the initial studies reported 25 patients in which the OverStitch device was utilized to reduce the GJ anastomotic diameter to <12 mm utilizing interrupted sutures (reduced from average of 26.4 mm to 6 mm). In 13/25 patients, sutures were also placed to reduce pouch size. Reported adverse events included nausea and vomiting, esophageal abrasion, bleeding during the procedure, hematemesis, one patient who required dilation of the gastrojejunal outlet, and one patient who had delayed bleeding requiring transfusion. At 12 months, there was a mean weight loss of 10.8 kg [78]. Patel et al. reported a series of 50 patients who underwent outlet reduction utilizing interrupted or a purse string suture technique. All patients achieved a GJ diameter of <10 mm after the procedure, with smaller outlets observed with the purse string suture technique. One year %EWL was 10% [79]. Similar weight loss results are noted in other series, with Gitelis et al. reporting 1 year %EWL of 17.1% in a series of 25 patients [7].

When comparing partial thickness outlet reduction with EndoCinch (59 patients) to full thickness outlet reduction with the OverStitch device (59 patients), mean weight loss and % excess weight loss were greater with full thickness suturing at 1 year of follow-up [63].

A prospective series of 150 patients was recently reported. This is one of the largest studies of endoscopic reduction of gastric outlet for weight regain after RYGB using a suturing platform. As similar to previous studies, argon plasma coagulation was first utilized to denude the mucosa along the entire margin of the gastrojejunostomy. Stoma diameter (and pouch reduction) was then completed utilizing the Overstitch system. Post-procedure, patients were kept on full liquids for 6 weeks. This study reported follow-up at 3 years. On average, stomal diameter was reduced from 24.1 mm to 9 mm. Adverse events included abdominal pain, bleeding, and nausea. Weight loss at 3 years was 9.5 kg, with an average loss of 3.4 BMI points lost. Percent EWL was 25% at 3 months, 28.8% at 6 months, 24.9% at 12 months, 20% at 24 months, and 19.2% at 36 months. No difference was noted in total weight loss (8.6% at 36 months) in patients who underwent plication of the gastric pouch versus those that did not [80].

This platform has also been utilized for attempted closure of GGFs. In a study of 56 patients with gastrointestinal fistulas (29 patients with gastrogastric fistulas), there was immediate technical success, but long-term success rate of closure of GGFs was much lower (approximately 17%) [81].

Conclusion

Treatment of weight regain after successful RYGB requires comprehensive evaluation of all potential contributing factors prior to determining an appropriate treatment strategy. This should include a thorough workup of possible anatomic factors. There are a number of strategies to assist these patients, including pharmacotherapy, surgical and endoscopic options. Endoscopic options appear to be most beneficial in patients with dilated gastrojejunal anastomotic diameter. The approach to endoscopic revision of RYGB has evolved with the improvements in the endoscopic suturing platforms. Full thickness suturing approaches appear to be more effective than partial thickness approaches, and reduction of stoma size to <10–12 mm appears crucial for long-term beneficial results. Overall the data surrounding the efficacy of endoscopic approaches is promising, but limited. Randomized trials and longer term reported outcomes will contribute to the further understanding of these procedures and assist with determination in appropriate patient

selection. Standardized reporting of actual weight loss as well as %EWL and TBWL will help in interpretation of the studies. Treatment plans encompassing surgical as well as nonsurgical treatments (i.e., AODs) are likely to result in increased success. Endoscopic treatments for GGF do not tend to have overall favorable long-term results, especially with fistulas >10 mm.

References

1. Brethauer SA, Aminian A, Romero-Talamas H, Batayyah E, Mackey J, Kennedy L, et al. Can diabetes be surgically cured? Long-term metabolic effects of bariatric surgery in obese patients with type 2 diabetes mellitus. Ann Surg. 2013;258(4):628–36; discussion 636–7.
2. Shah M, Simha V, Garg A. Review: long-term impact of bariatric surgery on body weight, comorbidities, and nutritional status. J Clin Endocrinol Metab. 2006;91(11):4223–31.
3. Brethauer SA, Chand B, Schauer PR. Risks and benefits of bariatric surgery: current evidence. Cleve Clin J Med. 2006;73(11):993–1007.
4. Peterli R, Wölnerhanssen BK, Vetter D, Nett P, Gass M, Borbély Y, et al. Laparoscopic sleeve gastrectomy versus Roux-Y-Gastric bypass for morbid obesity-3-year outcomes of the prospective randomized Swiss Multicenter Bypass or Sleeve Study (SM-BOSS). Ann Surg. 2017;265(3):466–73.
5. Sugerman HJ, Wolfe LG, Sica DA, Clore JN. Diabetes and hypertension in severe obesity and effects of gastric bypass-induced weight loss. Ann Surg. 2003;237(6):751–6; discussion 757–8.
6. Dakin GF, Eid G, Mikami D, Pryor A, Chand B, American Society for Metabolic and Bariatric Surgery (ASMBS) Emerging Technology and Procedures Committee. Endoluminal revision of gastric bypass for weight regain—a systematic review. Surg Obes Relat Dis. 2013;9(3):335–42.
7. Gitelis M, Ujiki M, Farwell L, Linn J, Wang C, Miller K, et al. Six month outcomes in patients experiencing weight gain after gastric bypass who underwent gastrojejunal revision using an endoluminal suturing device. Surg Endosc. 2015;29(8):2133–40.
8. Yimcharoen P, Heneghan HM, Singh M, Brethauer S, Schauer P, Rogula T, et al. Endoscopic findings and outcomes of revisional procedures for patients with weight recidivism after gastric bypass. Surg Endosc. 2011;25(10):3345–52.
9. Nedelcu M, Khwaja HA, Rogula TG. Weight regain after bariatric surgery-how should it be defined? Surg Obes Relat Dis. 2016;12(5):1129–30.
10. Haskins IN, Corcelles R, Froylich D, Boules M, Hag A, Burguera B, et al. Primary inadequate weight loss after Roux-en-Y gastric bypass is not associated

with poor cardiovascular or metabolic outcomes: experience from a single institution. Obes Surg. 2017;27(3):676–80.

11. Lo Menzo E, Szomstein S, Rosenthal RJ. Reoperative bariatric surgery. In: Nguyen NT, Blackstone RP, Morton JM, Ponce J, Rosenthal R, editors. The ASMBS textbook of bariatric surgery, vol. 1. New York: Springer; 2015. p. 269–82.

12. Christou NV, Look D, Maclean LD. Weight gain after short- and long-limb gastric bypass in patients followed for longer than 10 years. Ann Surg. 2006;244(5):734–40.

13. Hatoum IJ, Kaplan LM. Advantages of percent weight loss as a method of reporting weight loss after Roux-en-Y gastric bypass. Obesity (Silver Spring). 2013;21(8):1519–25.

14. Karmali S, Brar B, Shi X, Sharma AM, de Gara C, Birch DW. Weight recidivism post-bariatric surgery: a systematic review. Obes Surg. 2013;23(11):1922–33.

15. Magro DO, Geloneze B, Delfini R, Pareja BC, Callejas F, Pareja JC. Long-term weight regain after gastric bypass: a 5-year prospective study. Obes Surg. 2008;18(6):648–51.

16. Monaco-Ferreira DV, Leandro-Merhi VA. Weight regain 10 years after Roux-en-Y gastric bypass. Obes Surg. 2017;27(5):1137–44.

17. Hsu LK, Benotti PN, Dwyer J, Roberts SB, Saltzman E, Shikora S, Rolls BJ, Rand W. Nonsurgical factors that influence the outcome of bariatric surgery: a review. Psychosom Med. 1998;60(3):338–46.

18. Shantavasinkul PC, Omotosho P, Corsino L, Portenier D, Torquati A. Predictors of weight regain in patients who underwent Roux-en-Y gastric bypass surgery. Surg Obes Relat Dis. 2016;1(9):1640–5.

19. Kushner RF, Sorensen KW. Prevention of weight regain following bariatric surgery. Curr Obes Rep. 2015;4(2):198–206.

20. Maleckas A, Gudaityte R, Petereit R, Venclauskas L, Velickiene D. Weight regain after gastric bypass: etiology and treatment options. Gland Surg. 2016;5(6):617–24.

21. Yen YC, Huang CK, Tai CM. Psychiatric aspects of bariatric surgery. Curr Opin Psychiatry. 2014;27(5):374–9.

22. Rutledge T, Groesz LM, Savu M. Psychiatric factors and weight loss patterns following gastric bypass surgery in a veteran population. Obes Surg. 2011;21(1):29–35.

23. Stanford FC, Alfaris N, Gomez G, Ricks ET, Shukla AP, Corey KE, et al. The utility of weight loss medications after bariatric surgery for weight regain or inadequate weight loss: a multi-center study. Surg Obes Relat Dis. 2017;13(3):491–500.

24. Santo MA, Riccioppo D, Pajecki D, Kawamoto F, de Cleva R, Antonangelo L, et al. Weight regain after gastric bypass: influence of gut hormones. Obes Surg. 2016;26(5):919–25.

25. Roslin M, Damani T, Oren J, Andrews R, Yatco E, Shah P. Abnormal glucose tolerance testing following gastric bypass demonstrates reactive hypoglycemia. Surg Endosc. 2011;25(6):1926–32.

26. Brethauer SA, Nfonsam V, Sherman V, Udomsawaengsup S, Schauer PR, Chand B. Endoscopy and upper gastrointestinal contrast studies are complementary in evaluation of weight regain after bariatric surgery. Surg Obes Relat Dis. 2006;2(6):643–8; discussion 649–50.

27. Heneghan HM, Yimcharoen P, Brethauer SA, Kroh M, Chand B. Influence of pouch and stoma size on weight loss after gastric bypass. Surg Obes Relat Dis. 2012;8(4):408–15.

28. Pauli EM, Beshir H, Mathew A. Gastrogastric fistulae following gastric bypass surgery-clinical recognition and treatment. Curr Gastroenterol Rep. 2014;16(9):405.

29. Daneschvar HL, Aronson MD, Smetana GW. FDA-approved anti-obesity drugs in the United States. Am J Med. 2016;129(8):879.e1–6.

30. Khera R, Murad MH, Chandar AK, Dulai PS, Wang Z, Prokop LJ, et al. Association of pharmacological treatments for obesity with weight loss and adverse events: a systematic review and meta-analysis. JAMA. 2015;315(22):2424–34.

31. Pajecki D, Halpern A, Cercato C, Mancini M, de Cleva R, Santo MA. Short-term use of liraglutide in the management of patients with weight regain after bariatric surgery. Rev Col Bras Cir. 2013;40(3):191–5.

32. Jester L, Wittgrove AC, Clark W. Adjunctive use of appetite suppressant medications for improved weight management in bariatric surgical patients. Obes Surg. 1996;6(5):412–5.

33. Schwartz J, Chaudhry UI, Suzo A, Durkin N, Wehr AM, Foreman KS, et al. Pharmacotherapy in conjunction with a diet and exercise program for the treatment of weight recidivism or weight loss plateau post-bariatric surgery: a retrospective review. Obes Surg. 2016;26(2):452–8.

34. Tran DD, Nwokeabia ID, Purnell S, Zafar SN, Ortega G, Hughes K, Fullum TM. Revision of Roux-en-Y gastric bypass for weight regain: a systematic review of techniques and outcomes. Obes Surg. 2016;26(7):1627–34.

35. Iannelli A, Schneck AS, Hebuterne X, Gugenheim J. Gastric pouch resizing for Roux-en-Y gastric bypass failure in patients with a dilated pouch. Surg Obes Relat Dis. 2013;9(2):260–7.

36. Parikh M, Heacock L, Gagner M. Laparoscopic "gastrojejunal sleeve reduction" as a revision procedure for weight loss failure after roux-en-y gastric bypass. Obes Surg. 2011;21(5):650–4.

37. Al-Bader I, Khoursheed M, Al Sharaf K, Mouzannar DA, Ashraf A, Fingerhut A. Revisional laparoscopic gastric pouch resizing for inadequate weight loss after Roux-en-Y gastric bypass. Obes Surg. 2015;25(7):1103–8.

38. Hamdi A, Julien C, Brown P, Woods I, Hamdi A, Ortega G, Fullum T, Tran D. Midterm outcomes of revisional surgery for gastric pouch and gastrojejunal

anastomotic enlargement in patients with weight regain after gastric bypass for morbid obesity. Obes Surg. 2014;24(8):1386–90.

39. Bessler M, Daud A, DiGiorgi MF, Inabnet WB, Schrope B, Olivero-Rivera L, Davis D. Adjustable gastric banding as revisional bariatric procedure after failed gastric bypass—intermediate results. Surg Obes Relat Dis. 2010;6(1):31–5.

40. Chin PL, Ali M, Francis K, LePort PC. Adjustable gastric band placed around gastric bypass pouch as revision operation for failed gastric bypass. Surg Obes Relat Dis. 2009;5(1):38–42.

41. Vijgen GH, Schouten R, Bouvy ND, Greve JW. Salvage banding for failed Roux-en-Y gastric bypass. Surg Obes Relat Dis. 2012;8(6):803–8.

42. Sugerman HJ, Kellum JM, DeMaria EJ. Conversion of proximal to distal gastric bypass for failed gastric bypass for superobesity. J Gastrointest Surg. 1997;6:517–24; discussion 524–6.

43. Rawlins ML, Teel D 2nd, Hedgcorth K, Maguire JP. Revision of Roux-en-Y gastric bypass to distal bypass for failed weight loss. Surg Obes Relat Dis. 2011;7(1):45–9.

44. Srikanth MS, Oh KH, Fox SR. Revision to malabsorptive Roux-en-Y gastric bypass (MRNYGBP) provides long-term (10 years) durable weight loss in patients with failed anatomically intact gastric restrictive operations: long-term effectiveness of a malabsorptive Roux-en-Y gastric bypass in salvaging patients with poor weight loss or complications following gastroplasty and adjustable gastric bands. Obes Surg. 2011;21(7):825–31.

45. Brolin RE, Cody RP. Adding malabsorption for weight loss failure after gastric bypass. Surg Endosc. 2007;21(11):1924–6.

46. Scopinaro N, Gianetta E, Adami GF, Friedman D, Traverso E, Marinari GM, et al. Biliopancreatic diversion for obesity at eighteen years. Surgery. 1996;119(3):261–8.

47. Parikh M, Pomp A, Gagner M. Laparoscopic conversion of failed gastric bypass to duodenal switch: technical considerations and preliminary outcomes. Surg Obes Relat Dis. 2007;3(6):611–8.

48. Keshishian A, Zahriya K, Hartoonian T, Ayagian C. Duodenal switch is a safe operation for patients who have failed other bariatric operations. Obes Surg. 2004;14(9):1187–92.

49. Jirapinyo P, Dayyeh BK, Thompson CC. Gastrojejunal anastomotic reduction for weight regain in roux-en-y gastric bypass patients: physiological, behavioral, and anatomical effects of endoscopic suturing and sclerotherapy. Surg Obes Relat Dis. 2016;12(10):1810–6.

50. Spaulding L, et al. Obes Surg. 2003;13(2):254–7.

51. Spaulding L, Osler T, Patlak J. Long-term results of sclerotherapy for dilated gastrojejunostomy after gastric bypass. Surg Obes Relat Dis. 2007;3(6):623–6.

52. Catalano MF, Rudic G, Anderson AJ, Chua TY. Weight gain after bariatric surgery as a result of a large gastric stoma: endotherapy with sodium morrhuate may prevent the need for surgical revision. Gastrointest Endosc. 2007;66(2):240–5.

53. Loewen M, Barba C. Endoscopic sclerotherapy for dilated gastrojejunostomy of failed gastric bypass. Surg Obes Relat Dis. 2008;4(4):539–42; discussion 542–3.

54. Abu Dayyeh BK, Jirapinyo P, Weitzner Z, Barker C, Flicker MS, Lautz DB, Thompson CC. Endoscopic sclerotherapy for the treatment of weight regain after Roux-en-Y gastric bypass: outcomes, complications, and predictors of response in 575 procedures. Gastrointest Endosc. 2012;76(2):275–82.

55. Madan AK, Martinez JM, Khan KA, Tichansky DS. Endoscopic sclerotherapy for dilated gastrojejunostomy after gastric bypass. J Laparoendosc Adv Surg Tech A. 2010;20(3):235–7.

56. Giurgius M, Fearing N, Weir A, Micheas L, Ramaswamy A. Long-term follow-up evaluation of endoscopic sclerotherapy for dilated gastrojejunostomy after gastric bypass. Surg Endosc. 2014;28(5):1454–9.

57. Riva P, Perretta S, Swanstrom L. Weight regain following RYGB can be effectively treated using a combination of endoscopic suturing and sclerotherapy. Surg Endosc. 2017;31(4):1891–5.

58. Heylen AM, Jacobs A, Lybeer M, Prosst RL. The OTSC(R)-clip in revisional endoscopy against weight gain after bariatric gastric bypass surgery. Obes Surg. 2011;21(10):1629–33.

59. Niland B, Brock A. Over-the-scope clip for endoscopic closure of gastrogastric fistulae. Surg Obes Relat Dis. 2017;13(1):15–20.

60. Aly A. Argon plasma coagulation and gastric bypass—a novel solution to stomal dilation. Obes Surg. 2009;19(6):788–90.

61. Baretta GA, Alhinho HC, Matias JE, Marchesini JB, de Lima JH, Empinotti C, Campos JM. Argon plasma coagulation of gastrojejunal anastomosis for weight regain after gastric bypass. Obes Surg. 2015;25(1):72–9.

62. Abidi WM, Schulman A, Thompson CC. A large case series on the use of argon plasma coagulation for the treatment of weight regain after gastric bypass (abstract 1137). Gastroenterology. 2016;150(4 Suppl 1):S231.

63. Kumar N, Thompson CC. Comparison of a superficial suturing device with a full-thickness suturing device for transoral outlet reduction (with videos). Gastrointest Endosc. 2014;79(6):984–9.

64. Schweitzer M. Endoscopic intraluminal suture plication of the gastric pouch and stoma in postoperative Roux-en-Y gastric bypass patients. J Laparoendosc Adv Surg Tech A. 2004;14(4):223–6.

65. Thompson CC, Slattery J, Bundga ME, Lautz DB. Peroral endoscopic reduction of dilated gastrojejunal anastomosis after Roux-en-Y gastric bypass: a possible new option for patients with weight regain. Surg Endosc. 2006;20(11):1744–8.

66. Thompson CC, Roslin MS, Chand B, Chen YK, DeMarco DC, Miller LS, et al. Restore: randomized evaluation of endoscopic suturing transorally for anastomotic outlet reduction: a double-blind, sham-controlled multicenter study for treatment of inadequate weight loss or weight regain following

Roux-en-Y gastric bypass (abstract M1359). Gastroenterology. 2010;138(5 Suppl 1):S388.

67. Thompson CC, Chand B, Chen YK, Demarco DC, Miller L, Schweitzer M, et al. Endoscopic suturing for transoral outlet reduction increases weight loss after Roux-en-Y gastric bypass surgery. Gastroenterology. 2013;145(1):129–137.e3.

68. Fernandez-Esparrach G, Lautz DB, Thompson CC. Endoscopic repair of gastrogastric fistula after Roux-en-Y gastric bypass: a less-invasive approach. Surg Obes Relat Dis. 2010;6(3):282–8.

69. Mikami D, Needleman B, Narula V, Durant J, Melvin WS. Natural orifice surgery: initial US experience utilizing the StomaphyX device to reduce gastric pouches after Roux-en-Y gastric bypass. Surg Endosc. 2010;24(1):223–8.

70. Leitman IM, Virk CS, Avgerinos DV, Patel R, Lavarias V, Surick B, et al. Early results of trans-oral endoscopic plication and revision of the gastric pouch and stoma following Roux-en-Y gastric bypass surgery. JSLS. 2010;14(2):217–20.

71. Goyal V, Holover S, Garber S. Gastric pouch reduction using StomaphyX in post Roux-en-Y gastric bypass patients does not result in sustained weight loss: a retrospective analysis. Surg Endosc. 2013;27(9):3417–20.

72. Eid GM, McCloskey CA, Eagleton JK, Lee LB, Courcoulas AP. StomaphyX vs a sham procedure for revisional surgery to reduce regained weight in Roux-en-Y gastric bypass patients: a randomized clinical trial. JAMA Surg. 2014;149(4):372–9.

73. Ryou M, Mullady DK, Lautz DB, Thompson CC. Pilot study evaluating technical feasibility and early outcomes of second-generation endosurgical platform for treatment of weight regain after gastric bypass surgery. Surg Obes Relat Dis. 2009;5(4):450–4.

74. Mullady DK, Lautz DB, Thompson CC. Treatment of weight regain after gastric bypass surgery when using a new endoscopic platform: initial experience and early outcomes (with video). Gastrointest Endosc. 2009;70(3):440–4.

75. Thompson CC, Jacobsen GR, Schroder GL, Horgan S. Stoma size critical to 12-month outcomes in endoscopic suturing for gastric bypass repair. Surg Obes Relat Dis. 2012;8(3):282–7.

76. Raman SR, Holover S, Garber S. Endolumenal revision obesity surgery results in weight loss and closure of gastric-gastric fistula. Surg Obes Relat Dis. 2011;7(3):304–8.

77. Horgan S, Jacobsen G, Weiss GD, Oldham JS Jr, Denk PM, Borao F, et al. Incisionless revision of post-Roux-en-Y bypass stomal and pouch dilation: multicenter registry results. Surg Obes Relat Dis. 2010;6(3):290–5.

78. Jirapinyo P, Slattery J, Ryan MB, Abu Dayyeh BK, Lautz DB, Thompson CC. Evaluation of an endoscopic suturing device for transoral outlet reduction in patients with weight regain following Roux-en-Y gastric bypass. Endoscopy. 2013;45(7):532–6.

79. Patel LY, Lapin B, Brown CS, Stringer T, Gitelis ME, Linn JG, et al. Outcomes following 50 consecutive endoscopic gastrojejunal revisions for weight gain following Roux-en-Y gastric bypass: a comparison of endoscopic suturing techniques for stoma reduction. Surg Endosc. 2016. doi:10.1007/s00464-016-5281-3; [Epub ahead of print].

80. Kumar N, Thompson CC. Transoral outlet reduction for weight regain after gastric bypass: long-term follow-up. Gastrointest Endosc. 2016;83(4):776–9.

81. Mukewar S, Kumar N, Catalano M, Thompson C, Abidi W, Harmsen W, et al. Safety and efficacy of fistula closure by endoscopic suturing: a multi-center study. Endoscopy. 2016;48(11):1023–8.

Comprehensive Endoluminal Treatment of Sleeve Gastrectomy Complications

Manoel Galvao Neto and Natan Zundel

Bariatric endoscopy (BE) is a neologism created to define the interface of advanced therapeutic endoscopy with bariatric surgery (BS). Its interface deals with treating bariatric surgery complications, primary obesity therapy, and revising secondary obesity (postoperative weight loss failure or postoperative weight regain). Primary therapy for obesity and diabetes includes intragastric balloon, endoscopic suturing, duodenal mucosal resurfacing, and aspiration therapy. This chapter will focus on the comprehensive endoluminal treatment of sleeve gastrectomy complications.

The two main complications of sleeve gastrectomy at the reach of endoscopy are treating strictures/stenosis and leaks.

Throughout the world, the prevalence of Laparoscopic Sleeve gastroplasty (LSG) for morbid obesity has increased from 0 to 37% from 2003 to 2013 [1]. It is a widely accepted operation since proving to be safe and effective as a primary weight loss procedure. Furthermore, it seems easier and quicker to perform than other bariatric procedures [2], when comparing it to gastric bypass and duodenal switch. Nevertheless, it has its own set of complications. Bleeding, leaks, and fistula occur between 1 and 20%, and can be life-threatening [3]. Stenosis and mechanical obstructions have been reported to be between 0.7 and 4% of cases [2].

Stenosis

Sleeve gastrectomy stenosis is very peculiar when compared with other postsurgical stenosis. Most cases are sub-stenosis and will allow the endoscope to pass through. However, strictures after a gastric bypass will stop the scope at the gastrojejunostomy (Fig. 13.1). The challenge is to understand the type of "axis deviation," "helical or helix like path," or even a "functional stenosis" (Fig. 13.2). Those terms were not generally used before sleeve gastrectomy but are very useful and help to understand this specific complication. Dysphagia, regurgitation, vomiting, reflux, food intolerance, and rapid weight loss are usual symptoms when this condition occurs. Early strictures appear within the first few weeks and usually are due to gastric tube narrowing and twist. The location is typically at the level of incisura angularis. Obstructions can occur due to a tight bougie calibration during surgery, when stapling is performed too close to the incisura

M.G. Neto, M.D. (✉) • N. Zundel, M.D.
Department of General Surgery, Herbert Wertheim College of Medicine, Florida International University, 17038 West Dixie Hwy #210, Miami, FL 33160, USA
e-mail: galvaon@gmail.com; drnazuma99@yahoo.com

Fig. 13.1 Sleeve functional stenosis with axis deviation as seen in a gastrointestinal series and in computed tomography 3D reconstruction

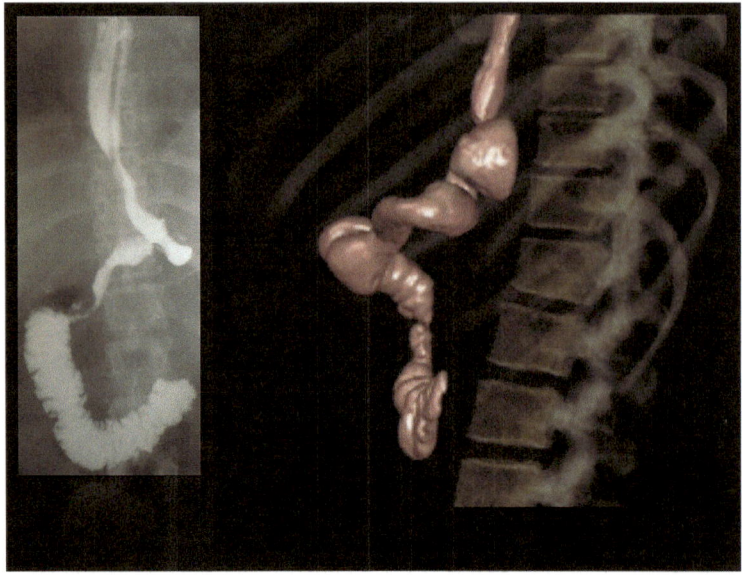

Fig. 13.2 Helical stenosis, which is with a helical twist at incisura level, as well as the presence of a persistently dilated gastric pouch above the kinking, as seen on the endoscopic image and X-ray

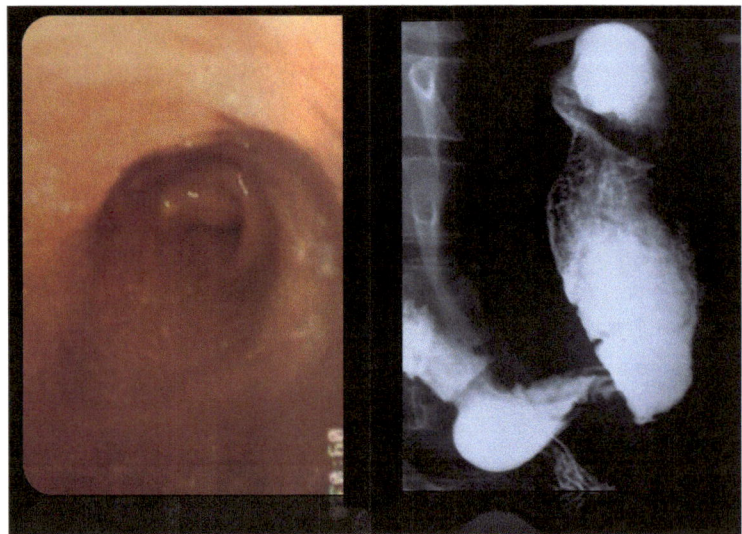

angularis, or even due to a helical staple line configuration [3, 4]. Edema and hematoma are also other causes of acute gastric tube narrowing [5]. On the other hand, late stenosis appears more than 1 month after primary surgery and is mostly functional due to a helix stricture, the so-called "twisted sleeve," defined by a clockwise rotation of the gastric sleeve. This mostly commonly occurs because of asymmetrical traction on the resected greater curve of the stomach and consequent misalignment while stapling [3].

Endoluminal treatment should be the initial approach and can be done with continuous radial expansion through the scope (CRE-TTS) balloons, pneumatic (achalasia) balloon dilation, stents, and possibly septotomy [6–9]. Dilation with CRE-TTS balloon seems to be the least effective. When endoscopy fails, surgical management is an option. Conversion to gastric bypass, seromyotomy, total gastrectomy, and loop gastrojejunostomy have all been described and offer acceptable options that should be considered. Each option depends on the individual patient scenario and the comfort level of the surgeon [10]. Short segment stenosis may respond to CRE-TTS hydrostatic dilation and is a simpler method to pneumatic dilation (Fig. 13.3). Pneumatic dilation is a more complex procedure, generates more pressure and a large diameter, and treats more mechanical obstructions; it also may have more success. Since described by Zundel et al. [6] in 2010, pneumatic dilation has been growing in popularity. Shnell [7] in 2014 described a series of 16 patients with sleeve stenosis based on symptoms and imaging studies. Most of the procedures were done using a 32FR bougie with no imbrication. All patients presented with a mid-sleeve stricture near the incisura and allowed the scope to pass. Three patients were successfully treated with pneumatic dilation, whereas 9 out of 13 (69.2%) failed hydrostatic CRE-TTS 20-mm balloon dilation. Ogra [8] in 2015 described a series of 23 patients with a fixed stenosis at the incisura angularis. Sixteen were

initially treated with dilatation by a CRE-TTS balloon. Seven were successfully dilated, although one needed two sessions. Of 9 (56.2%) failures, 6 were sequentially and successfully treated using a pneumatic 30-mm achalasia balloon and the other 3 required temporary placement of a self-expandable metal stent (SEMS). Seven other patients who presented with strictures at the incisura that were >3 cm long were initially started with pneumatic dilation. Five were successfully dilated and two required temporary placement of a SEMS. None of the 26 patients required a surgical procedure to correct their stenosis. The pneumatic dilation seems to have a therapeutic limitation when facing a functional helix stenosis (twisted sleeve) as described by Donatelli [9] in 2016. The 36 patients with functional helix stenosis in their series were initially pneumatically dilated to 30 mm in a stepwise manner. Thirteen out of thirty-five patients underwent a second dilation up to 35 mm, and eight patients underwent a third pneumatic dilation up to 40 mm. The stricture

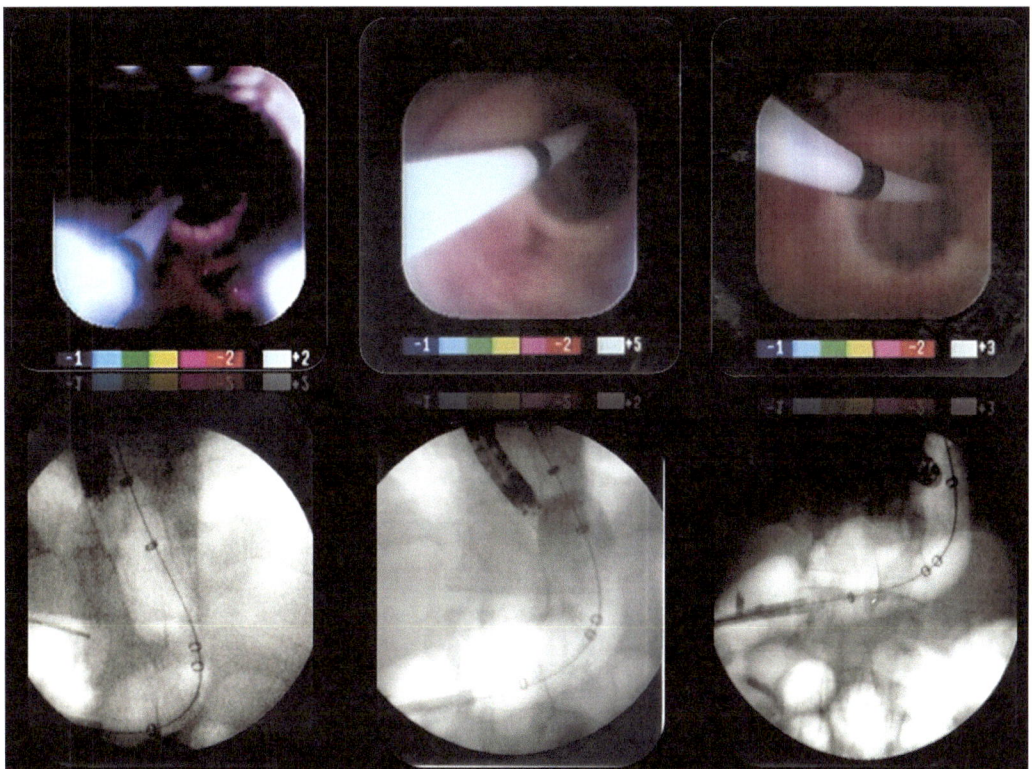

Fig. 13.3 Sequence of pneumatic dilation (*left to right*); (*top*) endoscopic images; (*bottom*) radiologic images

was located in mid-body in 32 patients and three had a narrowing adjacent to the cardia. Eleven twists formed an acute angle between the two segments of the stomach, while 24 angles were obtuse. Seven out of thirty-five patients presented with a persistent dilated pouch above the twist. Two patients were lost to follow-up. Overall results at an average follow-up of 15.5 months after primary surgery (7–49) were as follows: 12 clinical and 1 technical failure (40%), and (20 out of 33) (60%) with clinical success. Two severe complications were described: one perforation with a 30-mm balloon and one gastrointestinal bleed after 35-mm dilation. The authors conclude that pneumatic dilation of late functional helix twist is an effective technique for the majority of patients. A complete helix stricture, defined by the angle of the twist, as well as a persistently dilated gastric pouch above the kink, correlated with higher failure rates. The authors recommended surgical approach for these.

Leaks

Like sleeve stenosis, sleeve leaks also do not behave in the same manner as gastric bypass leaks. The sleeve is a higher-pressure system and leaks may become more chronic, when compared to leaks after gastric bypass. Leaks develop immediately below the angle of His in 90% of patients. This area may have a greater degree of ischemia secondary to less overall blood supply and because of the need to mobilize the short gastric arteries in order to create the sleeve. The usual endoscopic strategy involves early drainage—internal, external, or both, when necessary. Also, early stent placement is advocated. Stents can cover the leak and divert enteral flow, treat the gastric stricture, and decrease intragastric pressure. In LSG, stents also can correct the axis deviation and the helical stenosis as previously described. After initial sepsis control with antibiotics and resuscitation, specific endoscopic and surgical measures are taken. The endoscopic approach may provide decreased morbidity. It involves internal drainage, septotomy, dilations, endoscopic suturing, clips, and in most cases, endoscopic stenting [4, 10–16]. Early

diagnostic endoscopy allows proper evaluation of the leak internal orifice, identifies any strictures, helps in correct positioning of abdominal drains, and allows for internal abscess drainage. Endoscopic therapy can be used together with surgical therapy, especially with early onset leaks. The aims are to solve the three main issues perpetuating the leak: distal gastric stricture, increased intragastric pressure, and fistulous tract persistence. Specifically, in LSG there can be an axis deviation with associated increased intragastric pressure, which will benefit from an early and minimally invasive approach [7].

Among many treatment algorithms, the management may depend on the time of detection and the degree of illness of the patient. Rosenthal in 2012 [4] described several phases and options based on time of index surgery.

- Acute (<7 days): self-expandable metallic stents (SEMS) or pigtail drain
- Early (1–6 weeks): SEMS or pigtail drain followed by pneumatic balloon dilation + septotomy (rare)
- Late (6–12 weeks): septotomy + balloon dilation followed by SEMS (rare)
- Chronic (>12 weeks): septotomy + balloon dilation

In acute and early leaks, SEMS promote occlusion of the leak orifice, correct any pouch axis deviation and distal strictures, and also decrease intragastric pressure, facilitating leak closure [4, 16]. Traditionally, esophageal stents have been used, with a maximum length of 150–160 mm and a diameter of 23 mm. Stents can be either fully covered or partially covered and have both advantages and disadvantages. The totally covered stents have a higher migration rate but are easier to remove, while the partially covered stents migrate less but are more difficult to remove [12].

Recently, the so-called bariatric stents (Fig. 13.4) have been developed with specific designs customized for LSG. They can reach up to 240–280 mm in length with a maximum diameter of 30 mm, with promising initial results [13, 14, 17–20]. Stents should not be left in place for long periods secondary to increased complications,

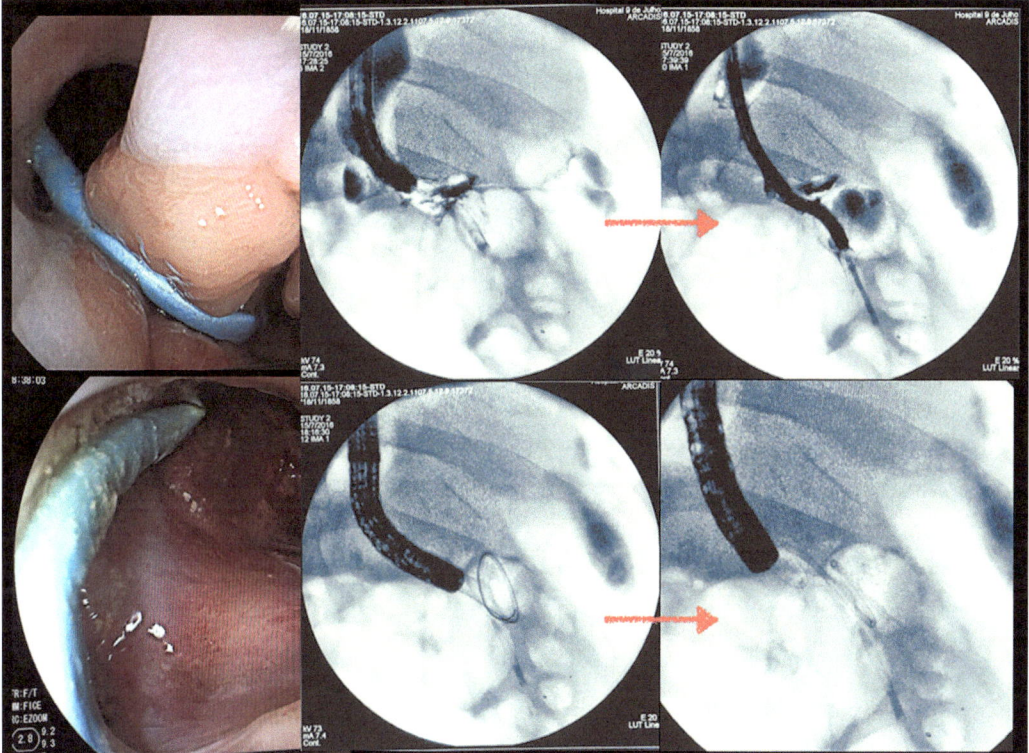

Fig. 13.4 Illustration of bariatric stent covering from the esophagus up to duodenum

Fig. 13.5 Internal drainage with a pigtail; (*left*) endoscopic images; (*right*) a radiologic sequence of the implant

from tissue ingrowth preventing removal to erosion into surrounding structures. Most require a stent surveillance protocol and remain in place for 1–2 months [10]. After initial leak control, even if complete remission is not achieved, endoscopic treatment can proceed with septotomy, stenotomy, and balloon dilations. Also, in early cases with associated perigastric abscess, internal drainage with pigtail drains (Fig. 13.5) has been described with success. This scenario is especially useful in small leaks with a diameter of less than 10 mm. This treatment should be used in conjunction with correction of any form of a distal stenosis [21]. Other endoscopic approaches include use of endoscopic clips such as the over-the-scope clip (OTSC System; Ovesco Endoscopy, Cary, NC, USA), biologic glues, and tissue sealants. Results have been varied [22, 23]. Endoscopic vacuum therapy has also been described for fistula treatment [24, 25].

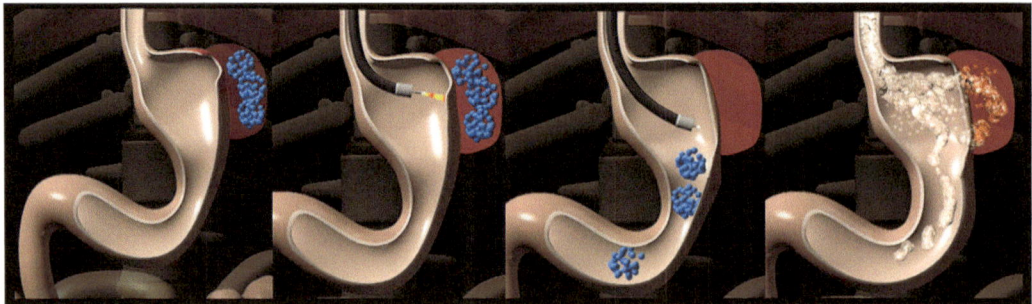

Fig. 13.6 Illustration of septotomy sequence

For late and chronic leaks, the literature is limited. Endoscopic treatment usually requires multiple sessions, employing all the above described techniques (multimodality). Septotomy (Fig. 13.6) can be performed when there is a septum between the gastric wall and adjacent fistulous orifice and associated abscess [26, 27]. Septotomy can be performed either with a needle knife or argon plasma coagulation (which may be associated with less bleeding), followed by gastric dilation. The goal is to allow digestive contents to flow back into the gastric lumen instead of staying in the abscess cavity. Stenotomy is performed with balloon dilation and can be performed when there is stenosis and fibrotic tissue. In LSG leaks, a 30-mm achalasia balloon is often used to correct this functional and anatomical deviation. More than one session is often required and can in many instances be done in an outpatient setting. The opening of the abscess to allow better internal drainage will eventually lead to leak closure [4]. Stents can be used in selected cases of late and chronic leaks, mainly when there are anatomical defects.

Gastrobronchial Fistula

In chronic cases, the leak can be associated with a subphrenic abscess, which may eventually lead to a pulmonary abscess and gastrobronchial fistula (GBF) formation. This complication has a high morbidity, especially if thoracic surgery is required. Endoscopic management can be an option in select cases; however, total gastrectomy may be required with separation of the fistula tract with the chest cavity [11].

GBF is usually related to a simple gastric leak that was not properly treated and eventually became a chronic tract. The most common symptoms of GBF are productive cough, fever, thoracic pain, recurrent pneumonia, vomiting, wheezing, hypoxemia, abdominal pain, and expectoration of food residues [11].

Diagnosis is usually late, made by computed tomography or contrast X-ray. Endoscopy is useful in identifying the internal orifice, in evaluating the gastric anatomy, and possibly in performing fistula treatment. Major abdominal and thoracic surgery are associated with greater morbidity, and in many cases may not promote complete remission [10, 11].

Endoscopic treatment aims to increase intragastric diameter, decrease pressure, and reduce the amount of fluids passing through the leak. It can be done through stent placement, septotomy, stenotomy, and balloon dilation as described previously [11]. Surgical treatment described in the literature involves total gastrectomy, splenectomy, pancreatectomy, and lung resection with the potential of significant morbidity [12].

References

1. Angrisani L, Santonicola A, Iovino P, Formisano G, Buchwald H, Scopinaro N. Bariatric surgery worldwide 2013. Obes Surg. 2015;25(10):1822–32.
2. Zellmer JD, Mathiason MA, Kallies KJ, Kothari SN. Is laparoscopic sleeve gastrectomy a lower risk bariatric procedure compared with laparoscopic

Roux-en-Y gastric bypass? A meta-analysis. Am J Surg. 2014;208(6):903–10; discussion 909–10.

3. Villalonga R, Himpens J, Van de Vrande S. Laparoscopic management of persistent stricture after laparoscopic sleeve gastrectomy. Obes Surg. 2013;23(10):1655–61.

4. Rosenthal RJ, International Sleeve Gastrectomy Expert Panel, Diaz AA, Arvidsson D, Baker RS, Basso N, et al. International sleeve Gastrectomy expert panel consensus statement: best practice guidelines based on experience of >12,000 cases. Surg Obes Relat Dis. 2012;8(1):8–19.

5. Burgos AM, Csendes A, Braghetto I. Gastric stenosis after laparoscopic sleeve gastrectomy in morbidly obese patients. Obes Surg. 2013;23(9):1481–6.

6. Shnell M, Fishman S, Eldar S, Goitein D, Santo E. Balloon dilatation for symptomatic gastric sleeve stricture. Gastrointest Endosc. 2014;79(3):521–4.

7. Zundel N, Hernandez JD, Galvao Neto M, Campos J. Strictures after laparoscopic sleeve gastrectomy. Surg Laparosc Endosc Percutan Tech. 2010;20(3):154–8.

8. Ogra R, Kini GP. Evolving endoscopic management options for symptomatic stenosis post-laparoscopic sleeve gastrectomy for morbid obesity: experience at a large bariatric surgery unit in New Zealand. Obes Surg. 2015;25(2):242–8.

9. Donatelli G, Dumont JL, Pourcher G, Tranchart H, Tuszynski T, Dagher I, et al. Pneumatic dilation for functional helix stenosis followings sleeve gastrectomy: long-term follow-up (with videos). Surg Obes Relat Dis. 2016;13(6):943–50. doi:10.1016/j.soard.2016.09.023.

10. Campos JM, Pereira EF, Evangelista LF, Siqueira L, Neto MG, Dib V, et al. Gastrobronchial fistula after sleeve gastrectomy and gastric bypass: endoscopic management and prevention. Obes Surg. 2011;21(10):1520–9.

11. Silva LB, Moon RC, Teixeira AF, Jawad MA, Ferraz ÁA, Neto MG, et al. Gastrobronchial fistula in sleeve gastrectomy and Roux-en-Y gastric bypass: a systematic review. Obes Surg. 2015;25(10):1959–65.

12. Puli SR, Spofford IS, Thompson CC. Use of self-expandable stents in the treatment of bariatric surgery leaks: a systematic review and meta-analysis. Gastrointest Endosc. 2012;75(2):287–93.

13. Basha J, Appasani S, Sinha SK, et al. Mega stents: a new option for management of leaks following laparoscopic sleeve gastrectomy. Endoscopy. 2014;46(Suppl 1):E49–50.

14. Shehab HM, Hakky SM, Gawdat KA. An endoscopic strategy combining mega stents and over-the-scope clips for the management of post-bariatric surgery leaks and fistulas (with video). Obes Surg. 2016;26(5):941–8.

15. Fischer A, Bausch D, Richter-Schrag HJ. Use of a specially designed partially covered self-expandable metal stent (PSEMS) with a 40-mm diameter for the treatment of upper gastrointestinal suture or staple line leaks in 11 cases. Surg Endosc. 2013;27(2):642–7.

16. Nedelcu M, Manos T, Cotirlet A, Noel P, Gagner M. Outcome of leaks after sleeve gastrectomy based on a new algorithm addressing leak size and gastric stenosis. Obes Surg. 2015;25(3):559–63.

17. Van Wezenbeek MR, de Milliano MM, Nienhuijs SW, Friederich P, Gillissen LP. A specifically designed stent for anastomotic leaks after bariatric surgery: experiences in a tertiary referral hospital. Obes Surg. 2016;26(8):1875–80.

18. Fishman MB, Sedov VM, Lantsberg L, et al. Vestn Khir Im I I Grek. 2008;167(1):29–32. (Article in Russian).

19. Galloro G, Magno L, Musella M, Manta R, Zullo A, Forestieri P. A novel dedicated endoscopic stent for staple-line leaks after laparoscopic sleeve gastrectomy: a case series. Surg Obes Relat Dis. 2014;10(4):607–11.

20. Galvao Neto M, Silva L, Quadros LG, de Souza G, MD RA, Ferraz AB, Campos J. Sleeve gastrectomy leak: endoscopic management through customized bariatric stent (A5028). Surg Obes Relat Dis. 2016;27(7 Suppl):S74–5.

21. Pequignot A, Fuks D, Verhaeghe P, Dhahri A, Brehant O, Bartoli E, et al. Is there a place for pigtail drains in the management of gastric leaks after laparoscopic sleeve gastrectomy? Obes Surg. 2012;22(5):712–20.

22. Caballero Y, López-Tomassetti E, Castellot A, Hernández JR. Endoscopic management of a gastric leak after laparoscopic sleeve gastrectomy using the over-the-scope-clip (Ovesco) system. Rev Esp Enferm Dig. 2016;108(11):746–50.

23. Keren D, Eyal O, Sroka G, Rainis T, Raziel A, Sakran N, et al. Over-the-scope clip (OTSC) system for sleeve gastrectomy leaks. Obes Surg. 2015;25(8):1358–63.

24. Seyfried F, Reimer S, Miras AD, Kenn W, Germer CT, Scheurlen M, Jurowich C. Successful treatment of a gastric leak after bariatric surgery using endoluminal vacuum therapy. Endoscopy. 2013;45(Suppl 2):E267–8.

25. Hwang JJ, Jeong YS, Park YS, Yoon H, Shin CM, Kim N, Lee DH. Comparison of endoscopic vacuum therapy and endoscopic stent implantation with self-expandable metal stent in treating postsurgical gastroesophageal leakage. Medicine (Baltimore). 2016;95(16):e3416.

26. Campos JM, Ferreira FC, Teixeira AF, Lima JS, Moon RC, D'Assunção MA, Neto MG. Septotomy and balloon dilation to treat chronic leak after sleeve gastrectomy: technical principles. Obes Surg. 2016;26(8):1992–3.

27. Mahadev S, Kumbhari V, Campos JM, Galvao Neto M, Khashab MA, Chavez YH, et al. Endoscopic septotomy: an effective approach for internal drainage of sleeve gastrectomy-associated collections. Endoscopy. 2017;49(5):504–8.

Hung P. Truong and Dean J. Mikami

Introduction

Obesity is a serious public health problem associated with increased morbidity and mortality and decreased quality of life. According to the World Health Organization in 2014, over 1.9 billion adults are overweight and 600 million are obese [1]. The prevalence of obesity has increased so rapidly over the last few decades that it is now considered a global epidemic, nicknamed "Globesity." As the obesity epidemic rapidly grows, national and global healthcare systems will have to absorb significant costs of managing comorbidities that follow, such as coronary artery disease, peripheral vascular disease, diabetes, nonalcoholic steatohepatosis, cirrhosis, pulmonary hypertension, obstructive sleep apnea, and hypercoagulability [2]. The estimated annual medical cost of obesity in the United States was $147 billion in 2008 according to the National Health and Nutrition Examination Surveys conducted by the Center for Disease Control.

The prevalence of obesity had more than doubled from 13.4% in 1960–1962 to 35.1% in 2005–2006 for adults aged 20–74 years [3],

and obesity rates have plateaued in recent years [4–6]. During those years between 2011 and 2014, obesity among US adults was 36.5%. However, when Ogden et al. [5] compared the distribution of BMI between 1976–1980 and 2005–2006, they observed that, among adults, the distribution of BMI shifted to the right, reflecting the change in prevalence of super-obesity (i.e., BMI $\geq 50 \text{ kg/m}^2$), which increased from 0.9% in 1960–1962 to 6.2% in 2005–2006 among adults.

Studies have indicated that obesity is responsible for more than 2.5 million deaths worldwide per year due to the underlying healthcare issues related to obesity. These comorbidities include type 2 diabetes, hyperlipidemia, hypertension, obstructive sleep apnea, heart disease, stroke, asthma, back and lower extremity weight-bearing degenerative problems, several forms of cancer, and depression [7–9]. Additionally, obesity is an independent risk factor for mortality. Currently, complications related to obese and overweight patients are one of the five leading global risks for mortality in the world along with high blood pressure, tobacco use, high blood glucose, and physical inactivity [10]. Previously, Fontaine et al. [11] demonstrated that compared with a normal weight individual, a 25-year-old morbidly obese man had a 22% reduction in life expectancy, representing approximately 12 years of life lost (YLL). Furthermore, a more recent study by Finkelstein et al. showed that in aggregate, excess BMI is responsible for approximately 95 million years of

H.P. Truong, M.D. • D.J. Mikami, M.D. (✉)
Department of Surgery, The Queen's Medical Center, University of Hawaii John A. Burns School of Medicine, 1356 Lusitania Street, 6th Floor, Honolulu, HI 96813, USA
e-mail: hptruong@hawaii.edu; dmikami2@hawaii.edu

lives lost [12]. A large prospective cohort study published in NEJM examined 10-year mortality rates in more than 500,000 Americans ages 50–71 years old, showed that middle-aged men and women who were nonsmokers and had no pre-existing illnesses had a 20–40% increased mortality in those who were overweight (i.e., BMI 25–30 kg/m^2) and a two- to threefold increased risk of mortality in individuals who were obese (BMI $\geq$ 30 kg/m^2) [13].

The frequency of weight lost and weight maintenance is very common practice in the United States [14]. More so, a recent systematic review and meta-analysis show that 42% of adults from the general population reported trying to lose weight [15]. However, it is well known that medical management of weight loss with diet modifications and pharmaceutical agents is ineffective in the long-term obesity treatment of obesity [16].

Current guidelines for the surgical management of morbid obesity is a BMI $\geq$ 40 kg/m^2 or BMI > 35 kg/m^2 in the presence of significant comorbidities (1991 National institutes of Health (NIH) consensus conference). This criteria was also supported by the American Society for Bariatric Surgery in 2004 [17–19]. The number of bariatric surgical procedures continues to dramatically increase from 20,000 procedures performed in 1999 to 144,000 obese individuals receiving surgical treatment in 2004, with current estimates by the American society for metabolic and bariatric surgery (ASMBS) of a total of 196,000 bariatric procedures in 2015 [20]. This dramatic increase in volume has been attributed to refinements in minimally invasive surgical techniques and better outcomes, an increase in media coverage, and an improvement of patient satisfaction. In 2004, Buchwald et al. systematic review and meta-analysis published in JAMA described bariatric surgery as the only effective long-term weight loss therapy for obese patients [21]. Subsequently, Colquitt et al. in a 2009 Cochrane review also concluded that surgery results in greater improvement in weight loss outcomes and obesity-associated comorbidities compared to nonsurgical methods [22].

Although current healthcare trends continue to focus on preventative measures, data continues to show that conservative management modalities such as diet and exercises have limited efficacy in treating obesity. As a result, bariatric surgery now plays a significant role in the treatment of obesity. Such bariatric surgical procedures can be categorized into restrictive, malabsorptive, or a combination of both. The restrictive category includes adjustable gastric banding, vertical banded gastroplasty, and sleeve gastrectomy. Whereas the malabsorptive category includes such procedure as the biliopancreatic diversion with/without duodenal switch and the combination of both which includes the well-known Roux-en-Y gastric bypass. Of the various procedures, Roux-en-Y gastric bypass (RNYGB) and now the gastric sleeve are the most commonly performed procedures [22]. The RNYGB is reportedly the most successful of these surgical treatments and has achieved 70% excess weight loss and maintenance at 1-year follow-up. Although these are promising outcomes, the reported estimates of "failure" RNYGB are up to 15–20% of patients (defined as either less than 50% estimated excess weight loss after a year or weight gain of more than 10% nadir) [23]. Furthermore, RNYGB follows with a set of known complications some of which include bleeding, wound infection, anastomotic leak, fistulas, internal and incisional hernias, and even deaths, with mortality rates of 0.28% (95% CI: 0.22–0.34) and 0.35% (95% CI: 0.12–0.58) at $\leq$30 day and >30 day, respectively [24].

Within the last 10 years, transoral techniques for preoperative, primary or stand-alone, and revisional bariatric procedures continue to be of emerging interest as the increasing demands for less invasive surgical weight loss modalities and the continuing advancements in surgical instruments and techniques continue to rise [25].

Endoscopic transoral procedures performed exclusively through the gastrointestinal (GI) tract with a flexible endoscope provide the possibility of ambulatory weight loss treatment with less invasiveness. Providing a more cost-effective approach, when compared to laparoscopic surgery, may also allow treatment for previous individuals who were precluded from surgery due to multiple comorbidities, older age, super-obesity (BMI $\geq$ 50 kg/m²), atypical anatomy, adhesions from previous abdominal surgery, and/or inflammatory bowel disease such as Crohn's disease. This chapter aims to review previous, current, and future available transoral techniques with a focus on those in human trials.

Transoral Devices Used as Primary Procedures

Primary transoral procedures can be divided similarly to laparoscopic approaches into restrictive, malabsorptive, and combination. The endoscopic restrictive devices include intragastric balloons, endoluminal suturing, endoluminal stapling, transoral restrictive implant system, aspiration therapy, and transpyloric shuttle. These devices are made to mimic restrictive laparoscopic procedures such as adjustable gastric banding, vertical banded gastroplasty, and sleeve gastrectomy. For malabsorptive transoral procedures, the duodenal-jejunal bypass sleeve is a device that mimics the biliopancreatic diversion with/without a duodenal switch or the RNYGB. The device may induce weight loss by bypassing the initial absorptive surfaces of the intestine or having an incretin affect.

Intragastric Balloon

One of the earliest endoscopic transoral restrictive devices was the intragastric balloon. Initially introduced in 1982, early generations of the intragastric balloons (i.e., Garren-Edwards, Ballobes, Taylor, and Wilson-Cook balloons, De Castrol, etc.) were abandoned due to significant complications, including premature balloon deflation, and failure to achieve meaningful weight loss. These balloons were riddled with issues such as low volume capacity and nondurable materials. Furthermore, serious complications such as erosion into gastric mucosa and gastric outlet syndrome resulted in less than desirable safety profiles. Since then, the intragastric balloon has gone through multiple revisions. Most notably, the BioEnteric intragastric balloon (BIB, Inamed,

Santa Barbara, CA, USA), developed in 1987, addressed previous major issues [26]. Today, there are currently several commercially available balloons such as MedSil, the Heliosphere Bag, Obalon system, and the Gastric Balloon. The BIB, however, remains the most widely researched procedure and was recently FDA approved for use in the United States and renamed as the Orbera system.

The Orbera balloon is a small, flexible balloon introduced in the collapsed state and expands into a spherical shape 10 cm in diameter when filled with 500 mL of saline solution. Volume adjustments range between 400 and 700 mL. The Orbera balloon shell is made of an inert, nontoxic silicone elastomer that is resistant to gastric acid and has a radiopaque self-sealing valve. Procedurally, they are endoscopically placed under conscious sedations or general anesthesia after a diagnostic endoscopy is performed to rule out any abnormalities that would preclude device placement [27]. The device assembly consists of the collapsed balloon attached to a balloon fill tube which is encased within a sheath. This assembly is introduced into the gastric fundus. A syringe is then used to fill the balloon under direct endoscopic visualization with 400–700 mL of saline solution. After the desired amount is achieved, gentle negative pressure exerted by withdrawing the plunger of the syringe seals the valve. The balloon is released by a quick pull on the fill tube which is then removed. The position of the free-floating balloon can then be confirmed radiographically (Fig. 14.1) [26]. Finally, removal of the Orbera balloon consists of removing as much fluid as possible before grasping the balloon with a snare or forceps. Both the endoscope and the grasped balloon are then gently removed. The Orbera balloon system is FDA approved to remain in the stomach for up to 6 months. The procedure is usually considered as outpatient with occasional overnight stay. Most common morbidities consist of nausea and vomiting and in some severe cases may require early removal due to premature deflation, gastric ulceration, and erosion [26]. Most patients are sent home with a proton pump inhibitor to help reduce and prevent reflux symptoms.

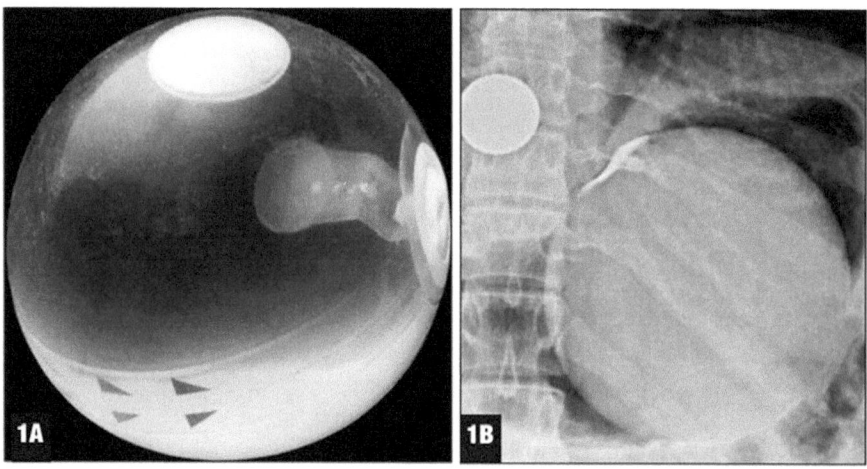

Fig. 14.1 (**a**, **b**) BioEnteric intragastric balloon (BIB), which is smooth and spherical (Inamed, Santa Barbara, CA, USA) (From Malthus-Vliegen et al. [26], with permission)

Intragastric balloons remain popular as a primary endoscopic transoral device because of its safety profile and ease of placement. Unlike laparoscopic procedures, intragastric balloon placement can occur as many times as needed which may be a better option in obese patients who are not surgical candidates. Although the mortality rate following intragastric balloon placement is less than 1%, the procedure still has its own set of complications [28].

According to Genco et al. study in 2005 on the BIB, proper positioning was achieved in all but two cases (0.08%) with associated overall complication rate of 2.8% (70/2515 patients). Of the noted five patients who had gastric perforation, four had previous gastric surgery. Balloon intolerance requiring balloon removal was the most common issue within the first week of insertion with 19 reported cases (0.76%). Balloon rupturing occurred in nine cases (0.36%). Esophagitis and gastric ulcers were seen in 32 patients (1.27%) and five patients (0.2%), respectively, which were both treated with medical therapy.

Furthermore, de Castro et al. reported that approximately half of the patients in their study had nausea and vomiting. Epigastric pain, nausea, and reflux symptoms were the next most common side effects which is why proton pump inhibitors are routinely prescribed. Also, de Castro's group had 13% of patients who required earlier removal secondary due to persistent nau-

sea and vomiting. Two patients developed gastrointestinal bleeding requiring balloon removal [27]. Interestingly, Alfredo et al. noted that nausea, vomiting, and epigastric pain were noticeably worst and lasted longer, approximately 4 days post second balloon insertion versus 2.5 days after the initial procedure.

On the contrary, air-filled balloons, such as the Heliosphere system, have a more tolerating profile as there is reduction in post-procedure nausea and emesis. A common complication with the Heliosphere balloons, however, was spontaneous deflation which resulted in complex retrieval methods ranging from uses of endoscopic forceps or snares to laparoscopic procedures [27]. Drozdowski et al. reported a case in which a deflated Heliosphere system eroded into the small intestine [29]. His group concluded that the balloon had likely deflated 3–4 days prior to the patient's presentation and was difficult to diagnose resulting in a delay.

When de Castro et al. compared the BIB versus the Heliosphere system, both had similar efficacies but as expected the Heliosphere system had a slightly higher incidence of balloon migration requiring laparoscopic or endoscopic retrieval. However, de Castro concluded that the higher risk of balloon migration favored the BIB, despite the higher post-procedural nausea and vomiting.

Intragastric balloons are commonly described as space occupying devices that result in weight loss and hormonal changes. Leptin is believed to be a pro-inflammatory and hypercoagulable molecule made by adipocytes. It is also believed to be associated with increasing cardiovascular risk in patients with obesity. As a result, post-bariatric surgery procedures target not only weight loss but also specifically decreasing body fat composition and leptin production. In a recent 2014 article, Buzga et al. reported a statistically significant increase in ghrelin and decreased levels of leptin at 1, 3, and 6 month intervals after placement of the MedSil intragastric balloon which correlates with previous studies [30]. It is also believed that the balloon induces a stretch response causing increased levels of CCK resulting in delayed gastric emptying and subsequently early satiety and weight loss.

Compared to medical management with diet and exercise, intragastric balloon devices offer a more effective treatment option. In 2006, a double-blinded, crossover study by Genco et al. showed statistically significant weight reduction over conservative management with only strict dietary and exercise regimens. The same group also conducted the most comprehensive retrospective analysis to assess the efficacy of the BIB in terms of weight loss and improvement in obesity-related comorbidities [2]. From 2002–2004, 2515 patients underwent endoscopic placement of the BIB with a mean BMI of 44.8 ± 7.8 kg/m^2. At 6-month follow-up, the percentage excess weight loss (%EWL) was 33.99 ± 18.7. Improvement in obesity-related comorbidities was seen with improvement or resolution of diabetes and hypertension in 86.9% and 93.7% patient, respectively. The same group also conducted a randomized, sham-controlled, crossover study of 32 patients that further supported previous studies [31].

Like other surgical weight loss procedures, long-term weight loss for intragastric balloons remains a concern. De Castro et al. prospective cohort analysis of 91 patients with intragastric balloon showed over 70% of patients showed significant weight loss compared to pre-procedure weight at time of device removal but poor weight

maintenance at 6- and 12-month follow-up post retrieval. The group's conclusion was that although the devices successfully provided effective initial weight loss, its effectiveness is only temporizing in nature [27]. Because of its temporary weight loss profile, some suggested repeated balloon placement to provide maximal long-term effectiveness. As a result, Alfredo et al. conducted a 6-year prospective study during which patients who gained more than 50% of their previous weight loss after the first balloon placement were automatically considered for another placement. In this study, all patients had at least 2 intragastric balloon placements with a considerable number of patients receiving 3 and up to 4 procedures. During this study, patients were able to maintain relatively consistent weight loss profile but there was weight gain seen between placements [32].

Conclusively, studies demonstrate that systems such as the BIB and Heliosphere in conjunction with the appropriate diet are a relatively safe, effective *short*-term weight loss procedures in patients without any previous gastric surgery. Furthermore, with long-term results showing these balloons are only temporalizing weight loss devices, its role of being a bridge to more definitive bariatric interventions has been proposed. Currently, the Orbera, Reshape, and Obalon intragastric balloons are approved for use in the United States [33].

TransPyloric Shuttle

The TransPyloric Shuttle (TPS$^®$) (BAROnova, Goleta, CA, USA) is a novel nonsurgical device that is delivered endoscopically into the stomach. According to Marinos et al., the transpyloric shuttle has a functional shape consistent of a large spherical bulb attached to a smaller cylindrical bulb by a flexible tether with consists of medical grade silicone. The primary function of the device is intended to create intermittent seals along the pylorus to reduce the rate of gastric outflow. This is achieved when the smaller bulb passes freely into the duodenum with peristalsis, self-orienting the larger bulb to assume its proper position. A prospective, open-label, non-randomized, single center study was conducted in 20 patients to evaluate the safety and efficacy of the procedure and device. Mean BMI was 36.0 kg with primary outcomes measuring % of EWL. Marinos et al. reported all 20 patients underwent successful deployment and retrieval of the device without immediate complications. Mean procedure times for delivery and retrieval was 10 min and 13 min, respectively. At 3 and 6 months, mean %EWL was 31.3% ± 15.7% and 50.0% ± 26.4% [34]. Complications included gastric ulceration requiring removal of device with subsequent resolution in some patients.

The initial studies of the transpyloric shuttle show it to be a safe and a reliable nonsurgical method to weight loss. It is still, however, undergoing appropriate trials. Further studies will be needed to see the feasibility and associated improvement in comorbidities.

Endoluminal Suturing

Bard EndoCinch. The Bard EndoCinch Suturing System (C.R. Bard, Murray Hill NJ, USA) was the first endoscopic suturing device used in the treatment of obesity. It was initially created for treating gastroesophageal reflux disease, but due to lack of durability, its role in control of gastroesophageal reflux disease (GERD) was abandoned [35–37]. As a result, its focus was transitioned to creating endoluminal vertical gastroplasty (EVG) for primary intervention of morbid obesity.

Initial studies for applications of treatment of obesity were described by Fogel et al. [38] which used the EndoCinch system in 64 patients. The primary objectives were to determine safety and feasibility of the EVG with secondary goals of assessment of weight loss efficacy.

Using the EndoCinch device to create a vertical gastroplasty, the authors placed one continuous polypropylene suture through 5–7 full-thickness plications in a cross-linked fashion from the proximal fundus to distal body [38]. The system is described as a metal capsule that is placed on the end of a diagnostic endoscope to deploy the continuous suture. Suction is applied

to the gastric wall by the endoscope. This allows the gastric wall to be suctioned into the chamber of the device. Fogel et al. describes placing the first stitch in the nearest fold on the anterior face of the gastric fundus at approximately 40–43 cm from the mouth. The second purchase is then applied as far down on the anterior most distal rugae, proximal to the antrum and about 10–13 cm from the first stitch. This is approximately 53 cm from the mouth. Subsequently suture placement is about 1–2 cm proximal to the second stitch in an alternating fashion between the posterior and anterior surface of the stomach. The pattern continues in a proximal fashion until the last stitch is about 1–2 cm proximal to the initial stitch [38]. The vertical gastroplasty is created by tightening of the suture, which brings the two faces of the stomach together. During the 1-year study in 64 patients, Fogel et al. [38] had a mean procedure time of 45 min with postprocedure recovery time ranging between 1 and 2 h. All 64 patients were discharged on the same day without any serious adverse events. Common complications consisted of nausea and reflux-like symptoms that resolved within 24 h.

Follow-up at 1 year was in 59 of 64 patients. Likewise, data outcomes with weight loss showed significant reduction in BMI at 12 months with a mean BMI of 30.6 ± 4.7 kg/m^2 compared to a baseline of 39.9 ± 5.1 kg/m^2; $P < 0.001$. The average %EWL were 21.1 ± 6.2, 39.6 ± 11.3, and 58.1 ± 19.9 at 1, 3, and 12 months, respectively, with greater %EWL in lower BMI patients [38]. Repeat endoscopy was performed randomly in 14 of 64 patients after plateauing weight loss or return of sensation of feeling hungry. Eleven patients had intact gastroplasty with three having disrupted sutures requiring repeat procedure.

Brethauer et al. also conducted a pilot study called TRIM (transoral gastric volume reduction) with 18 patients showing 12-month %EWL of 27.7 ± 21.9. Their average procedure time was 125 ± 23 min without again any serious procedure-related complications. Patients experienced mild nausea, vomiting, and abdominal discomfort. However, all patients in this trial underwent an upper endoscopy at 12 months showing loss of plications in 72% (13 patients) [39].

Long-term durability and reproducing ability of the Endocinch plication continued to be of concern for this procedure and led to its removal from the market. However, the technique and concept paved the way to subsequent more robust devices.

Apollo OverStitch. OverStitch (Apollo Endosurgery, Austin TX, USA) is a very promising full-thickness endoscopic suturing device that can apply interrupted and running sutures with real-time suture reloading. This device can be used for numerous other applications such as stent fixation and endoscopic perforation repair [40–42]. The Overstitch device comprises an endoscopic needle driver attached to the tip of a double lumen endoscope. An actuating handle is attached to the endoscope handle and a catheter is introduced through one channel of the endoscope functioning as a suture anchor. A tissue helix is inserted into the other lumen to allow tissue acquisition [40]. Kumar et al. performed an international procedure development trial with the first five patients completed in India as a pilot study and 23 other patients in Panama and Dominican Republic to determine the efficacy and feasibility of the technique [43]. This technique consists of using the OverStitch to perform running sutures in a triangular fashion with approximately 6 stitches each from the anterior gastric wall to the greater curvature and to the posterior wall. Placement starts from the antrum and migrates proximally to the fundus.

Sharaiha et al. conducted a series of 10 patients with mean BMI of 45.2 showing excess weight loss of 18, 26, and 30% at 1, 3, and 6 months, respectively [44]. Furthermore, Abu Dayyeh et al. conducted a prospective study with 25 patients with a mean BMI of 38.5 ± 4.6 with $53\% \pm 17\%$, $56\% \pm 23\%$, $54\% \pm 40\%$, and $45\% \pm 41\%$ of excess body weight at 6, 9, 12, and 20 months, respectively ($P < 0.05$) [45]. In this study, patients showed a decrease in 59% of caloric consumption and slowing gastric emptying of solids. Of note, 3 patients had serious adverse events including a perigastric inflammatory collection, pulmonary embolism, and small pneumothorax. The authors contribute these secondary to the initial technique and with further refinements have had no further serious adverse events.

Furthermore, López-Nava et al. also completed a single center, prospective study in 25 patients with 1-year follow-up. Mean % total body weight loss at 1 year was 18.7 ± 10.7 [46]. Mean procedure time was 80 min with all patients undergoing successful gastroplasty with no associated major adverse events.

Kumar et al. also conducted an international multicenter trial consisting of 126 patients with a decrease in BMI of 30.9–29.8 at 6 months to 1 year. Also, overall weight changed from a baseline of 101.6 ± 2.3 kg to 86.9 ± 3.3 kg at 6 months and subsequently to 81.8 ± 3.8 at 1 year.

The OverStitch device appears to be a feasible system with multiple uses and can possibly offer a primary treatment for morbid obesity. Further studies regarding long-term weight loss with improvement in comorbidities are currently ongoing.

Endoluminal Stapling

The Transoral Gastroplasty System (TOGa, Satiety, Palo Alto, CA, USA) was the first endoscopic stapling device used to create a gastric sleeve with full-thickness plications along the lesser curve of the stomach [47]. The TOGa stapling device is a flexible 18-cm stapler that is passed over a guide wire after upper endoscopy and placement of a 60 Fr dilating bougie. Once the stapling device is introduced, the guide wire is removed and a 8.6 endoscope is introduced through the device channel, advanced into the stomach, and retroflexed for direct visualization of the stapling procedure. Once device is laid along the lesser curvature in the proper position, a retraction wire is deployed to spread and orient the stomach allowing capture of the tissue within the device. Suction is used to acquire the two walls of the stomach into the two vacuum pods of the stapler. The stapler is closed and fired creating full-thickness staple lines with three rows of 11 titanium staples. This process is repeated to achieve a sleeve approximately 8–9 cm in length parallel to the lesser curvature. A TOGa restrictor is used, a single-suction-pod stapler that creates pleats of tissue, to narrow the distal sleeve outlet to less than 20 mm. The entire procedure mimics the surgical vertical gastroplasty commonly performed in the 1980s.

Devière et al. conducted the first human prospective, multicenter, single-arm trial studying the safety and feasibility of the TOGa system in 21 patients with a mean starting BMI of 43.3 (35–53 kg/m²). No serious complications were noted besides postoperative nausea, vomiting, abdominal pain, and transient dysphagia. Primary outcomes were safety, endoscopic appearance of the gastric pouch, and %EWL at 6 months.

At 6 months, endoscopic assessment of the pouch showed partial or fully intact sleeves. However, staple line gaps were seen in 13 of 21 patients with 3 patients showing incomplete distal sleeves. Five patients were seen to have normal pouch anatomy with intact sleeves and staple lines. Mean %EWL were 16.2%, 22.6%, and 24.4% at 1, 3, and 6 months. The mean BMI decreased from 43.3 pretreatment to 37.8 at 6 months ($P < 0.0001$) [47].

A single-arm prospective follow-up study was also created by Devière et al. studying the safety and feasibility of a second-generation TOGa system. The device was modified with an adjustable septum that allowed closer apposition of the two staple lines to address gaps. The trial consisted of 11 patients. No serious adverse events were noted besides procedure-related complications of transient epigastric pain, nausea, esophagitis, and mild dysphagia. 6-month endoscopic examination showed 4 of 11 patients had a less than 1 cm gap between the first and second staple line. %EWL were 19.2%, 33.7%, and 46.0% at 1, 3, and 6 months, respectively ($P < 0.05$). Mean BMI were 38.1 kg/m², 35.4 kg/m², and 33.1 kg/m² at 1, 3, and 6 months, respectively compared to a baseline of 41.6 kg/m² ($P < 0.01$) [48]. This second version of the device did address some of the technical limitations of the earlier version.

Familiari et al. published a subsequent European trial in 2011 which consisted of 67 patients. 53 patients had 1-year follow-up. Three-, 6-, and 12-month follow-up showed 33.9%, 42.6%, and 44.9% excess BMI loss, respectively. Hemoglobin A1C and triglycerides levels had significant decreases of 7.0 to 5.7%

and 142.8 to 98 mg/dL, respectively. Two major complications occurred and were respiratory insufficiency and asymptomatic pneumoperitoneum [49].

All together, these studies showed the TOGa system to be feasible, safe and induce significant weight loss in the short-term follow-up. A multicenter, randomized controlled FDA trial was terminated prematurely secondary to lack of efficacy. The company dissolved and the device was never approved in the US market.

Transoral Endoscopic Restrictive Implant System (TERIS)

The transoral endoscopic restrictive implant system (TERIS) (BaroSense, Redwood City, CA, USA) is an endoscopic system that implants a prosthetic restricting device to create a gastric reservoir at the level of the cardia. Implantation entails creation of 5 gastric plications with the placement of 5 silicone anchors followed by deployment of the gastric restrictor [50]. The plications are created 3 cm distal to the GE junction at the level of the cardia. The initial full-thickness gastric plication is just above the lesser curvature using an articulating suctioning endoscopic circular stapler. The stapling device compresses the tissue to create 2 concentric 3.5-mm reinforced staple rings. A 2-lumen cannulation guide is used to place the silicone anchors through the plications under direct endoscopic visualization using an anchor grasper. The procedure is repeated until 5 anchors are placed. Once all anchors are in place, attachment to the gastric restrictor is then performed under direct visualizations [50].

A randomized, uncontrolled, open-label, single group Phase I human trial by Biertho et al. [50] was used to describe the initial feasibility and safety of the TERIS system in 20 human subjects. Their study showed no intra- or postoperative complications with patients being discharged home on post-procedural day two tolerating a soft diet. Three- and 6-month %EWL were 21% and 26%, respectively. Ryou et al. in 2011 also published a Phase 1 trial consisting of

13 patients. Implant of the system was successful in 12 of 13 patients. Short-term follow-up showed 12.3% and 22.2% EWL at 1 and 3 months [51].

The TERIS system requires further investigation and FDA approval prior to use in the United States.

Duodenal-Jejunal Bypass Sleeve

The duodenal-jejunal bypass sleeve (DJBS) (EndoBarrier, GI Dynamics, Lexington MA, USA) is an endoscopically placed barrier device using a 60-cm long fluoropolymer liner anchored in the duodenum. The device prevents mixture of pancreaticobiliary secretions with food. The device is delivered under both fluoroscopy and endoscopy. The device is deployed using a combination of an over-the-wire catheter system with a capsule at the distal end of the catheter containing the sleeve. First the capsule is placed in the proximal duodenum, then an inner catheter is released allowing placement of the sleeve into the proximal jejunum using the aid of an atraumatic ball attached at the distal end of the catheter. Once the sleeve is fully deployed, the anchor is deployed from the capsule to sit within the duodenal bulb. The anchor is self-expanding with barbs that latches onto the surrounding tissue to prevent migration. Position is confirmed using contrast flushed into the sleeve to ensure patency of the sleeve. Once proper positioning is achieved, the sleeve and ball are detached from the catheter which is removed, leaving the implant in place [33, 52, 53].

In 2008, a pilot study performed by Rodriguez-Grunert et al. [52] reported on the first human experience, delivering and retrieving the DJBS in 12 patients with a 12-week endpoint. Primary outcomes were to identify and describe the severity of adverse events, while secondary outcomes focused on %EWL and changes in comorbid status. All 12 patients had successful deployment of the sleeve; however, only 10 of 12 patients completed the 12-week course. Two patients had intractable abdominal pain, nausea, and vomiting requiring early retrieval. Mean implant and explant times were 26.6 and 43.3 min, respectively.

Most complications occurred within 2 weeks of implantation which included abdominal pain, nausea, and vomiting. Of note, there was one partial pharyngeal tear and one esophageal tear during explantations. Furthermore, localized inflammation at the duodenal bulb anchoring site was seen in all patients.

The average percent excess weight loss at 12 weeks was 23.6% with all patients achieving a minimum of 10%EWL [52]. The trial showed that the four diabetic patients had normal fasting plasma glucose levels for the entire duration of the study without the need for oral hypoglycemics. Also 75% of the diabetic patients showed a HbA1c of ≥0.5% improvement at 12 weeks.

Tarnoff et al. [54] conducted a second open-label, multicenter, prospective randomized control trial comparing the effect of the DJBS with a low-fat diet versus a low-fat diet alone for 12 weeks. The study consisted of 25 patients in the experiment arm versus 14 patients within the diet alone control arm. Prior to the procedure, both group received counseling on a low-calorie diet with recommendations on exercise and behavior modifications. In the experiment arm, 20 of 25 device subjects maintained the sleeve for 12 weeks with average %EWL of 22% and 5% for the device and control groups, respectively. Five of twenty-five patients required early device explantation due to three GI bleeding, one anchor migration, and one sleeve obstruction. A total of four patients had type 2 diabetes in the study, 1 in the control group and 3 in the device group. All four patients had improved HbA1c levels with one complete resolution at 12 weeks in the device group.

A recent multicenter randomized control trial was conducted by Schouten R et al. to study the use of the EndoBarrier device in 41 preoperative bariatric surgery patients. Thirty patients were randomized to the treatment arm and 11 patients were randomized to the diet control group. A total of 26 devices were successfully implanted for 12 weeks. There were four device failures, one had dislocation of the anchor, another had obstruction of the sleeve, another had migration of the sleeve, and the last patient had intractable epigastric pain. All complications required early removal of the device. Mean excess weight loss was 19% for the treatment group and 6.9% for the control group at 12 weeks. Lower hemoglobin A1c and decrease hypoglycemic medication requirement were seen in 7 of 8 diabetic patients at 12 weeks [55].

A pivotal US trial was prematurely halted secondary to significant liver abscess formation. This was thought to be secondary to translocation of bacteria via the fixation barbs in the duodenum. Modifications to the fixation platform are currently underway and hope to revive the pivotal US trial.

Future studies are needed to elucidate the safety and feasibility of the DJBS in both the short and long term. Currently, major adverse events range from 10–20% in most studies with this version of the device. This device has much more promise in the type II diabetic population and focus on the metabolic affects of endoluminal therapies is outweighing the weight loss changes.

ValenTx Sleeve

The ValenTx endoluminal bypass (ValenTx, Maple Grove, MN, USA) attempts to mimic the Roux-en-Y gastric bypass (RNYGB). The implantable 120-cm sleeve is placed endoscopically starting at the GE junction and extends into the proximal mid-jejunum with the goal of bypassing the stomach and duodenum. This results in a similar property to the RNYGB [56]. Currently the technique requires both endoscopic deployment and suturing under laparoscopic visualization [51]. Sandler et al. in 2011 conducted the first pilot study consisting of a single center prospective human trial in 22 patients. Only 17 patients completed the 12-week trial period with 5 patients (23%) requiring device removal all due to odynophagia. No major complications occurred during the placement or retrieval of the device. The average %EWL was 39.7% at 12 weeks. Improvement in diabetes was seen in seven patients with significant reduction in hemoglobin A1c. All seven patients were off oral hypoglycemic agents while the sleeve was in place. Furthermore, two patients had complete resolution of their hypertension and three patients had normal lipid profiles at the end of the 12 weeks [57].

The ValenTx sleeve appears to be a very promising device in the treatment of metabolic derangements. The device and technique are still undergoing refinements prior to the pivotal US FDA trial.

Magnetic Endoscopic Incisionless Anastomosis System

The self-assembling magnetic endoscopic incisionless anastomosis system known as either IAS (incisionless anastomosis system) or SAMSEN (Smart Self-Assembling MagnetS for ENdoscopy) is a new device created by GI Windows (West Bridgewater, MA, USA). It consists of two self-assembling magnets which are placed by simultaneous enteroscopic and colonoscopic guidance into the distal ileum and mid-jejunum [40, 58]. The compressive forces between the two rings create a large compression side-to-side anastomosis over several days. Once the anastomosis is formed, the magnets automatically pass spontaneously through the GI tract [58]. Two porcine trials have been described one creating a large jejuno-colonic anastomosis [59] and the other creating jejunoileal bypass [60] both of which showed promising results. As a result, the technology was piloted in a human trial consisting of 10 patients with an average BMI of 41 kg/m^2. All 10 subjects had successful device placement and creation of the compression anastomosis [61]. Reported complications were mainly transient nausea and diarrhea. Mean %EWL was 28.3%. Of the 4 patients with type II diabetes, all patients were able to discontinue oral hypoglycemic in 6 months with decreasing HbA1c and fasting glucose levels.

The device is now undergoing evaluation for a pivotal US trial. The benefits from the side-to-side anastomosis may be secondary to early entry of food into the distal small bowel therefore altering the hormonal affect of incretins to hunger and satiety.

AspireAssist

AspireAssist (Aspire Bariatrics, King of Prussia, PA, USA) is a device that eliminates food and liquid from the stomach. This procedure uses a 30-French percutaneous endoscopic gastrostomy (PEG) tube. The device consists of a valve port placed at the skin level to assist in aspirating gastric contents. The technique includes infusing water into the stomach 20 min after a meal and then manual gastric content drainage. The efficacy of aspiration therapy was demonstrated in three separate studies [40].

The AspireAssist was studied by Sullivan et al. in a randomized clinical trial of 18 patients which consisted of 11 AspireAssist and 7 control patients. Total weight loss was 18.6% at 12 months in the device group, compared to 5.9% in the control group [62]. Ten of eleven patients in the device group completed the trial, whereas 4 of 7 completed the trial in the control group. Both groups had similar initial BMI, 42.0 ± 1.4 and 39.3 ± 1.1, respectively, in the device and control group. Furthermore, 7 of the remaining 10 patients in the device group continued for 12 months and had an average total body weight loss of 20.1% ± 3.5%. Unfortunately, glucose and lipid values remained unchanged from baseline. Patients in this trial did not exhibit any maladaptive eating behavior during the study.

In another study by Forssell et al. with 25 patients with a BMI of 39.8 ± 0.9, patients were placed on a very low calorie diet for 4 weeks before aspiration therapy. These patients exhibited a total excess weight loss of 40.8 ± 19.8% after 6 months and 14.8% ± 6.3% total body weight loss. Furthermore, patients exhibited a trend to improved fasting glucose and hemoglobin A1c. Most notably, 3 of 5 patients with type II diabetes mellitus were able to discontinue their diabetes medication [63].

Finally, the multicenter PATHWAY trial compared weigh loss among patients who used AspireAssist with lifestyle counseling with an only lifestyle counseling group in a 2:1 ratio and found a 37.2 ± 27.5% excess weight loss in the AspireAssist patients compared to 13% ± 17.6% in the lifestyle counseling group alone at 52 weeks [64]. This pivotal trial allowed for FDA approval of the device in the United States.

No major complications were seen in the Sullivan et al. study. Complications were related to the PEG tube and included 3 skin infections and one persistent fistula, which closed without intervention after removal of the system. Patients also noted abdominal pain from the device that was successfully remedied by redesigning the device [35]. Similarly Forssell et al. also only noted abdominal pain and skin infection. However, this study also had patients with intra-abdominal fluid collection and skin breakdown around the stoma. Notably, 52% of patients experienced moderate abdominal pain during the first week with 12% experiencing severe pain [40, 63]. Finally, in the multicenter PATHWAY trial, the most common complication was having similar abdominal pain, postoperative granulation tissue, and peristomal irritation [64].

Currently, the AspireAssist appears to have promising short- and mid-term data and currently has obtained FDA approval. Further results relating to changes in comorbidities should continue to be evaluated.

Transoral Surgery for Revisional Bariatric Procedures

Even though the Roux-en-Y gastric bypass surgery remains the gold standard for bariatric surgical procedures, with %EWL at 2 years up to 61.6% [21], early and late mortality rates range around 0.16% and 0.09%, respectively [24]. More significantly, inadequate weight loss with also weight regain is reported up to 25–30% after gastric bypass or other bariatric weight loss surgery [65, 66]. Failure of bariatric surgery and weight regain is multifactorial which can include inadequate long-term management of multiple factors such as psychological, dietary, or medical issues, as well as anatomical aberrancies [67].

Anatomic issues are usually seen on an esophagogastroduodenoscopy (EGD) or upper GI study to evaluate for gastro-gastric fistula, gastric pouch dilation, and/or anastomotic dilation. Enlargement of the gastrojejunal anastomosis and/or gastric pouch enlargement are common reasons for weight regain. Patients with these anatomic findings may experience a loss of satiety and a greater degree of rapid emptying of contents into the small bowel. Once enlargement of the gastric pouch or GJ anastomosis is seen, discussion of revisional surgery may be necessary. However, recent studies show a complication rate of 5%–13% for major complications in re-operative surgery [68] with potential serious complications including anastomotic leaks, wound dehiscence, incisional hernias, and pulmonary complications.

Given the frequency of weight regain and risk of revisional surgery, endoscopic revisions of gastric bypass have also become a trending technique. Multiple techniques and technologies include revisional obesity surgery endolumenal (ROSE), transoral outlet reduction TORe, argon plasma coagulation, StomaphyX, endoscopic sclerotherapy, and over the scope clips. Results of each device and technique vary widely [40, 69].

Transoral Outlet Reduction (TORe)

Transoral outlet reduction is a technique that uses an endoscopic suturing device that places endoluminal full-thickness stitches around the gastrojejunal anastomosis thereby reducing its aperture. The procedure is done under general anesthesia with the stomach inflated using carbon dioxide. A standard upper endoscopy is performed to examine the esophagus, gastric pouch, GJ anastomosis, and both limbs of the small bowel. Argon plasma coagulation is then used to ablate a 5-mm thick margin on the gastric anastomotic side. Interrupted or a continuous suture is then placed at the margin of the anastomosis crossing its lumen and tightened to oppose the sides of the anastomosis.

Interestingly, TORe with the OverStitch device appears to provide more promising results when compared to the older EndoCinch device. This newer technology has allowed more full-thickness tissue purchase which then leads to greater suture and plication durability. According to Kumar et al. [70], the OverStitch group lost 8.6 ± 2.5 kg at 1 year versus 2.9 ± 1.0 kg with the EndoCinch device and saw further successful excess weight loss in a long-term study up to 3 years for the TORe Overstitch [71].

Although the TORe technique is feasible and appears to be safer than surgical approaches, durability of the technique still needs to be further studied.

StomaphyX

Mikami et al. [72] investigated reduction of dilated gastric pouches to its original inner diameter and/or volume by utilizing the StomaphyX™ device (EndoGastric Solutions, Redmond, WA, USA). It is an endoscopic device that deploys 7-mm, 3–0 polypropylene H-fasteners to create full-thickness, serosal-to-serosal tissue approximation. Under general anesthesia, the apparatus is passed into the efferent jejunal limb to allow passage of the StomaphyX™ device through the gastro-jejunostomy anastomosis. Using a combination of suction and scope manipulation, H-fasteners are deployed in a circular pleat 1 cm proximal to the anastomosis with an additional second row 1 cm proximal to the first. Repeat endoscopy is completed to assess the reduction of the gastric pouch and anastomosis (Fig. 14.2).

During Mikami et al.'s study, a total of 39 patients were enrolled in a trial [72]. The average procedure time was 35 min (16–62 min) and between 12 and 41 H-fasteners were used in each case. A total of 37 of 39 patients were discharged on the same day with 2 patients kept overnight as a result of the procedure being performed later in the day. No immediate major adverse events occurred. Minor complications included sore throats and epigastric pain resolved within a few days. Resolution of late dumping syndrome was seen in 3 patients and at 1 month follow-up, 8 patients with gastric esophageal reflux noted improvement in their symptoms.

In terms of weight loss, at 1 month it was 10.6% EBWL, at 3 months it was 13.1% EBWL, at 6 months it was 17.0% EBWL, and at 12 months it was 19.5% EBWL [72].

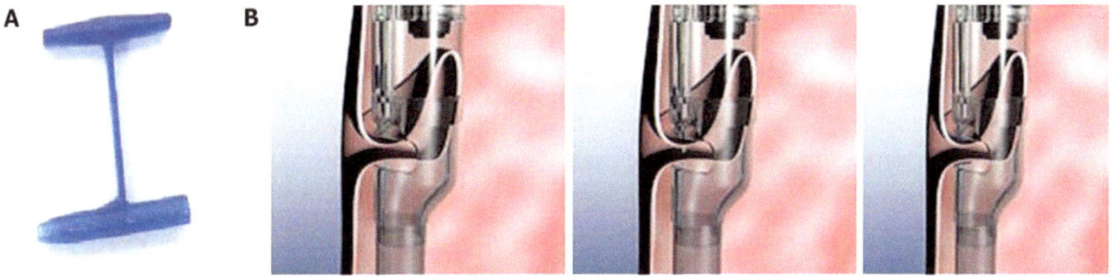

Fig. 14.2 StomaphyX device (EndoGastric Solutions, Redmond, WA). (**a**) Polypropylene fastener. (**b**) StomaphyX™ mechanism of tissue approximation (From Mikami et al. [72], with permission)

This trial demonstrates that the StomaphyX™ procedure may offer a safe, effective revisional bariatric procedure; however, enrollment in a randomized sham-controlled trial was terminated due to failure to reach endpoints [73]. The device is currently not available in the United States.

Conclusion

Given the growing prevalence of obesity in the United States and increasing numbers of bariatric procedures annually, there is a growing demand for less invasive approaches. Endoscopic transoral techniques as primary intervention, bridging to bariatric surgery, and revisional procedures continue to grow and offer promising results.

However, like other therapies, transoral techniques need to be rigorously tested to determine their short- and long-term safety and efficacy. Furthermore, transoral procedures should demonstrate equivalent or lower morbidity and mortality rates when compared to current laparoscopic therapies while also offering meaningful weight loss and improvement in comorbid states. Currently, only laparoscopic surgical therapies for morbid obesity are effective in achieving significant weight loss and improvements in obesity-related comorbidities. However, these laparoscopic approaches are not without risk and have limited use in patients with multiple significant comorbidities, older age, super-obesity, and atypical anatomy [74, 75].

Currently, several techniques and devices have been approved by the FDA with more endoscopic devices under human trial and FDA review (Table 14.1) [40]. With advancements in these transoral techniques, weight loss procedures can be safer and less invasive compared to surgical approaches. Also, these procedures can circumvent permanent surgical procedures. This would allow patients who were previously not surgical candidates to undergo potentially life impacting procedures. Furthermore, transoral techniques could also be a bridge for more definitive weight loss procedures. This will help allow patients

Table 14.1 Summary of the regulatory status of transoral procedures [40]

Device	Procedure	Mechanism	Regulatory status
Orbera (BIB)	Intragastric balloon	Restrictive	FDA-approved
TransPyloric shuttle	Intragastric balloon	Restrictive	Human trials
OverStitch	Endoscopic sleeve gastroplasty	Restrictive/gastric remodeling	FDA-approved
AspireAssist	Aspiration therapy	Aspiration	FDA-approved
Self-assembling magnets	Endoscopic enteral anastomosis	Dual-path enteral bypass	Human trials
TORe OverStitch and TORe Endocinch	Transoral outlet reduction for revision of gastric bypass	Anastomotic reduction	FDA-approved
Endobarrier sleeve	Pancreaticobiliary bypass	Malabsorption	Human trials
ValenTx sleeve	Malabsorptive and restrictive	Restrictive and malabsorptive	Human trials

who were unable to obtain definitive weight loss surgery due to comorbidities such as extreme BMIs. Finally, there is an emerging field of transoral techniques that can provide safer means of revising bariatric procedures in individuals that have reached their weight loss plateau or have started regaining weight.

References

1. World Health Organization. Fact sheet: obesity and overweight. Updated Jun 2016. http://www.who.int/mediacentre/factsheets/fs311/en/print.html. Accessed 31 May 2017.
2. Genco A, Bruni T, Doldi SB, Forestieri P, Marino M, Busetto L, et al. BioEnterics intragastric balloon: the Italian experience with 2,515 patients. Obes Surg. 2005;15(8):1161–4.
3. Ogden CL. Disparities in obesity prevalence in the United States: black women at risk. Am J Clin Nutr. 2009;89(4):1001–2.
4. Ogden CL, Carroll MD, Curtin LR, McDowell MA, Tabak CJ, Flegal KM. Prevalence of overweight and obesity in the United States, 1999-2004. JAMA. 2006;295(13):1549–55.
5. Ogden CL, Carroll MD, McDowell MA, Flegal KM. Obesity among adults in the United States — no statistically significant chance since 2003-2004. NCHS Data Brief. 2007;(1):1–8.
6. Bessesen DH. Update on obesity. J Clin Endocrinol Metab. 2008;93(6):2027–34.
7. World Health Organization. World Health Report 2002 — reducing risks, promoting healthy life. http://www.iotf.org. Accessed 31 May 2017.
8. Must A, Spadano J, Coakley EH, Field AE, Colditz G, Dietz WH. The disease burden associated with overweight and obesity. JAMA. 1999;282(16):1523–9.
9. National Task Force on the Prevention and Treatment of Obesity. Overweight, obesity, and health risk. Arch Intern Med. 2000;160(7):898–904.
10. WHO. Global health risks: mortality and burden of disease attributable to selected major risks. Geneva, Switzerland: World Health Organization; 2009. http://www.who.int/healthinfo/global_burden_disease/GlobalHealthRisks_report_part2.pdf. Accessed 4 Jun 2017.
11. Fontaine KR, Redden DT, Wang C, Westfall AO, Allison DB. Years of life lost due to obesity. JAMA. 2003;289(2):187–93.
12. Finkelstein EA, Brown DS, Wrage LA, Allaire BT, Hoerger TJ. Individual and aggregate years-of-life-lost associated with overweight and obesity. Obesity (Silver Spring). 2010;18(2):333–9.
13. Adams KF, Schatzkin A, Harris TB, Kipnis V, Mouw T, Ballard-Barbash R, et al. Overweight, obesity, and

mortality in a large prospective cohort of persons 50 to 71 years old. N Engl J Med. 2006;355:763–78.
14. Serdula MK, Mokdad AH, Williamson DF, Galuska DA, Mendlein JM, Heath GW. Prevalence of attempting weight loss and strategies for controlling weight. JAMA. 1999;282(14):1353–8.
15. Santos I, Sniehotta FF, Marques MM, Carraça EV, Teixeira PJ. Prevalence of personal weight control attempts in adults: a systematic review and meta-analysis. Obes Rev. 2017;18(1):32–50.
16. National Institutes of Health. North American Association for the Study of Obesity; National Heart, Lung, and Blood Institute. The practical guide to the identification, evaluation, and treatment of overweight and obesity in adults. Bethesda, MD: National Institutes of Health; Oct 2000. NIH publication 00–4084. http://www.nhlbi.nih.gov/guidelines/obesity/prctgd_c.pdf. Accessed 4 Jun 2017.
17. NIH conference. Gastrointestinal surgery for severe obesity. Consensus Development Conference Panel. Ann Intern Med. 1991;115(12):956–61.
18. Gastrointestinal surgery for severe obesity. Proceedings of a National Institutes of Health Consensus Development Conference. March 25–27, 1991, Bethesda, MD. Am J Clin Nutr. 1992;55(2 Suppl):487S–619S.
19. American Society for Metabolic and Bariatric Surgery. Estimates of bariatric surgery numbers, 2011–2015. 2016. https://asmbs.org/resources/estimate-of-bariatric-surgery-numbers. Accessed 4 Jun 2017.
20. Parker M, Loewen M, Sullivan T, Yatco E, Cerabona T, Savino JA, Kaul A. Predictors of outcome after obesity surgery in New York state from 1991 to 2003. Surg Endosc. 2007;21(9):1482–6.
21. Buchwald H, Avidor Y, Braunwald E, Jensen MD, Pories W, Fahrbach K, Schoelles K. Bariatric surgery: a systematic review and meta-analysis. JAMA. 2004;292(14):1724–37.
22. Colquitt JL, Pickett K, Loveman E, Frampton GK. Surgery for weight loss in adults. Cochrane Database Syst Rev. 2014;8:CD003641.
23. Thompson CC, Slattery J, Bundga ME, Lautz DB. Peroral endoscopic reduction of dilated gastro-jejunal anastomosis after Roux-en-Y gastric bypass: a possible new option for patients with weight regain. Surg Endosc. 2006;20(11):1744–8.
24. Buchwald H, Estok R, Fahrbach K, Banel D, Sledge I. Trends in mortality in bariatric surgery: a systematic review and meta-analysis. Surgery. 2007;142(4):621–35; discussion 632–5.
25. Hazey JW, Dunkin BJ, Melvin WS. Changing attitudes toward endolumenal therapy. Surg Endosc. 2007;21(3):445–8.
26. Mathus-Vliegen EM, Tytgat GN. Intragastric balloon for treatment-resistant obesity: safety, tolerance, and efficacy of 1-year balloon treatment followed by a 1-year balloon-free follow-up. Gastrointest Endosc. 2005;61(1):19–27.

27. de Castro ML, Morales MJ, Martínez-Olmos MA, Pineda JR, Cid L, Estévez P, et al. Safety and effectiveness of gastric balloons associated with hypocaloric diet for the treatment of obesity. Rev Esp Enferm Dig (Madrid). 2013;105(9):529–36.

28. Adrianzén Vargas M, Cassinello Fernández N, Ortega SJ. Preoperative weight loss in patients with indication of bariatric surgery: which is the best method? Nutr Hosp. 2011;26(6):1227–30.

29. Drozdowski R, Wyleżoł M, Frączek M, Hevelke P, Giaro M, Sobański P. Small bowel necrosis as a consequence of spontaneous deflation and migration of an air-filled intragastric balloon—a potentially life-threatening complication. Wideochir Inne Tech Maloinwazyjne. 2014;9(2):292–6.

30. Bužga M, Evžen M, Pavel K, Tomáš K, Vladislava Z, Pavel Z, Svagera Z. Effects of the intragastric balloon MedSil on weight loss, fat tissue, lipid metabolism, and hormones involved in energy balance. Obes Surg. 2014;24(6):909–15.

31. Genco A, Cipriano M, Bacci V, Cuzzolaro M, Materia A, Raparelli L, et al. BioEnterics intragastric balloon (BIB): a short-term, double-blind, randomised, controlled, crossover study on weight reduction in morbidly obese patients. Int J Obes. 2006;30(1):129–33.

32. Alfredo G, Roberta M, Massimiliano C, Michele L, Nicola B, Adriano R. Long-term multiple intragastric balloon treatment—a new strategy to treat morbid obese patients refusing surgery: prospective 6-year follow-up study. Surg Obes Relat Dis. 2014;10(2):307–11.

33. Majumder S, Birk J. A review of the current status of endoluminal therapy as a primary approach to obesity management. Surg Endosc. 2013;27(7):2305–11.

34. Marinos G, Eliades C, Raman Muthusamy V, Greenway F. Weight loss and improved quality of life with a nonsurgical endoscopic treatment for obesity: clinical results from a 3- and 6-month study. Surg Obes Relat Dis. 2014;10(5):929–34.

35. Schwartz MP, Wellink H, Gooszen HG, Conchillo JM, Samsom M, Smout AJ. Endoscopic gastroplication for the treatment of gastro-oesophageal reflux disease: a randomised, sham-controlled trial. Gut. 2007;56(1):20–8.

36. Mahmood Z, McMahon BP, Arfin Q, Byrne PJ, Reynolds JV, Murphy EM, Weir DG. Endocinch therapy for gastro-oesophageal reflux disease: a one year prospective follow up. Gut. 2003;52(1):34–9.

37. Rothstein RI, Filipi CJ. Endoscopic suturing for gastroesophageal reflux disease: clinical outcome with the bard EndoCinch. Gastrointest Endosc Clin N Am. 2003;13(1):89–101.

38. Fogel R, De Fogel J, Bonilla Y, De La Fuente R. Clinical experience of transoral suturing for an endoluminal vertical gastroplasty: 1-year follow-up in 64 patients. Gastrointest Endosc. 2008;68(1):51–8.

39. Brethauer SA, Chand B, Schauer PR, Thompson CC. Transoral gastric volume reduction as intervention for weight management: 12 month follow up of TRIM trial. Surg Obes Relat Dis. 2012;8(3):296–303.

40. Kumar N. Weight loss endoscopy: development, applications, and current status. World J Gastroenterol. 2016;22(31):7069–79. Review.

41. Fujii LL, Bonin EA, Baron TH, Gostout CJ, Wong Kee Song LM. Utility of an endoscopic suturing system for prevention of covered luminal stent migration in the upper GI tract. Gastrointest Endosc. 2013;78(5):787–93.

42. Kumar N, Thompson CC. A novel method for endoscopic perforation management by using abdominal exploration and full-thickness sutured closure. Gastrointest Endosc. 2014;80(1):156–61.

43. Kumar N, Sahdala HN, Shaikh S, Wilson EB, Manoel GN, Zundel N, Thompson CC. Endoscopic sleeve gastroplasty for primary therapy of obesity: initial human cases (abstract MO1155). Gastroenterology. 2014;146(5):S-571–2.

44. Sharaiha RZ, Kedia P, Kumta N, DeFilippis EM, Gaidhane M, Shukla A, et al. Initial experience with endoscopic sleeve gastroplasty: technical success and reproducibility in the bariatric population. Endoscopy. 2015;47(2):164–6.

45. Abu Dayyeh BK, Acosta A, Camilleri M, Mundi MS, Rajan E, Topazian MD, Gostout CJ. Endoscopic sleeve gastroplasty alters gastric physiology and induces loss of body weight in obese individuals. Clin Gastroenterol Hepatol. 2017;15(1):37–43.e1.

46. Lopez-Nava G, Galvao M, Bautista-Castaño I, Fernandez-Corbelle JP, Trell M. Endoscopic sleeve gastroplasty with 1-year follow-up: factors predictive of success. Endosc Int Open. 2016;4(2):E222–7.

47. Devière J, Ojeda Valdes G, Cuevas Herrera L, Closset J, Le Moine O, Eisendrath P, et al. Safety, feasibility and weight loss after transoral gastroplasty: first human multicenter study. Surg Endosc. 2008;22(3):589–98.

48. Moreno C, Closset J, Dugardeyn S, Baréa M, Mehdi A, Collignon L, et al. Transoral gastroplasty is safe, feasible, and induces significant weight loss in morbidly obese patients: results of the second human pilot study. Endoscopy. 2008;40(05):406–13.

49. Familiari P, Costamagna G, Blero D, Le Moine O, Perri V, Boskoski I, et al. Transoral gastroplasty for morbid obesity: a multicenter trial with 1 year outcome. Gatrointest Endosc. 2011;74(6):1248–58.

50. Biertho L, Hould FS, Lebel S, Biron S. Transoral endoscopic restrictive implant system: a new endoscopic technique for the treatment of obesity. Surg Obes Relat Dis. 2010;6(2):203–5.

51. Ryou M, Ryan MB, Thompson CC. Current status of endoluminal bariatric procedures for primary and revision indications. Gastrointest Endosc Clin N Am. 2011;21(2):315–33.

52. Rodriguez-Grunert L, Galvao Neto MP, Alamo M, Ramos AC, Baez PB, Tarnoff M. First human experience with endoscopically delivered and retrieved duodenal-jejunal bypass sleeve. Surg Obes Relat Dis. 2008;4(1):55–9.

53. Narula VK, Mikami DJ, Hazey JW. Endoscopic consideration in morbid obesity. In: Marks JM, Dunkin B,

editors. Principles of flexible endoscopy for surgeons. New York: Springer; 2013. p. 139–55.

54. Tarnoff M, Rodriguez L, Escalona A, Ramos A, Neto M, Alamo M, et al. Open label, prospective, randomized controlled trial of an endoscopic duodenal-jejunal bypass sleeve versus low calorie diet for pre-operative weight loss in bariatric surgery. Surg Endosc. 2009;23(3):650–6.

55. Schouten R, Rijs CS, Bouvy ND, Hameeteman W, Koek GH, Janssen IM, Greve JW. A multicenter, randomized efficacy study of the EndoBarrier gastrointestinal liner for presurgical weight loss prior to bariatric surgery. Ann Surg. 2010;251(2):236–43.

56. ValenTx Endo Bypass System. http://www.valentx.com/technology.php. Accessed 4 Jun 2017.

57. Sandler BJ, Rumbaut R, Swain CP, Torres G, Morales L, Gonzales L, et al. Human experience with an endoluminal, endoscopic, gastrojejunal bypass sleeve. Surg Endosc. 2011;25(9):3028–33.

58. Ryou M, Cantillon-Murphy P, Azagury D, Shaikh SN, Ha G, Greenwalt I, et al. Smart Self-Assembling MagnetS for ENdoscopy (SAMSEN) for transoral endoscopic creation of immediate gastrojejunostomy (with video). Gastrointest Endosc. 2011;73(2):353–9.

59. Ryou M, Agoston AT, Thompson CC. Endoscopic intestinal bypass creation by using self-assembling magnets in a porcine model. Gastrointest Endosc. 2016;83(4):821–5.

60. Ryou M, Aihara H, Thompson CC. Minimally invasive entero-enteral dual-path bypass using self-assembling magnets. Surg Endosc. 2016;30(10):4533–8.

61. Machytka E, Buzga M, Ryou MK, Lautz DB, Thompson CC. Endoscopic dual-path enteral anastomosis using self-assembling magnets: first-in-human clinical feasibility (abstract 1139). Gastroenterology. 2016;150(4):S232.

62. Sullivan S, Stein R, Jonnalagadda S, Mullady D, Edmundowicz S. Aspiration therapy leads to weight loss in obese subjects: a pilot study. Gastroenterology. 2013;145(6):1245–1252.e5.

63. Forssell H, Norén E. A novel endoscopic weight loss therapy using gastric aspiration: results after 6 months. Endoscopy. 2015;47(1):68–71.

64. Thompson CC, Abu Dayyeh BK, Kushner K, Sullivan S, Schorr AB, Amaro A, et al. The AspireAssist is an effective tool in the treatment of class II and class III

obesity: results of a one-year clinical trial (abstract 381). Gastroenterology. 2016;150(4):S86.

65. Yale CE. Gastric surgery for morbid obesity. Complications and long-term weight control. Arch Surg. 1989;124(8):941–6.

66. Sugerman HJ, Kellum JM, Engle KM, Wolfe L, Starkey JV, Birkenhauer R, et al. Gastric bypass for treating severe obesity. Am J Clin Nutr. 1992;55(2 Suppl):560S–6S.

67. Christou NV, Look D, Maclean LD. Weight gain after short- and long-limb gastric bypass in patients followed for longer than 10 years. Ann Surg. 2006;244(5):734–40.

68. Martin MJ, Mullenix PS, Steele SR, See CS, Cuadrado DG, Carter PL. A case-match analysis of failed prior bariatric procedures converted to resectional gastric bypass. Am J Surg. 2004;187(5):666–71; discussion 670–1.

69. Gallo AS, DuCoin CG, Berducci MA, Nino DF, Almadani M, Sandler BJ, Horgan S, Jacobsen GR. Endoscopic revision of gastric bypass: holy grail or epic fail? Surg Endosc. 2016;30(9):3922–7.

70. Kumar N, Thompson CC. Comparison of a superficial suturing device with a full-thickness suturing device for transoral outlet reduction (with videos). Gastrointest Endosc. 2014;79(6):984–9.

71. Kumar N, Thompson CC. Transoral outlet reduction for weight regain after gastric bypass: long-term follow-up. Gastrointest Endosc. 2016;83(4):776–9.

72. Mikami D, Needleman B, Narula V, Durant J, Melvin WS. Natural orifice surgery: initial US experience utilizing the StomaphyX device to reduce gastric pouches after Roux-en-Y gastric bypass. Surg Endosc. 2010;24(1):223–8.

73. Eid GM, McCloskey CA, Eagleton JK, Lee LB, Courcoulas AP. StomaphyX vs a sham procedure for revisional surgery to reduce regained weight in Roux-en-Y gastric bypass patients: a randomized clinical trial. JAMA Surg. 2014;149(4):372.

74. Maggard MA, Shugarman LR, Suttorp M, Maglione M, Sugerman HJ, Livingston EH, et al. Meta-analysis: surgical treatment of obesity. Ann Intern Med. 2005;142(7):547–59.

75. Allen JW. Laparoscopic gastric band complications. Med Clin North Am. 2007;91(3):485–97, xii.

76. Colquitt JL, Picot J, Loveman E, Clegg AJ. Surgery for obesity. Cochrane Database Syst Rev. 2009;(2):CD003641.

Endoluminal Small Bowel Procedures for Obesity and Metabolic Diseases

Pichamol Jirapinyo and Christopher C. Thompson

Introduction

The small bowel is an important organ where the majority of nutrient absorption takes place. In addition, it also plays a major role in glucose homeostasis via gut hormone incretins. To date, there are two key incretin hormones that have been identified: glucose-dependent insulinotropic polypeptide (GIP), which is secreted by K cells located predominantly in the duodenum and jejunum [1, 2], and glucagon-like peptide-1 (GLP-1), which is secreted by L cells found primarily in the ileum and proximal colon [3–5]. The incretin effect refers to a phenomenon when there is increased stimulation of insulin secretion with oral glucose intake compared to intravenous infusion of the same amount of glucose [6, 7]. This effect is thought to be due to incretin hormones, the function of which is enhanced by a contact between ingested nutrients and the small bowel. In addition to their effect on glucose homeostasis, GIP and GLP-1 also induce satiety and lead to delayed gastrointestinal motility.

Given the role of small bowel on nutrient absorption and glucose homeostasis as described above, endoluminal small bowel procedures appear to have an effect on not only weight loss but also glycemic improvement. To date, there are several small bowel endoscopic bariatric and metabolic therapies (EBMTs). However, none have been FDA-approved for use in the USA. This chapter reviews the currently available small bowel EBMTs, their safety and efficacy data from the pilot and pivotal studies (if available), and the current status of each device as of 2017.

EndoBarrier

The EndoBarrier (GI Dynamics, Boston MA, USA), also known as duodenal-jejunal bypass liner (DJBL), is a 60-cm fluoropolymer sleeve that is attached to the duodenal bulb and ends at the proximal jejunum (Fig. 15.1a) [8]. The device is placed and removed endoscopically. Ingested food passes from the stomach into the sleeve and goes directly into the jejunum without contacting the duodenum. Bile and pancreatic juice flow down between the sleeve and the small bowel wall, and mix with chyme in the jejunum. Similar to Roux-en-Y gastric bypass (RYGB), DJBL excludes the proximal small bowel from being in

P. Jirapinyo, M.D. • C.C. Thompson, M.D., M.Sc., F.A.C.G., F.A.S.G.E., A.G.A.F. (✉)
Division of Gastroenterology, Hepatology and Endoscopy, Brigham and Women's Hospital/Harvard Medical School, 75 Francis Street, Thorn 1404, Boston, MA 02115, USA
e-mail: pjirapinyo@bwh.harvard.edu; cthompson@hms.harvard.edu

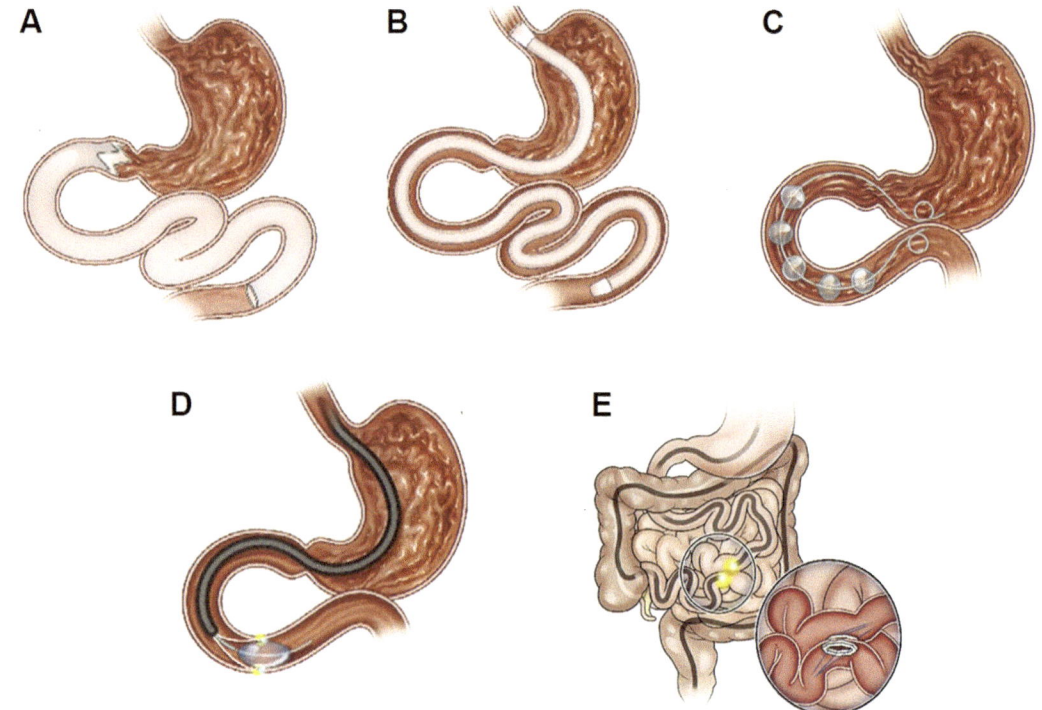

Fig. 15.1 Small bowel endoscopic bariatric and metabolic therapies. (**a**) EndoBarrier, (**b**) endoluminal bypass, (**c**) SatiSphere, (**d**) duodenal mucosal resurfacing, (**e**) incision-less magnetic anastomotic system (From Jirapinyo and Thompson [8], with permission)

contact with chyme, which likely leads to an increase in postprandial GLP-1 and a decrease in GIP [9–11]. These likely contribute to weight loss and improvement in glycemic control after the procedure.

In 2008, a pilot study was conducted in 12 patients with obesity with a mean BMI of 43 kg/m². Of these, four had type 2 diabetes mellitus (T2DM). Of the 12 patients, 10 were able to maintain the device for the entire study period of 12 weeks. Two underwent early explantation due to poor device placement. At 12 weeks, the mean excess weight loss (EWL) was 23.6% among the ten patients with the device in place. Additionally, all four patients with T2DM had normal fasting glucose without being on any hypoglycemic medication for the entire study period. Three of the four patients experienced a decrease in hemoglobin A1c (HbA1c) by ≥0.5% [12].

The ENDO trial was a multicenter, randomized, sham-controlled pivotal trial of Endobarrier in the USA. The study met efficacy end points with 60% of the patients achieving at least 5% of total body weight loss (TWL) and 34.8% reaching hemoglobin A1c (HbA1c) goal of 7% or less at 12 months (compared to 20% and 9.8% in the sham group, respectively). The trial was, however, stopped early by the company due to a hepatic abscess rate of 3.5%, which was higher than the known 1% incidence rate from outside the US experience. All cases were managed conservatively and did not require intensive care unit stay [13].

A meta-analysis of 4 randomized controlled trials (RCTs) with 151 patients with obesity demonstrated that DJBL-treated patients experienced 5.1 kg greater weight loss, which corresponded to an additional 12.6% EWL compared with control intervention [14]. In another meta-analysis which included 123 patients with obesity and concomitant

T2DM from 4 RCTs, DJBL group experienced a significantly greater decrease in HbA1c by 0.9% compared to the control group [15].

Endoluminal Bypass

The endoluminal bypass (ValenTx, Carpinteria CA, USA), also known as gastro-duodeno-jejunal bypass sleeve (GJBS), is a 120-cm sleeve that is attached to the gastroesophageal (GE) junction to create an endoluminal gastro-duodeno-jejunal bypass (Fig. 15.1b). Ingested food passes from the distal esophagus into the sleeve and goes directly into the jejunum without contacting the stomach and first 100 cm of the small bowel. The sleeve is implanted and retrieved endoscopically. Therefore, similar to DJBL, GJBS preserves the gastrointestinal anatomy, while mimicking the permanent anatomical changes of RYGB.

In 2009, a pilot study was conducted on 13 patients with obesity with a mean BMI of 42 kg/m^2. One patient was excluded at the time of endoscopy due to inflammation at the GE junction. Two patients required early explantation of the device due to intolerance. Out of the remaining 10 patients, technical success rate of device implantation was 100%. At 1 year, 6 of the 10 patients had fully attached and functional devices, and the remaining 4 had partial cuff detachment seen on follow-up endoscopy. The mean EWL was 54% in the group with fully attached sleeve, and lower in those with partial cuff detachment. Comorbidities including hypertension, diabetes, and hyperlipidemia improved at 1 year [16]. More investigational studies are ongoing.

SatiSphere

SatiSphere (EndoSphere, Columbus OH, USA) consists of a 1-mm nitinol wire and several mesh spheres mounted along its course with two pigtails at each end (Fig. 15.1c). It is placed endoscopically, and fluoroscopy may be used to confirm the location of the device after implantation. The device conforms to the duodenal C-shape configuration and thereby self-anchors.

It is thought that this device works by delaying transit time of nutrients through the duodenum, which may lead to changes in gut hormones and glucose metabolism.

In 2012, a pilot study was conducted on 31 patients with obesity with a mean BMI of 41.3 kg/m^2. Of these, 21 were randomized to the SatiSphere arm and the remainder 10 were randomized to the control arm. Device migration occurred in 10 of 21 study arm patients, with two necessitating emergent surgery, which led to termination of the study. At 3 months, the mean EWL was 18.4% in those who completed the trial compared to 4.4% in the control arm. This study also showed that the device was associated with delayed glucose absorption and altered kinetics of GLP-1 levels [17].

Duodenal Mucosal Resurfacing

Duodenal mucosal resurfacing (DMR) (Fractyl Laboratories, Lexington MA, USA), also known as the Revita procedure, is an endoscopic procedure that involves hydrothermal ablation of the duodenal mucosa and subsequent mucosal healing (Fig. 15.1d). The procedure consists of intestinal luminal sizing, submucosal expansion with saline (to protect the deeper tissue layers), and circumferential thermal ablation of the duodenum. Although the exact mechanism of the procedure remains unknown, it is thought that mucosal remodeling may reset the diseased duodenal enteroendocrine cells. This then leads to restoration of the normal glycemic signaling through the incretin effect.

In 2013, a proof-of-concept study was conducted on 39 patients with poorly controlled T2DM, defined as HbA1c > 7.5% on at least 1 oral antidiabetic medication. Technical success rate was 100%. Out of the 39 patients, 28 had long segment ablation (LS-DMR, ≥9 cm of ablation) and 11 had a short segment ablated (SS-DMR, <6 cm of ablation). At 6 months, HbA1c decreased from 9.5 to 8.3% for the entire cohort. More potent glycemic effect was seen in the LS-DMR group (a decrease in HbA1c of 2.5%) compared to the SS-DMR group (a decrease in HbA1c of 1.2%), which suggested a dose-dependent treatment effect from DMR. Three patients experienced duodenal stenosis treated successfully with balloon dilation [18]. Currently, a randomized, double-blinded, sham-controlled trial (the Revita-1 study) is being conducted in Europe and Brazil to assess the safety and efficacy of DMR in patients with poorly controlled T2DM. Additionally, a US pivotal trial is underway.

Incisionless Magnetic Anastomotic System

The incisionless magnetic anastomotic system (IMAS) (GI Windows, Bridgewater MA, USA) uses miniature self-assembling magnets to create an entero-enteral bypass. This technology has many applications including the treatment of obstruction, obesity, and metabolic diseases. During the bariatric dual-path bypass procedure, enteroscopy and colonoscopy are performed simultaneously. The IMAS is then deployed from the working channel of each endoscope forming magnetic octagons in the jejunum and ileum (Fig. 15.1e). After several days, the coupled magnets are naturally expelled leaving behind a patent jejunal-ileal anastomosis. With this anastomosis, nutrients and bile acids are thought to reach the distal small bowel sooner, which may result in stimulation of the incretin effect and subsequent improvement in glycemic control [19, 20].

In 2015, a proof-of-concept study was conducted on ten patients with obesity. Technical success rate was 100%. At 12 months, average weight loss was 14.6% EWL. The HbA1c level decreased from 6.6 to 5.4%. The postprandial GLP-1 level increased at 2 months; however, longer term results are needed to draw further conclusions [21].

Summary

Given a rapid increase in the prevalence of obesity and concomitant T2DM, effective treatment options for these two metabolic diseases are urgently needed. In this chapter, small bowel EBMTs are reviewed as a potentially more effective option than lifestyle modification and pharmacotherapy, with less invasiveness than bariatric surgery. Moving forward, studies to assess the effect of combination therapy, such as gastric and small bowel EBMTs or drug-device combination therapy, may enhance the efficacy of endoluminal bariatric therapies. Furthermore, because obesity and metabolic diseases are chronic conditions, these minimally invasive and reversible procedures may allow sequential therapy to further enhance their durability.

References

1. McIntosh CHS, Widenmaier S, Kim SJ. Glucose-dependent insulinotropic polypeptide (gastric inhibitory polypeptide; GIP). Vitam Horm. 2009;80:409–71.
2. Meier JJ, Hücking K, Holst JJ, Deacon CF, Schmiegel WH, Nauck MA. Reduced insulinotropic effect of gastric inhibitory polypeptide in first-degree relatives of patients with type 2 diabetes. Diabetes. 2001;50(11):2497–504.
3. Nauck MA, Niedereichholz U, Ettler R, Holst JJ, Orskov C, Ritzel R, Schmiegel WH. Glucagon-like peptide 1 inhibition of gastric emptying outweighs its insulinotropic effects in healthy humans. Am J Phys. 1997;273(5 Pt 1):E981–8.
4. Creutzfeldt WO, Kleine N, Willms B, Orskov C, Holst JJ, Nauck MA. Glucagonostatic actions and reduction of fasting hyperglycemia by exogenous glucagon-like peptide I(7-36) amide in type I diabetic patients. Diabetes Care. 1996;19(6):580–6.
5. Punjabi M, Arnold M, Geary N, Langhans W, Pacheco-López G. Peripheral glucagon-like peptide-1 (GLP-1) and satiation. Physiol Behav. 2011;105(1):71–6. Review.
6. Kazafeos K. Incretin effect: GLP-1, GIP, DPP4. Diabetes Res Clin Pract. 2011;93(Suppl 1):S32–6.
7. Herrmann C, Göke R, Richter G, Fehmann HC, Arnold R, Göke B. Glucagon-like peptide-1 and glucose-dependent insulin-releasing polypeptide plasma levels in response to nutrients. Digestion. 1995;56(2):117–26.
8. Jirapinyo P, Thompson CC. Endoscopic bariatric and metabolic therapies: surgical analogues and mechanisms of action. Clin Gastroenterol Hepatol. 2017;15(5):619–30.
9. de Jonge C, Rensen SS, Verdam FJ, Vincent RP, Bloom SR, Buurman WA, et al. Endoscopic duodenal-jejunal bypass liner rapidly improves type 2 diabetes. Obes Surg. 2013;23(9):1354–60.

10. de Jonge C, Rensen SS, Verdam FJ, Vincent RP, BLoom SR, Buurman WA, et al. Impact of duodenal-jejunal exclusion on satiety hormones. Obes Surg. 2016;26(3):672–8.

11. Kaválková P, Mráz M, Trachta P, Kloučková J, Cinkajzlová A, Lacinová Z, et al. Endocrine effects of duodenal-jejunal exclusion in obese patients with type 2 diabetes mellitus. J Endocrinol. 2016;231(1):11–22.

12. Rodriguez-Grunert L, Galvao Neto MP, Alamo M, Ramos AC, Baez PB, Tarnoff M. First human experience with endoscopically delivered and retrieved duodenal-jejunal bypass sleeve. Surg Obes Relat. 2008;4(1):55–9.

13. Kaplan LM, Buse JB, Mullin C, Edmundo-Wicz S, Bass E, Visintainer P, et al. EndoBarrier therapy is associated with glycemic improvement, weight loss and satiety issues in patients with obesity and type 2 diabetes on oral antihyperglycemic agents (abstract 362-LB). Diabetes. 2016;65(6 Suppl 1A). https://professional.diabetes.org/content/late-breaking-abstracts. Accessed 6 Jun 2017.

14. Rohde U, Hedbäck N, Gluud LL, Vilsbøll T, Knop FK. Effect of the EndoBarrier gastrointestinal liner on obesity and type 2 diabetes: a systematic review and meta-analysis. Diabetes Obes Metab. 2016;18(3):300–5.

15. Jirapinyo P, Haas AV, Thompson CC. Effect of the duodenal-jejunal bypass liner on glycemic control in type-2 diabetic patients with obesity: a meta-analysis with secondary analysis on weight loss and hormonal changes (abstract 594). Gastrointest Endosc. 2017;85(5):AB82–3. doi:10.1016/j.gie.2017.03.112.

16. Sandler BJ, Rumbaut R, Swain CP, Torres G, Morales L, Gonzales L, et al. One-year human experience with a novel endoluminal, endoscopic gastric bypass sleeve for morbid obesity. Surg Endosc. 2015;29(11):3298–303.

17. Sauer N, Rösch T, Pezold J, Reining F, Anders M, Groth S, et al. A new endoscopically implantable device (SatiSphere) for treatment of obesity—efficacy, safety, and metabolic effects on glucose, insulin, and GLP-1 levels. Obes Surg. 2013;23(11):1727–33.

18. Rajagopalan H, Cherrington AD, Thompson CC, Kaplan LM, Rubino F, Mingrone G, et al. Endoscopic duodenal mucosal resurfacing for the treatment of type 2 diabetes: 6-month interim analysis from the first-in-human proof-of-concept study. Diabetes Care. 2016;39(12):2254–61.

19. Mason EE. The mechanisms of surgical treatment of type 2 diabetes. Obes Surg. 2005;15(4):459–61.

20. Meek CL, Lewis HB, Reimann F, Gribble M, Park AJ. The effect of bariatric surgery on gastrointestinal and pancreatic peptide hormones. Peptides. 2016;77:28–37.

21. Machytka E, Buzga M, Ryou M, Lautz DB, Thompson CC. Endoscopic dual-path enteral bypass using a magnetic incisionless anastomosis system (IAS) (abstract 1044). Gastrointest Endosc. 2016;83(5):AB196. doi:10.1016/j.gie.2016.03.214.

Index